WORKBOOK of EPIDEMIOLOGY

WORKBOOK of EPIDEMIOLOGY

Staffan E. Norell

New York   Oxford
OXFORD UNIVERSITY PRESS
1995

Oxford University Press

Oxford   New York
Athens   Auckland   Bangkok   Bombay
Calcutta   Cape Town   Dar es Salaam   Delhi
Florence   Hong Kong   Istanbul   Karachi
Kuala Lumpur   Madras   Madrid   Melbourne
Mexico City   Nairobi   Paris   Singapore
Taipei   Tokyo   Toronto

and associated companies in
Berlin   Ibadan

Published by Oxford University Press, Inc.,
200 Madison Avenue, New York, New York 10016

Oxford is a registered trademark of Oxford University Press

ISBN 0-19-507490-4—ISBN 0-19-507491-2 (pbk)

9 8 7 6 5 4 3 2 1

Printed in the United States of America
on acid-free paper

To Helena

PREFACE

"There are two kinds of epidemiology," a senior colleague told me, "theoretical epidemiology and real epidemiology." Some years later, when I began teaching, students reminded me of the gap between principles, as presented in many textbooks, and their application in the planning and critical evaluation of epidemiologic studies. In an attempt to bridge this gap, general principles and their applications are presented together in this workbook. The contents are influenced by efforts to find a common basis for epidemiologic studies: the principal sources of error, their impact on the results, and the research strategies available to prevent or control different errors. These strategies may be viewed as the building blocks used in the design of epidemiologic studies, with the overall objective of obtaining accurate results with limited resources.

Chapter 1 may be read as an introductory text in epidemiology, where basic concepts and principles are presented and illustrated by examples. In the following chapters, these principles are applied to the different steps in the planning and conduct of an epidemiologic study: asking the questions (Chapter 2), selecting the study population and follow-up period (Chapter 3), and obtaining information on exposure (Chapter 4) and disease (Chapter 5). The principles and methods discussed in these chapters are similar in experimental and nonexperimental studies—and in different kinds of nonexperimental studies. Some strategies are specific to case-referent studies* (Chapter 6) or to experimental studies (Chapter 7). In Chapters 2 to 7, following a short introduction, the principles and methods are presented in the form of exercises based on studies published in international journals. Exercises are not critical reviews, and the studies are selected to illustrate specific problems and possibilities and to cover a wide range of exposures and outcomes. General exercises are used for an overall review of the different aspects of study design (Chapter 8). Answers to exercises are presented in a separate section (Chapter

*The term "referents" is preferred to "controls" which has been used for both noncases (in "case-control" studies) and nonexposed (e.g., in experimental studies).

9). At least some of the answers may be used as a basis for further discussion, rather than as the final answer. This is a workbook of epidemiology, not of statistics; other books are available on the use of statistical methods in the analysis of data from epidemiologic studies.

I wish to thank Lars Erik Rutqvist, Lorann Stallones, and Gunnar Steineck for reading the manuscript and offering their constructive criticism. I asked Lars Alfredsson, Sander Greenland, and Helena Silfverhielm to read an early version of Chapter 1, and I appreciate their thoughtful comments and suggestions. I am grateful to Jeffrey House at Oxford University Press for encouragement and support. Finally, I am indebted to over 1,000 authors of papers used as a background for the exercises, and to the many colleagues and students who have provided me with ideas and suggestions for exercises. Preliminary versions of the text have been used in a couple of courses, and students have been helpful in pointing out ambiguities. Any remaining need for clarification or correction is, of course, my responsibility and I would appreciate it if it were brought to my attention (Address for correspondence: S.E. Norell, Kungsklippan 12, S-112 25 Stockholm, Sweden).

All exercises are based on actual studies (references in Chapter 9) and I am grateful for permissions to use information from the following journals: *American Journal of Epidemiology, American Journal of Public Health, British Medical Journal* (BMJ), *Epidemiology, European Heart Journal, Gut, International Journal of Cancer, International Journal of Epidemiology, Journal of the American Medical Association* (JAMA), *Journal of Clinical Epidemiology* (former *Journal of Chronic Diseases*), *Journal of Internal Medicine* (former *Acta Medica Scandinavica*), *Journal of the National Cancer Institute* (JNCI), *Journal of Occupational Medicine, Lancet, New England Journal of Medicine, Occupational and Environmental Medicine* (former *British Journal of Industrial Medicine*), and *Thorax*.

Stockholm   S.E.N.

CONTENTS

WORKBOOK of EPIDEMIOLOGY

1 *Basic Concepts*

■■■ **DISEASE OCCURRENCE AND CAUSATION**

In 1753, James Lind described the occurrence of scurvy in relation to environmental conditions and dietary habits onboard the ship *Salisbury*. On the basis of these observations, he conducted experimental studies showing that scurvy could be prevented and successfully treated by adding oranges and lemons to the diet (Lind 1753). But long before Lind's discovery, Hippocrates (about 460–377 B.C.) in his famous "Airs, waters, and places" mentioned observations about environmental factors and disease occurrence as a basis for making predictions and securing health (Jones 1948).

Early studies of the occurrence, causation, and prevention of disease dealt with infectious diseases, including smallpox (Jenner 1798), cholera (Snow 1855) and childbed fever (Semmelweis 1861), and with nutritional deficiencies, including beriberi (Fletcher 1907) and pellagra (Goldberger et al. 1926). In more recent years, attention has been paid to diseases such as cancer and cardiovascular disease, and to the role of lifestyle and environmental factors such as tobacco, alcohol, diet, drugs, ionizing radiation, and occupational exposures.

Epidemiology is the study of disease occurrence. *Disease* is defined broadly to include, for instance, injuries and causes of death (World Health Organization 1992–1993). The *purpose* of an epidemiologic study may be to describe the occurrence of disease (*descriptive epidemiology*), or to explore the causation (etiology) of disease (*etiologic epidemiology*). Descriptive studies may include variations in disease occurrence according to time (e.g., season, year, decade), place (e.g., region, urban/rural area), and person (e.g., age, sex, occupation). Descriptive data are used as a basis for the planning of health services, and may give rise to questions about disease causation. Etiologic studies are designed to explore disease causation by evaluating the effect of an "exposure" on the risk of developing disease. *Exposure* may be defined broadly to include any characteristic or event that could possibly affect the risk of developing a disease. An exposure may increase or reduce the risk of disease. Important applications of etiologic epidemiology are found in preventive medicine and public health.

Studies of disease causation may be classified as experimental or nonexperimental ("observational"), depending upon whether or not exposure is assigned with the purpose of improving accuracy. In an experimental study, random assignment of exposure may be viewed as a strategy used to avoid certain sources of error. Other strategies include the use of placebo and blinding. Similarly, strategies used in the selection of a study population and follow-up period, and in obtaining information on the subjects, are aimed at avoiding or controlling different sources of error. These strategies are, to a large extent, similar in experimental and nonexperimental studies—and in different kinds of nonexperimental studies. The overall objective of an etiologic study is to obtain an accurate estimate of the effect of an exposure on the risk of developing a disease. In the design of epidemiologic studies, research strategies are combined with the purpose of achieving this objective.

■■■ MEASURES OF DISEASE OCCURRENCE

The occurrence of a disease can be described in terms of prevalence or incidence. The *prevalence* is the proportion of a population that has the disease. The *incidence* is the frequency of development of new cases of the disease in a population (Morgenstern et al. 1980). A *case* is a disease episode, or a subject representing a disease episode. A *prevalent case* is the state of having the disease, or a subject representing such a state. An *incident case* is the event of developing the disease, or a subject representing such an event. Subjects who have not (yet) developed the disease are sometimes referred to as *noncases*.

In order to identify incident cases (disease onsets), each subject has to be followed over a period of time. However, the development of a disease episode is usually a gradual process and any particular episode of the disease may become more or less advanced. Some episodes may give rise to symptoms severe enough to make the subject see a doctor, while other episodes of the same disease may not produce any symptoms and may or may not be detectable at screening examinations. Thus, the occurrence

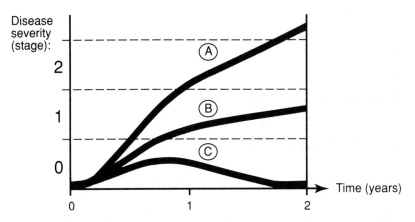

Figure 1-1 Defining the disease according to severity (stage). Three subjects (A, B, and C) followed over a 2-year period: When the disease is defined as *stage 1+*, subjects A and B, but not subject C, are incident cases (by crossing the line to stage 1 during follow-up). But when the disease is defined as *stage 2+*, only subject A is an incident case (by crossing the line to stage 2 during follow-up).

of a disease will depend upon how it is defined in terms of severity or stage of development (Morrison 1979). The disease under study should be defined in this respect, and an incident case is the event when the disease reaches that particular stage of development (as illustrated in Fig. 1–1). A study is often limited to first cases of the disease since the risk of developing a disease usually depends heavily upon whether or not the subject had the disease earlier. If so, subjects who have had the disease are not included since they are not at risk of developing the disease for the first time. Three measures of disease occurrence will be presented below: prevalence proportion, incidence proportion, and incidence rate.

Prevalence Proportion

The *prevalence proportion,* (PP) is the proportion of subjects who have the disease at a point in time. To calculate PP, the number of individuals who have the disease at a specific time (prevalent cases) is divided by the number of individuals in the population at that point in time. This is illustrated in Figure 1–2.

> *Example:* Of 1,500 middle-aged women 30 had diabetes on January 1, 1990. The prevalence proportion of diabetes was PP = 30/1,500 = 0.02 (or 2%).

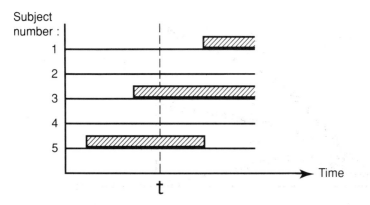

Figure 1–2 Prevalence proportion (PP). At time "t", 2 out of 5 subjects had the disease: PP = 2/5 = 0.4. (Each subject is represented by a horizontal line, and a disease episode by a bar).

The prevalence proportion is determined at a specific point in time. This could be a point in calendar time, such as January 1, 1990. But it could also be a point in life, for instance, at the time of birth. For example, of 2,000 babies born during the period January 1, 1990 to December 31, 1992, 60 had malformations at birth. The proportion of babies who had malformations at the time of birth, that is, the prevalence proportion of malformations at birth, was PP = 60/2,000 = 0.03. Similarly, the prevalence proportion of diabetes in middle-aged women could be determined at the time when they entered the study even if, for some reason, the women entered the study at different points in calendar time. The prevalence proportion is determined by examining each subject once, for the presence of preexisting (prevalent) disease. Since PP is a proportion, it is dimensionless and can never take on values less than 0 or greater than 1 (100%).

Incidence Proportion

The *incidence proportion* (IP) (also called *cumulative incidence*) is the proportion of subjects who develop the disease during a certain period of time. To calculate IP, the number of individuals who develop the disease during a certain period is divided by the number of individuals in the population at the beginning of the period. All individuals should initially be free from the disease, and thus at risk to get it. This is illustrated in Figure 1–3.

> *Example:* Of 20,000 middle-aged men (with no previous myocardial infarction), 60 developed a myocardial infarction during a 6-month period.

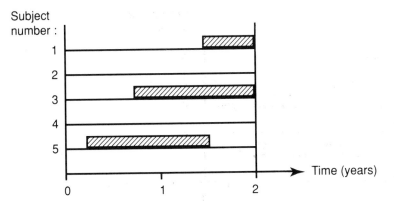

Figure 1-3 Incidence proportion (IP). During a 2-year period, 3 out of 5 subjects developed the disease: IP = 3/5 = 0.6 during a 2-year period. (Each subject is represented by a horizontal line, and a disease episode by a bar.)

The incidence proportion of myocardial infarction was IP = 60/20,000 = 0.003 (or 0.3%) during a 6-month period.

The length of the time period should always be mentioned, since the incidence proportion during, for example, a 12-month period would be about twice that during a 6-month period. In order to determine the incidence proportion, each subject should be followed for a similar period of time (e.g., 6 months). This period could begin, for example, on January 1, 1990 (i.e., at a point in calendar time), at age 55, or at any time when a subject enters the study. Since IP is a proportion, it is dimensionless and can never take on values less than 0 or greater than 1 (100%).

Incidence Rate

The *incidence rate,* (IR) (also called *incidence density*) is the number of incident cases divided by the person-time, usually the number of person-years, at risk (Miettinen 1976, Morrison 1979). One *person-year* is equivalent to one subject followed for 1 year (or two subjects followed for ½ year, etc). During follow-up the subjects are considered to be *at risk* as long as they are free from the disease. This is illustrated in Figure 1–4.

Example: In the previous example, 20,000 middle-aged men were followed for ½ year. During that time, 60 developed a myocardial infarction. Disregarding a relatively small number of person-years lost in this way, there were 20,000 * ½ = 10,000 person-years at risk. If only first cases of myocardial infarction are considered, there were 60 cases and the inci-

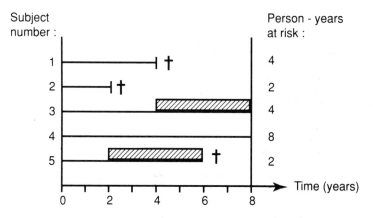

Figure 1–4 Incidence rate (IR). During (4 + 2 + 4 + 8 + 2 =) 20 person-years at risk, there were 2 incident cases (disease onsets): IR = 2/20 = 0.1 cases per person-year. (Each subject is represented by a horizontal line, and a disease episode by a bar; † = death).

dence rate was 60/10,000 = 0.006 cases per person-year, or simply 0.006 per year.

Since time is taken into account, the incidence rate (unlike the incidence proportion) is independent of the length of the follow-up period. The denominator is the person-time (usually the number of person-years) at risk. Subjects do not contribute person-time at risk when they have the disease under study—and thereafter if the study is limited to first cases of the disease. But this will make little or no difference if only a small proportion of the subjects develop the disease during follow-up (as in the above example with myocardial infarction). More important, subjects who die are no longer at risk. During long periods of follow-up, a substantial proportion of the subjects may die or be lost to follow-up for other reasons. This should be taken into account when calculating the number of person-years at risk. Finally, individual follow-up periods may, by definition, be of different lengths. For example, the incidence of myocardial infarction may be studied among residents in a town during a 5-year period (with people moving in and out during that period). An approximation of the total number of person-years at risk can sometimes be obtained by multiplying the length of the period by the average of the population size at the beginning and end of the period. The incidence rate is not a proportion like the two previous measures, since it is the number of cases per unit of person-time. It can never take on values less than 0, but there is no upper limit. (For instance, the incidence rate of common cold may be one case per person-month, 12 cases per person-year, or 120 cases per person-decade).

Table 1-1 Three measures of disease occurrence

Prevalence proportion

$$PP = \frac{\text{no. of subjects having the disease}}{\text{total no. of subjects}} \text{ at a point in time}$$

Incidence proportion

$$IP = \frac{\text{no. of subjects who get the disease during a period}}{\text{no. of subjects at risk at the beginning of the period}}$$

Incidence rate

$$IR = \frac{\text{no. of disease onsets}}{\text{person-time at risk}}$$

Comments

The three measures of disease occurrence are summarized in Table 1-1. When studying the causation and prevention of disease, there is primarily an interest in incident cases and measures of disease incidence. The incidence proportion is an estimate of the risk of developing the disease during a certain period of time. When only a small proportion of the subjects develop the disease during follow-up (and only one case in each subject is considered), IP is approximately equal to $IR * t$ (where t = time of follow-up). The time of follow-up will often be of different length for different subjects. This should be taken into account by considering the person-time at risk contributed by each subject (using the incidence rate), or by adjusting for differences in the length of follow-up in the data analysis (when using the incidence proportion). The incidence proportion is often used if all subjects are followed for a similar period of time. Sometimes, for example, in studies of congenital malformations or some chronic diseases, only information on prevalent cases is available. When studies are based on prevalence, it should be recognized that the prevalence depends not only on the incidence but also on the average duration of the disease, that is, the time it takes to get well or die after developing the disease (Freeman, Hutchinson 1980). In addition, the prevalence is influenced by any migration of cases (or noncases) into or out of the population. For descriptive purposes, there is sometimes a primary interest in the prevalence of disease as well as in different measures of disease incidence.

■■■ MEASURES OF EFFECT

A cause of a single disease episode may be thought of as a factor in the absence of which the subject would not have developed the disease at that time. In epidemiology, causes of disease may be viewed as exposures in the absence of which there would be a lower risk of disease as measured by the incidence during short periods of time (where $IP = IR * t$). Conversely, preventive factors may be viewed as exposures in the absence of which the risk would be higher. Exposed and unexposed subjects are said to be comparable (or exchangeable) when, in the absence of the exposure, the risk would be the same in the exposed as in the unexposed. If so, the effect of an exposure may be estimated by comparing the disease occurrence in the exposed and unexposed.

Relative Effect

The *relative effect* is measured by the *ratio* between the disease occurrence in the exposed and that in the unexposed, using one of the measures of disease occurrence described previously. Thus, the *IR ratio* (also called *rate ratio*) is the incidence rate (IR) in the exposed divided by that in the unexposed. Similarly, the *IP ratio* (also called *risk ratio*) is the incidence proportion (IP) in the exposed divided by that in the unexposed, and the *PP ratio* (also called *prevalence ratio*) is the prevalence proportion (PP) in the exposed divided by that in the unexposed. When only a small proportion of the subjects develop the disease during follow-up (and only one case in each subject is considered), the IR ratio is approximately equal to the IP ratio. When the exposure is unrelated to the duration of the disease, the PP ratio may sometimes be used as an approximation of the IR ratio (in a stable situation, where the PP ratio is not influenced by migration into or out of the population). The single term *relative risk (RR)* is often used to refer to any of the three measures of relative effect.

As an example, consider maternal smoking during pregnancy and infant mortality. Suppose that of 2,000 babies to mothers who smoked at least 15 cigarettes per day, 60 died during their first year of life (IP = 60/2,000 = 0.030), and of 4,000 babies to mothers who did not smoke during pregnancy 80 died during their first year of life (IP = 80/4,000 = 0.020). The relative risk (or IP ratio) is 0.030/0.020 = 1.50. Thus, infant mortality was 50% higher in the exposed than in the unexposed. To the extent that the exposed and unexposed infants were comparable, the relative risk reflects the relative effect of the exposure, that is, maternal smoking of at least 15 cigarettes per day increased the risk of infant death by 50%.

The relative risk can take on any value from zero (RR = 0 if only unexposed subjects develop the disease) to infinity (RR = ∞ if only exposed subjects develop the disease). Using the relative risk as an estimate of effect, RR = 1 means that the exposure did not affect the risk of disease. A relative risk above RR = 1 means that the risk of disease is increased by the exposure: the stronger the relative effect, the higher the relative risk. For instance, RR = 2 means that the exposure doubled the risk of disease. A relative risk below RR = 1 means that the risk of disease is reduced by the exposure: the stronger the relative effect, the lower (closer to RR = 0) the relative risk. For instance, RR = 0.60 means that the exposure reduced the risk of disease by $(1 - 0.60) = 0.40$ or 40%.

Absolute Effect

The *absolute effect* is measured by the *difference* between the disease occurrence in the exposed and that in the unexposed, using one of the measures of disease occurrence described previously. Thus, the *IR difference* (also called *rate difference*) is the difference between the incidence rate (IR) in the exposed and that in the unexposed. Similarly, the *IP difference* (also called *risk difference*) is the difference between the incidence proportion (IP) in the exposed and that in the unexposed, and the *PP difference* (also called *prevalence difference*) is the difference between the prevalence proportion (PP) in the exposed and that in the unexposed. In the previous example of maternal smoking and infant mortality, the proportion of babies who died during their first year of life was 0.030 in the exposed and 0.020 in the unexposed. The risk difference (or IP difference) is $0.030 - 0.020 = 0.010$. To the extent that the exposed and unexposed infants were comparable, the risk difference reflects the absolute effect of the exposure, that is, maternal smoking of at least 15 cigarettes per day increased the risk of infant death by $0.010 = 10$ per 1,000 babies.

Attributable Fraction

The *attributable fraction* (AF) is the proportion of cases that is attributable to an exposure (Miettinen 1974, Greenland, Robins 1988). Provided that the exposed and unexposed are comparable, the attributable fraction among the exposed is the difference between the disease occurrence in the exposed and that in the unexposed divided by the disease occurrence in the exposed. The attributable fraction among the exposed may also be calculated as AF = (RR − 1)/RR, where RR is the relative risk. The attributable fraction may be based on different measures of disease occurrence, such as the incidence rate (IR fraction) or the incidence proportion (IP fraction or "excess fraction"). In the example of maternal smoking and infant mortality, the proportion of babies who died during their first year of life was 0.030 in the exposed and 0.020 in the unexposed. Provided that the exposed and unexposed infants were comparable, the attributable fraction among the exposed is (0.030–0.020)/0.030 = 0.33. In other words, 33% of the infant deaths that occurred among the exposed were due to maternal smoking during pregnancy.

Comments

The relative risk is by far the most commonly used measure of effect. But the absolute effect provides useful information on the size of the public health problem involved. When there are two or more levels (or categories) of an exposure, for example smoking 1–14 cigarettes per day or 15+ cigarettes per day, each level (category) is compared with the unexposed. When the effects of two or more different exposures (e.g., smoking and alcohol intake) are being studied, the unexposed should not be exposed to any of these factors. The attributable fraction may provide valuable information provided that there is strong evidence of a cause-effect relationship.

■■ CAUSATION OF DISEASE

In the design and interpretation of epidemiologic studies, attention should be paid to some basic principles of disease causation. These include the difference between association and causation, the concept of contributing cause (risk factor), the overlapping of attributable fractions, and the induction time.

Association and Causation

In epidemiology, the causation of disease is investigated by comparisons of disease occurrence in exposed and unexposed subjects. If the disease occurs more (or less) often in the exposed than in the unexposed, there is an *association* between exposure and disease. There are, in principle, three possible explanations for such associations: 1) the exposure is a cause of the disease; 2) the exposure and disease have a common cause; 3) the disease is a cause of the exposure. Only the two first alternatives apply if the exposure occurred (or was present) prior to the disease. If so, the exposure is a *risk indicator* for the disease. For example, residence, occupation, and smoking are risk indicators for many diseases. A risk indicator may or may not be a *cause* of the disease, and alternative 2 illustrates an important source of error (so-called confounding) in epidemiologic studies.

Causes

Causes of disease are rarely, if ever, *sufficient causes* (Rothman 1976 and 1986). For example, smoking is not a sufficient cause of lung cancer since many smokers do not develop lung cancer, and exposure to rubella virus is not a sufficient cause of rubella (german measles) since many exposed do not develop the disease (e.g., due to aquired immunity). Thus, most (if not all) causes of disease are *contributing causes*, often called *risk factors* (although the term "risk factor" has also been used as a synonym for risk indicator). Some causes of disease are *necessary causes*. For example, exposure to rubella virus is (by definition) necessary for the development of rubella, but smoking is not necessary for the development of lung cancer.

Overlapping of Attributable Fractions

Each risk factor contributes a certain proportion of the cases of a disease, the attributable fraction. But since a risk factor is only a contributing cause of disease, two or more risk factors are required to bring about a single case of disease. For example, many cases of myocardial infarction are due to the joint effect of smoking, hypertension, elevated serum cholesterol, and other risk factors. Thus, there is considerable overlapping between the attributable fractions. The sum of the attributable fractions for all causes (risk factors) of a certain disease is therefore not 100%, but much higher (there is, in principle, no upper limit). For instance, in the causation of myocardial infarction in a certain population, the attributable fraction for smoking, hypertension, and elevated serum cholesterol could each be about 60%. This means that 60% of the cases would not occur in the absence of smoking, *or* in the absence of hypertension, *or* in the absence of elevated serum cholesterol. (But the joint effect of avoiding both smoking and hypertension would be considerably less than the sum of the two separate effects due to overlapping of the attributable fractions).

Induction Time

The *induction time* (or induction period) is the time from exposure until its effect on the occurrence of disease. The length of the induction time varies considerably between different exposure-disease associations. For example, the induction time for smoking in the causation of lung cancer is several years. But the time from exposure to rubella virus to the onset of disease (rubella) is only 2 to 3 weeks. (For infectious agents this time is also called the incubation period. The "latent period" is the time interval between disease onset and detection (Rothman, 1981), but the term has also been used as a synonym for induction time.)

■■■ STUDY POPULATION AND FOLLOW-UP PERIOD

Epidemiology is the study of disease occurrence, and the *study population* is the subjects investigated with regard to disease occurrence. When the effect of an exposure is investigated, the study population should include both exposed and unexposed individuals. In studies based on incidence, the study population should only include subjects who are at risk of developing the disease under study. Subjects are not at risk if they have the disease—or if they have had the disease, when the study is limited to first cases of the disease.

The *follow-up period* is the time during which a subject in the study population is followed with regard to disease onset (in studies based on incidence). When the effect of an exposure is being studied, the induction time should be taken into account in selecting the follow-up period. The *study period* is the time during which the study subjects (i.e., the subjects in the study population) are examined for disease occurrence. For example, in a study of 2,000 babies born between January 1, 1990 and December 31, 1992, 60 had malformations at birth (PP = 60/2,000 = 0.03). The study period was 3 years, but individual follow-up periods were zero (prevalent cases at the time of birth). In studies based on incidence, individual follow-up periods may be defined to cover the entire study period or parts thereof. For instance, individual follow-up periods may be limited to the part of the study period when a subject is aged 50–69 years, is employed in a certain company, or lives in a certain area.

In studies based on incidence rates, the results may be presented according to Table 1–2A. The incidence rate (IR), calculated separately for the exposed and the unexposed, is the number of incident cases divided by the number of person-years at risk. The IR ratio (= $a*D/b*C$) is the incidence rate in the exposed divided by that in the unexposed.

In studies based on incidence proportions, the results may be presented according to Table 1–2B. The incidence proportion (IP), calculated separately for the exposed and the unexposed, is the number of subjects who developed the disease during the follow-up period (cases) divided by the number of subjects at the beginning of the period. The IP ratio (= $a'*D'/b'*C'$) is the incidence proportion in the exposed divided by that in the unexposed. The so-called *incidence odds ratio*, IOR = $a'*(D' - b')/b'*(C' - a')$, may be used as an estimate of the IP ratio if the disease is

Table 1–2 Tables of results

A) Incidence rate:

	Exposed	Unexposed
Cases	a	b
Person-time	C	D
Incidence rate (IR)	a/C	b/D

$$\text{IR ratio} = \frac{a/C}{b/D} = \frac{a*D}{b*C}$$

B) Incidence proportion:

	Exposed	Unexposed
Cases	a'	b'
Noncases	C'−a'	D'−b'
All subjects	C'	D'
Incidence proportion (IP)	a'/C'	b'/D'

$$\text{IP ratio} = \frac{a'/C'}{b'/D'} = \frac{a'*D'}{b'*C'}$$

"rare" in the sense that only a small proportion of the subjects developed the disease during follow-up (i.e., if (D' - b') is approximately equal to D', and (C' - a') is approximately equal to C'). The noncases are the subjects who did not develop the disease during follow-up.

In studies based on prevalence proportions (sometimes called prevalence studies or cross-sectional studies), each subject is examined for the presence of the disease at one point in time (i.e., individual follow-up periods are equal to zero). The results may be presented in a table similar to Table 1–2B. The prevalence proportion (PP), calculated separately for the exposed and the unexposed, is the number of prevalent cases divided by the number of subjects examined for the presence of the disease. The PP ratio is the prevalence proportion in the exposed divided by that in the unexposed. The so-called *prevalence odds ratio*, POR (calculated in the same way as the incidence odds ratio), may be used as an estimate of the PP ratio if the disease prevalence is low. In certain situations, a POR may be used as an estimate of the IR ratio (Miettinen 1976, Rothman 1986).

The single term *relative risk (RR)* is often used to refer to any of the measures of relative effect. Information should then be provided on the measure of disease occurrence (and whether the odds ratio is used as an estimate of the relative risk). In addition, the absolute effect and the attributable fraction may be calculated as described previously.

The *study base* is the study population during follow-up, that is, the total person-time at risk (Miettinen 1982, 1985). The *accuracy* of the result is the extent to which the measured effect (e.g., relative risk) reflects the true effect of the exposure in the study base. The *generalizability* of the result is the extent to which it applies outside the study base.

■ ACCURACY AND SOURCES OF ERROR

The purpose of an etiologic study is to estimate the effect of an exposure on the risk of developing a disease. In the design and conduct of a study, the overall objective is to measure this effect as accurately as possible with the limited resources available. The *accuracy* of the result is the degree of absence of error in the measurement of the effect. An *error* is a discrepancy between the measured and true effect. Knowledge of the different sources of error, their impact on the accuracy of the results, and the strategies used to deal with them are the basis for the design and evaluation of epidemiologic studies.

Two types of errors are usually considered: systematic error and random error (Table 1–3). *Systematic error (bias)* may be due to: 1) lack of comparability between the exposed and unexposed with regard to other factors that affect the risk of developing the disease (confounding), 2) errors in the classification of subjects according to exposure or disease (misclassification), and 3) the selection of subjects for, or their participation in, a study being influenced by the disease (outcome) under study (selection bias). *Random error* may be described as an uncertainty introduced by small numbers of observations. Each type of error will be discussed in a separate section.

To a large extent, the accuracy of the results is determined by strategies used in the design and conduct of a study. Several strategies are available to prevent confounding, misclassification, and selection bias, and to reduce random error. In the data analysis, there are methods to control confounding, and to evaluate random error. The *accuracy* of a result is determined by the degree of absence of systematic error (*validity*), and the degree of absence of random error (*precision*). In addition, accuracy depends upon the absence of error in the analysis and presentation of data.

Table 1–3 Subdivision of errors.

A. Systematic error (= bias)
   1. Confounding bias
   2. Misclassification bias
   3. Selection bias
B. Random error

CONFOUNDING BIAS

In any study, the exposed and unexposed may differ with regard to other factors that affect the risk of developing the disease. Such a factor may introduce an error, when estimating the effect of the exposure by comparing the disease occurrence in the exposed and unexposed. If so, the factor is called a *confounder* (confounding factor), and the bias that it introduces is called *confounding* (Miettinen, Cook 1981, Rothman 1986). To introduce confounding, a factor must be:

1. a risk factor among the unexposed, and
2. associated with the exposure in the study base.

If a factor affects the risk of disease only among the exposed, no bias is introduced but the effect of the exposure is modified (as will be discussed later). Confounding is not introduced by a factor that is simply an intermediate step in the causal path between the exposure and the disease, that is, a mediator of the effect of the exposure.

The relative risk may be overestimated (biased towards $RR = \infty$) or underestimated (biased towards $RR = 0$) by confounding, depending upon whether the confounding factor is more or less common in the exposed than in the unexposed, and whether it increases or reduces the risk of the disease. The confounding effect introduced by one factor may or may not be balanced by that introduced by other factors.

As an example of confounding, consider a study of the effect of alcohol intake on the risk of myocardial infarction. Middle-aged people with a moderate alcohol intake (exposed) or no alcohol intake (unexposed) were followed for their first myocardial infarction. The results, shown in Table 1–4, suggest that moderate alcohol intake increased the risk of myocardial infarction by 40% ($RR = 1.40$).

But sex is a possible confounder, since sex may be associated with alcohol intake and affects the risk of myocardial infarction. Table 1–5, presenting the results from Table 1–4 for men and women separately, shows that moderate alcohol intake had no effect on the risk of myocardial infarction, neither in men nor in women. The proportion of men was higher in the exposed than in the unexposed, and myocardial infarction was more common in men than in women. Thus, confounding by sex resulted in an overestimation of the relative risk (bias towards $RR = \infty$) in Table 1–4. Figure 1–5 summarizes the information in Tables 1–4 and 1–5.

In principle, confounding could even change the direction of the asso-

Table 1–4 Alcohol intake and myocardial infarction—an illustration of confounding (cf. Table 1–5)

	Exposed	Unexposed
Cases	140	100
Person-years	30,000	30,000
Incidence rate		
(per 1,000 years)	4.67	3.33
	RR = 4.67/3.33 = 1.40	

ciation. For instance, smoking could be another confounder in the present study. Smoking may be more common in people who drink alcohol than in those who do not, and smoking increases the risk of myocardial infarction. Thus, if smoking was taken into account by considering the effect of alcohol intake in smokers and nonsmokers separately (in each sex), the results might show that moderate alcohol intake actually reduced the risk of myocardial infarction. (As an illustration, consider the findings among men in Table 1–5 with the following subdivision into smokers and nonsmokers. Exposed: 120 cases = 80 smokers + 40 nonsmokers; 20,000 person-years = 10,000 smokers + 10,000 nonsmokers. Unexposed: 60 cases = 20 smokers + 40 nonsmokers; 10,000 person-years = 2,000 smokers + 8,000 nonsmokers. Using this information in one table for smokers and another for nonsmokers, would give RR = 0.80 among smokers and RR = 0.80 among nonsmokers).

Sources of Confounding

Any risk factor for the disease could be associated with the exposure in the study base, and thus introduce confounding. Consequently all risk factors for the disease under study should be listed as potential confounders. However, many risk factors are unknown and risk indicators are used in their place. (Such risk indicators may be viewed as indicators or "proxy variables" of true confounders). Age, sex, residence, and other

Table 1–5 The results in Table 1–4, presented for men and women separately

	Men:		Women:	
	Exposed	Unexposed	Exposed	Unexposed
Cases	120	60	20	40
Person-years	20,000	10,000	10,000	20,000
Incidence rate				
(per 1,000 years)	6.00	6.00	2.00	2.00
	RR = 6.00/6.00 = 1		RR = 2.00/2.00 = 1	

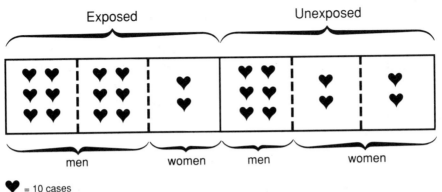

Exposed   Unexposed

men   women   men   women

♥ = 10 cases
Each square represents 10,000 person - years

Figure 1–5 Confounding (by sex). The proportion of men is higher in the exposed than in the unexposed, and the disease is more common in men than in women. Thus, when sex is not taken into account, the disease appears to be more common in the exposed than in the unexposed.

sociodemographic variables are risk indicators for many diseases, and are usually considered as potential confounders. To the extent that there are associations between confounders in the study base, there will be overlapping between their confounding effects.

An association between the exposure and a risk factor (or risk indicator) for the disease may arise in different ways. The exposure may be more common among certain kinds of people. For example, alcohol intake may be more common in men than in women, and more common in smokers than in nonsmokers. When studying the effect of occupational exposures, it has been found that the exposure may be more common in people who are selected for, and remain in, certain jobs due to their good general state of health. Since a good general state of health reduces the risk of many diseases, it may introduce confounding: so-called healthy worker effect, bias towards RR = 0 (McMichael 1976). In addition, confounding may be introduced if the exposure under study is associated with other occupational exposures in the same job (bias towards RR = ∞). Similarly, in studies where the exposure of interest is a drug treatment, confounding may be introduced by the health condition of subjects who receive the drug ("unhealthy patient effect," bias towards RR = ∞) as well as by other treatments or examinations used for the same condition. An association between the exposure and a risk factor for the disease may also be introduced by the way in which the study population is selected, or the way in which subjects are lost from the study.

The risk of developing a disease usually depends heavily upon whether or not the subject had the disease earlier. Thus, if associated with the exposure, previous episodes of the disease under study may be a strong confounder. For example, in a study of coffee intake and gastric ulcer, a previous ulcer (or other gastric complaint) may tend to reduce coffee intake and increase the risk of gastric ulcer (and thus introduce confounding with a bias towards RR = 0).

Strategies in Dealing with Confounding

Confounding may be avoided by *restriction* when selecting the study population. For instance, confounding by sex is avoided if only men (or only women) are included in the study, and confounding by smoking is avoided if only nonsmokers are included. Similarly, a "healthy worker effect" may be avoided by including only healthy workers (exposed and unexposed), and an "unhealthy patient effect" may be avoided by including only patients (exposed and unexposed) with similar health conditions. In order to avoid confounding by previous episodes of the disease, studies are often restricted to subjects who have not had the disease previously. Confounding by a continuous variable such as age may be reduced by restricting the study to a certain age interval, and confounding by age within that interval may be dealt with in the data analysis. In some studies, confounding by several factors have been avoided by restrictions with regard to, for example, age, sex, occupation, residence, and ethnic background. Any restrictions should be made according to strict criteria, determined in advance. Restriction is a useful way of avoiding confounding, its only principal limitation being a possible shortage of study subjects.

Matching of unexposed to exposed subjects, when selecting the study population, is another way of avoiding confounding. For example, confounding by sex is avoided if, for every exposed subject, an unexposed subject of the same sex is selected. But matching of unexposed to exposed subjects is usually too costly to be used in large scale epidemiologic studies. (Matching of unexposed to exposed subjects should not be confused with matching of referents to the cases, discussed in Chapter 6).

Confounding may also be *controlled in the data analysis* (Breslow, Day 1980 and 1987). Just as confounding is avoided by restrictions when selecting the study population, it can be dealt with by restrictions in the data analysis. For instance, confounding by sex is avoided if the effect is estimated in men and women separately (cf. Table 1–5). This is the basis for methods used for adjustment or control of confounding in the data analysis. In a *stratified analysis*, the effect of an exposure is evaluated within each stratum of the confounder (e.g., in each sex or age group) and the results are combined into a single overall estimate of the effect. In a *multivariate analysis*, adjustment for confounding is achieved through mathematic modeling. To be able to control confounding, the association between exposure and confounder should not be perfect. (For instance, it would not be possible to control confounding by sex if all exposed were men and all unexposed were women). In addition, information on potential confounders is required. If the information is inaccurate ("confounder misclassification"), the adjustment may leave residual confounding or even introduce bias.

The above methods can only be used to avoid or control confounding by factors that have been recognized as potential confounders and identified in the study. The possibility of confounding by unidentified factors is a major limitation in nonexperimental research. Such confounding may, in principle at least, be avoided in *experimental studies* by random assignment of the exposure, and by the use of placebo (sham treatment) and blinding. These strategies are discussed in Chapter 7.

■■■ MISCLASSIFICATION BIAS

In a study population, subjects are examined and classified with regard to exposure and disease. *Exposure misclassification* occurs when exposed subjects are incorrectly classified as unexposed, or vice versa. Similarly, *disease misclassification* occurs when diseased subjects are incorrectly classified as nondiseased, or vice versa.

Suppose that a study is planned to investigate the effect of passive smoking on the risk of myocardial infarction. Passive smoking may be defined as the "inhalation of tobacco smoke from other people's smoking," and myocardial infarction may be defined as the "necrosis (death) of heart muscle tissue." These are *theoretical definitions* in the sense that they describe the kind of information we would like to have. But in practice, there is no direct way of measuring the inhalation of tobacco smoke or the occurrence of myocardial necrosis in a large scale study. Thus, *empirical definitions* are introduced as an aid for the data collection. Such definitions are based on variables that are associated with the exposure or disease of interest (sometimes called "indicators" or "proxy variables"). For instance, passive smoking may be defined on the basis of the time spent with smokers, and myocardial infarction may be defined on the basis of certain criteria (including chest pain, enzyme levels, and signs on electrocardiograms). These definitions are empirical in the sense that they are based on the information we may be able to collect. However, empirical definitions can be more or less accurate in reflecting the theoretical definitions.

A *measurement error* is the gap between the measured and true value of a variable. Several variables may be used to classify subjects with regard to exposure and disease, respectively. Measurement errors are a source of misclassification, but do not always result in misclassification ("measurement error without misclassification"). Any gap between the theoretical and empirical definition is another source of misclassification ("misclassification without measurement error"). Both sources of misclassification should be taken into account (Fig. 1–6). For example, in a study of serum nutrients and cancer, the nutrient level was measured in a serum sample from each subject. However, there may be considerable variations in nutrient levels over time. Thus, even if there was no measurement error, the nutrient level in a single serum sample (empirical definition) may not reflect the level over an etiologically relevant period of time (theoretical definition). A theoretical definition of an exposure should involve both the duration of exposure and the time of exposure in relation to the study period (taking the induction time into account). Failure to take the induction time into account may be regarded as a source of exposure misclassification.

Sensitivity and Specificity

The *sensitivity* is the probability that an exposed subject will be classified as exposed (or the probability that a diseased subject will be classified as diseased). The sensitivity is estimated as the number of exposed subjects classified as exposed divided by the number of exposed subjects (or the number of diseased subjects classified as diseased divided by the number of diseased subjects). This is exemplified in Table 1–6.

The *specificity* is the probability that an unexposed subject will be classified as unexposed (or the probability that a nondiseased subject will be classified as nondiseased). The specificity is estimated as the number of unexposed subjects classified as unexposed divided by the number of unexposed subjects (or the number of nondiseased subjects classified as nondiseased divided by the number of nondiseased subjects). This is exemplified in Table 1–6.

Sensitivity and specificity are not properties of a method of examination and classification, but rather of such a method applied in a certain way to a certain kind of population. For example, when using a dietary questionnaire, the misclassification with regard to nutrient intake may be quite different in men and women. Thus, when using a method, the

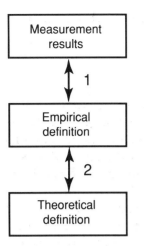

Figure 1–6 Two sources of misclassification: measurement errors (1), and any gap between the empirical and theoretical definition (2).

sensitivity and specificity may vary considerably with age, sex, and other characteristics of the population. It may be argued that the sensitivity and specificity cannot be measured, since the true (theoretical) exposure or disease status of subjects remains unknown. But sometimes the sensitivity and specificity can be estimated by comparing two different methods used to classify the same subjects: a simple method to be evaluated, and an accurate reference method (that may be too complex or expensive for use in large-scale epidemiologic studies).

The amount of exposure misclassification depends on the sensitivity and specificity, but also on the occurrence of the exposure. For instance, a sensitivity of 0.50 would result in misclassification of 25% of all subjects if 50% are exposed, but only of 5% of all subjects if 10% are ex-

Table 1–6 Sensitivity and specificity (a numerical example)

	Exposed	*Unexposed*
Classified as:		
Exposed	150	30
Unexposed	50	170

Sensitivity = 150/(150 + 50) = 0.75 (or 75%).
Specificity = 170/(170 + 30) = 0.85 (or 85%).

"True positives" = 150	"False positives" = 30
"False negatives" = 50	"True negatives" = 170

posed. The same principles apply to methods used to classify subjects with regard to disease.

Nondifferential Exposure Misclassification

Exposure misclassification is *nondifferential* if the misclassification (sensitivity and specificity) does not differ between the cases and noncases (Kleinbaum et al. 1982, Flegal et al. 1986). In general, nondifferential exposure misclassification results in a "dilution" of the effect, that is, a bias towards RR = 1. (There are some exceptions to this general rule, as discussed in Chapter 4.)

Nondifferential exposure misclassification may be introduced by a gap between the theoretical and empirical definition of the exposure or by a measurement error that is independent of the disease under study. When the induction time is not adequately taken into account, the consequences are usually similar to those of a nondifferential exposure misclassification (bias towards RR = 1).

As an example, consider a study of the effect of X-ray exposure on the risk of breast cancer. A total of 120 cases of breast cancer occurred during 2 years' follow-up of 50,000 middle-aged women. With no misclassification, the results would be as in Table 1–7, with RR = 2.00. However, there was a tendency to overestimate X-ray exposure from interview data. Suppose that 75% of those who had not received X-ray exposure of their breasts were correctly classified as unexposed (specificity = 0.75), regardless of whether or not they developed a breast cancer (nondifferential misclassification). The remaining 25% were incorrectly classified as exposed, which would give the results presented in Table 1–8 with RR = 1.50. Thus, a nondifferential misclassification of unexposed as exposed (specificity < 1) resulted in a bias towards RR = 1 (from the true effect RR = 2.00 to RR = 1.50). This "dilution" of the effect is illustrated in Figure 1–7, summarizing the information in Tables 1–7 and 1–8. If exposed women had been misclassified as unexposed (sensitivity < 1),

Table 1–7 Data on X-ray exposure and breast cancer (no misclassification)

	Exposed	Unexposed	Sum
Breast cancer	40	80	120
No breast cancer	9,960	39,920	49,880
All women	10,000	40,000	50,000
Incidence proportion (* 1,000)	4.00	2.00	
	RR = 4.00/2.00 = 2.00		

Table 1–8 Nondifferential exposure misclassification (sensitivity = 1.00, specificity = 0.75). Based on the data in Table 1–7.

	Classified as:		
	Exposed	Unexposed	Sum
Breast cancer	60	60	120
No breast cancer	19,940	29,940	49,880
All women	20,000	30,000	50,000
Incidence proportion (* 1,000)	3.00	2.00	
	RR = 3.00/2.00 = 1.50		

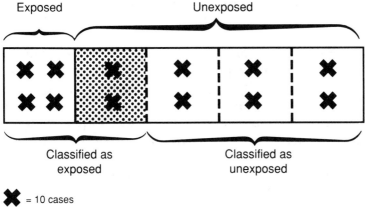

Figure 1–7 Nondifferential exposure misclassification resulting in a "dilution" of the effect—that is, a bias towards RR = 1. A similar proportion of the unexposed cases (20/80 = 25%) and of all unexposed women (10,000/40,000 = 25%) are misclassified as exposed (i.e., specificity = 75%, both among the cases and noncases).

this would also result in a bias towards RR = 1, as long as the misclassification is nondifferential.

Differential Exposure Misclassification

Exposure misclassification is *differential* if the misclassification (sensitivity or specificity) differs between the cases and noncases. Differential exposure misclassification introduces a bias towards RR = 0 or RR = ∞.

In studies where exposure information is collected only after the cases have appeared, differential exposure misclassification may be introduced if the information is influenced by the disease. This may occur when exposure information is collected (or handled) after the cases have been identified, or their disease has reached the stage of development where it can influence the exposure information. Compared with other study subjects, those who have developed the disease could be more (or less) likely to recall and report past exposure ("*recall bias*"). Similarly, the interviewer may be influenced by awareness of the presence or absence of disease in a subject ("*interviewer bias*"). Measurements and observations can also be influenced by awareness of disease status, and by changes in exposure status induced by the disease. A differential exposure misclassification may be introduced if different methods of data collection, or different sources of exposure information, are used for cases and noncases.

Regardless of the timing of the data collection, a differential exposure misclassification may be introduced if the exposure information is influenced by a risk indicator for the disease. For example, age is a risk indicator for many diseases and may influence the accuracy of exposure information. Such misclassification is nondifferential within strata, for example, within each age group. When the risk indicator is controlled in the data analysis, the remaining bias is towards RR = 1. (But the "adjusted" RR is not always closer to the true relative risk. Greenland, Robins 1985).

As an example, consider again the study of X-ray exposure and breast cancer. The relative risk was RR = 2.00 with no misclassification (Table 1-7), and RR = 1.50 with a nondifferential exposure misclassification (specificity = 0.75, Table 1-8). Suppose that, for those who developed a breast cancer, accurate information on their X-ray exposure could be retrieved from the medical records. If this information was used, there would be no exposure misclassification among those who developed a breast cancer, but there would still be an exposure misclassification (specificity = 0.75) among the others. This is an example of differential exposure misclassification, since the specificity is different in those who did (1.0) and those who did not (0.75) develop the disease. The results would be as shown in Table 1-9 with RR = 0.75. When compared with Table 1-8, it may seem awkward that an improvement in the accuracy of exposure information (no misclassification among those who developed breast cancer in Table 1-9) actually reduced the accuracy of the result. This is because the misclassification in Table 1-8 is nondifferential (introducing a bias towards RR = 1), whereas the misclassification in Table 1-9 is differential (which may introduce a bias towards RR = 0 or RR = ∞). Thus, epidemiologists are usually more concerned with the *comparability*

Table 1–9 Differential exposure misclassification (sensitivity = 1.00, specificity = 1.00 among cases; sensitivity = 1.00, specificity = 0.75 among noncases). Based on the data in Table 1–7.

	Classified as:		Sum
	Exposed	Unexposed	
Breast cancer	40	80	120
No breast cancer	19,940	29,940	49,880
All women	19,980	30,020	50,000
Incidence proportion (∗ 1,000)	2.00	2.66	
	RR = 2.00/2.66 = 0.75		

of exposure information (avoiding differential misclassification) than with improving the accuracy of the information.

Nondifferential Disease Misclassification

Disease misclassification is *nondifferential* if the misclassification (sensitivity and specificity) does not differ between the exposed and unexposed (Kleinbaum et al. 1982, White 1986). Nondifferential disease misclassification may not bias the relative risk (sensitivity < 1), or result in a bias towards RR = 1 (specificity < 1).

Nondifferential disease misclassification may be introduced by a gap between the theoretical and empirical definition of the disease, for instance, by using too narrow or too wide diagnostic criteria (the symptoms, signs, and test results required for a certain diagnosis). Nondifferential disease misclassification may also be introduced by a measurement error that is independent of the exposure.

As an example, consider a study of the effect of oral contraceptive use on the risk of deep venous thrombosis. A total of 200 cases occurred during 3 years' follow-up of 80,000 women aged 30–39 years. With no misclassification, the results would be as in Table 1–10 with RR = 1.50. However, all cases of deep venous thrombosis were not identified. Suppose that 75% of the cases were identified (sensitivity = 0.75), regardless of whether or not they were exposed (nondifferential misclassification). This would give the results presented in Table 1–11 with RR = 1.50. Thus, a nondifferential misclassification of diseased as nondiseased (sensitivity < 1) did not bias the relative risk.

A nondifferential disease misclassification with specificity < 1 would, however, introduce a bias towards RR = 1. For instance, a specificity of 0.99 would mean that a thrombosis was incorrectly diagnosed in 1% of

Table 1-10 Data on oral contraceptive use and deep venous thrombosis (no misclassification)

	Exposed	Unexposed	Sum
Thrombosis	120	80	200
No thrombosis	39,880	39,920	79,800
All women	40,000	40,000	80,000
Incidence proportion (* 1,000)	3.00	2.00	
	RR = 3.00/2.00 = 1.50		

Table 1-11 Nondifferential disease misclassification with a reduced sensitivity (sensitivity = 0.75, specificity = 1.00). Based on the data in Table 1-10.

	Classified as:		
	Exposed	Unexposed	Sum
Thrombosis	90	60	150
No thrombosis	39,910	39,940	79,850
All women	40,000	40,000	80,000
Incidence proportion (* 1,000)	2.25	1.50	
	RR = 2.25/1.50 = 1.50		

those who did not develop a thrombosis. In Table 1–10, this would add 399 false positives to the 120 exposed cases (incidence proportion = 13.0 per 1,000 women), and 399 false positives to the 80 unexposed cases (incidence proportion = 12.0 per 1,000 women):

$$RR = 13.0/12.0 = 1.08$$

Differential Disease Misclassification

Disease misclassification is *differential* if the misclassification (sensitivity or specificity) differs between the exposed and unexposed. Differential disease misclassification introduces a bias towards RR = 0 or RR = ∞.

Differential disease misclassification is introduced if the exposure influences the follow-up and identification of cases. For instance, exposed subjects may be more (or less) likely than unexposed subjects to report symptoms of disease or to visit a doctor. Similarly, the staff involved in the follow-up and diagnosis of disease may be influenced by awareness of the exposure status of subjects. A differential disease misclassification may be introduced if different follow-up methods, or different sources of information, are used for the exposed and unexposed.

Differential disease misclassification may also be introduced if a factor associated with the exposure influences the follow-up and identification of cases. For example, age is associated with many exposures and may influence the accuracy of information on disease. Such misclassification is nondifferential within strata, for example, within each age group. When the factor is controlled in the data analysis, the remaining bias is towards RR = 1. (But the "adjusted" RR is not always closer to the true relative risk. Greenland, Robins 1985).

As an example, consider again the study of oral contraceptives and venous thrombosis. The relative risk was RR = 1.50 (Table 1–10), and was not biased by a nondifferential disease misclassification with a reduced sensitivity (Table 1–11). Suppose that both the women and their physicians knew that oral contraceptives may increase the risk of thrombosis and that, as a consequence, a venous thrombosis was identified in all women on oral contraceptives who developed a thrombosis. If so, there would be no disease misclassification among the exposed, but there would still be a disease misclassification (sensitivity = 0.75) among the unexposed. The results would be as shown in Table 1–12 with RR = 2.00. Compared with Table 1–11, an improvement in the accuracy of information on disease introduced a bias of the relative risk. Thus, epidemiologists are usually more concerned with the *comparability of disease information* (avoiding differential misclassification) than with improving the accuracy of the information.

Strategies in Dealing with Misclassification

Research strategies should be used with the purpose of reducing misclassification bias, and not only improving the accuracy of information. The direction of a bias may influence the interpretation of the results.

A high priority should be given to preventing differential misclassification. In studies where exposure information is collected or handled after the cases have appeared, differential exposure misclassification may sometimes be avoided by *blinding*, that is, by keeping those involved in

Table 1–12 Differential disease misclassification (sensitivity = 1.00, specificity = 1.00 among exposed; sensitivity = 0.75, specificity = 1.00 among unexposed). Based on the data in Table 1–10.

	Classified as:		
	Exposed	*Unexposed*	*Sum*
Thrombosis	120	60	180
No thrombosis	39,880	39,940	79,820
All women	40,000	40,000	80,000
Incidence proportion (∗ 1,000)	3.00	1.50	
	RR = 3.00/1.50 = 2.00		

the collection and handling of data unaware of the subjects' disease status. The same examination methods and data sources should be used for cases and noncases. If differential exposure misclassification (e.g., recall bias or interviewer bias) is likely to be an important source of error, it may be useful to consider the possibility of using exposure information collected before the cases appear.

In order to avoid differential disease misclassification, the follow-up of disease occurrence should be made in the same way, using the same methods and sources of information, for the exposed and unexposed. Sometimes it is possible to use *blinding*, that is, to keep those involved in the follow-up and identification of cases unaware of the subjects' exposure status. This may be facilitated by the use of placebo (sham treatment) in experimental studies or, in nonexperimental studies, by selecting the unexposed among people perceived as being similar to the exposed (e.g., in the same occupation as the exposed). Diagnostic criteria should, of course, be independent of the exposure. For example, in a study of smoking and chronic bronchitis, smoking should not be used as a criterion in the diagnosis of chronic bronchitis.

Nondifferential misclassification (with regard to exposure and disease) is an important source of underestimation of effects, and a large amount of nondifferential misclassification may conceal an effect. In order to avoid such bias, efforts should be made to avoid not only measurement errors but also any gap between the empirical and the theoretical definition of a specific exposure or disease.

The comparability and accuracy of information on exposure and disease that can be obtained in any particular study is determined by the choice of study population and follow-up period, by the definitions used, and by the methods used in the collection of information and classification of subjects.

■■■ SELECTION BIAS

Selection bias is defined here as the error that is introduced if the participation in (selection of subjects into or out of) a study is influenced by the disease (outcome) under study. The relative risk may be overestimated (biased towards RR = ∞) or underestimated (biased towards RR = 0) if the selection is differential, that is, if the disease influences study participation differently in the exposed and unexposed. Otherwise there is usually little or no bias of the relative risk for "rare" diseases (no bias of the odds ratio). But the absolute effect is biased (overestimated or underestimated), even if the selection is nondifferential, that is, similar in the exposed and unexposed. (Selection is nondifferential if $p_1/p_2 = p_3/p_4$

where the proportion participating is p_1 and p_2 in exposed cases and noncases, and p_3 and p_4 in unexposed cases and noncases, respectively. But in practice, this information is not likely to be available).

As an example, consider a study of irradiation and cataracts. At the beginning of their employment, all employees at certain laboratories participated in a health examination, including screening for cataracts. Subsequently, some employees were exposed to an occupational source of irradiation; others were not. After several years, all employees who were free from cataracts at the initial examination were invited to a follow-up examination. The purpose was to identify subjects who had developed cataracts since the time of the first examination. Suppose that 50 of 10,000 exposed and 100 of 20,000 unexposed employees developed cataracts (true RR = 50*20,000/100*10,000 = 1). Depending upon the circumstances, attention should be paid to the following sources of selection bias:

1. Selection bias is introduced if the disease under study influences the loss of subjects to follow-up. Suppose that, in the above example, the study population was defined as all subjects who were free from cataracts at the beginning of their employment. A considerable proportion of these subjects may have been lost to follow-up. But, at least among the exposed, people may be more inclined to attend a follow-up examination if they have experienced symptoms of cataracts (visual loss). If the follow-up examination was attended by all exposed cases, but only by 40% of unexposed cases and of all exposed and unexposed employees, then RR = 50*(0.40*20,000)/(0.40*100)*(0.40*10,000) = 2.5 (true value: RR = 1). Thus, the relative risk was overestimated by this selective loss to follow-up.

2. Whenever a study population is defined only after the cases have appeared, selection bias is introduced if the disease under study influences the selection of subjects for the study. This may occur when subjects enter a study after the cases have been identified, or their disease has reached the stage of development where it can influence the selection of subjects. Suppose that, in the above example, the study population was defined as all subjects who participated in the follow-up examination and were free from cataracts at the beginning of their employment. The same selection bias as above (1) would, of course, be present. But now it appears as a biased selection of subjects for the study.

3. Selection bias is introduced if the disease under study influences the loss of information. Suppose that, in the above example, individual exposure information was recorded continuously and stored at a department of occupational health. But some of these records may be lost. For instance, when subjects with a history of occupational exposure develop

visual loss, their physician may send for the record of occupational exposure. If some of these records (of exposed cases) were lost because they were not returned, selective loss of information would result in underestimation of the relative risk.

4. Whenever exposure information is collected only after the cases have appeared, selection bias is introduced if the disease under study influences the extent to which exposure information is obtained. Suppose that, in the above example, no exposure records were available and that, after follow-up, exposure information was collected by interview. Some subjects may, however, refuse to participate in these interviews. If exposed cases were more likely than others to provide exposure information, selective lack of exposure information would result in overestimation of the relative risk.

In a study, there may be selection bias even if the total loss of cases and noncases is similar. This is because the disease may influence the loss of subjects (or information) differently in the exposed and unexposed. To see this, in the above example, suppose that 40 percent of the exposed cases and 70 percent of the unexposed cases went to see their own physician and that only the remaining 60 percent of the exposed cases and 30 percent of the unexposed cases attended the follow-up examination. If so, there would be 0.60 * 50 = 30 exposed cases and 0.30 * 100 = 30 unexposed cases, and the total number of cases would be 30 + 30 = 60 or 40 percent of all 150 cases. With participation of 40 percent of all exposed and unexposed subjects (as above, 1), RR = 30*(0.40*20,000)/ 30*(0.40*10,000) = 2.0 (true value: RR = 1). Thus, a selection bias was introduced by a loss of 60 percent of all cases and 60 percent of all noncases.

In practice, the bias introduced by a loss of subjects cannot be calculated since information is missing about the occurrence of the exposure or disease (or both) among the subjects that were lost. But if information is available on the number of cases and noncases lost, the possible magnitude of a selection bias can be estimated by making more or less extreme assumptions about the occurrence of the exposure among the cases and noncases that were lost. Similarly, if information is available on the number of exposed and unexposed subjects lost, the possible magnitude of a selection bias can be estimated by making more or less extreme assumptions about the occurrence of the disease among the exposed and unexposed subjects that were lost.

Strategies in Dealing with Selection Bias

In general, selection bias cannot be controlled in the data analysis (although selection may sometimes be less differential after controlling factors associated with the exposure). The focus is on strategies to prevent selection bias. The different sources of selection bias may be avoided in defining the study population, in obtaining exposure information, and in the follow-up of disease occurrence.

The study population should be defined independently of the disease (outcome) of interest. When the study population is defined only after the cases have appeared, selection bias is introduced if the disease influences the selection of subjects for the study. Such definitions tend to conceal a selection bias, and possibilities of avoiding selection bias may be overlooked. Thus, whenever possible, the study population should be defined prior to follow-up (or from a list of subjects prepared prior to follow-up). In studies of prevalent cases, selection bias may be avoided by investigating asymptomatic disease or by selecting a study population that is likely to be defined independently of the disease. This may be achieved if the study population is defined as, for example, all men living within a certain area (unless the area happens to be, e.g., a health resort for exposed workers who have developed the disease under study—or the area from which they moved).

Selection bias is also introduced if the disease influences the availability of information. In studies where exposure information is collected only after the cases have appeared, the possibility of avoiding selection bias by obtaining information from all subjects is influenced by the choice of study population as well as by the methods used in the collection of exposure information. Regardless of the timing of the data collection, all information on the subjects should be secured to avoid selective loss of information.

Finally, selection bias is introduced if the disease influences the loss of study subjects during follow-up. Loss to follow-up may be prevented by selecting a suitable study population and follow-up period, and by appropriate routines for follow-up. In addition, various techniques have been used to trace subjects and increase their motivation for continued follow-up. Special attention should be paid to the possibility of selective withdrawals. In principle, it may be possible to examine each subject for the presence of disease at the time of withdrawal. In experimental studies, randomization, placebo, and blinding may be used to avoid any differences between the exposed and unexposed with regard to selective loss to follow-up.

■■■ RANDOM ERROR

Random error may be described as an uncertainty introduced by small numbers of observations. Suppose that a study was conducted among employees in some companies to investigate the effect (if any) of video display terminal (VDT) use during pregnancy on the risk of certain malformations in the newborn child. The results are presented in Table 1–13, showing a total of three cases among 800 babies and RR = 2.

Should we conclude that VDT use doubles the risk of malformations? Few, if any, epidemiologists would do so, even if great care was taken to avoid any sources of systematic error in the study. Some would argue that the number of cases is so small that the difference between the exposed (two cases) and the unexposed (one case) could very well be due to "chance." Others would say that the number of cases is so small that the difference could very well be due to a minor, unrecognized systematic error. According to both views (sometimes referred to as "probabilistic" and "deterministic", respectively), the result is uncertain due to the small number of cases in the study. (Besides, in a study where 50 percent of the babies are exposed, and only three cases occur, the relative risk could never be RR = 1).

Confidence Intervals

If the size of the study is increased, the number of observations (cases) will increase and the uncertainty due to small numbers will decrease. Usually a *confidence interval* is used to describe the degree of uncertainty (Rothman 1986, Bulpitt 1987). This is based on the view that the uncertainty is introduced by random variation ("chance"). A 95 percent confidence interval is constructed in such a way that the probability is 95 percent that the interval would contain the "true" value (e.g., the true RR), if there were no systematic errors. Thus, the confidence interval only reflects the uncertainty due to small numbers (random error) and does not account for systematic errors (confounding, misclassification, selection bias).

In a study of the effect of X-ray exposure on the risk of breast cancer in middle-aged women, the relative risk (with 95 percent confidence interval) was 1.6 (1.1–2.2). Thus, if there were no systematic errors, the probability is 95 percent that the true effect was between RR = 1.1 and RR = 2.2. (The probability that the true relative risk was below 1.1 is 2.5

Table 1–13 VDT use and malformations—an illustration of random error

	Exposed	*Unexposed*
Cases	2	1
Babies	400	400
Prevalence proportion (* 1,000)	5.0	2.5
	RR = 5.0/2.5 = 2.0	

percent, and the probability that it was above 2.2 is also 2.5 percent). However, the true value is more likely to be close to RR = 1.6, than close to RR = 1.1 or RR = 2.2. This could be illustrated by calculating a series of confidence intervals, for example 80, 90, 95, and 99 percent confidence intervals, where the 99 percent interval is the widest and the 80 percent interval is the tightest. The choice of a 95 percent interval is, disregarding tradition, an arbitrary choice. Thus, its limits (1.1 and 2.2, in the above example) should not be regarded as rigid. Should the lower limit be 0.9 rather than 1.1, this would not dramatically change the interpretation of the results. A critical discussion of the confidence interval and the role of statistics in epidemiology is provided by Greenland (1990).

Precision and Study Size

Precision is the degree of absence of random error. Precision can be improved by increasing the *study size*, that is, the size of the study population, or the duration of follow-up, or both. The greater the number of observations, the higher precision (tighter confidence interval).

The size of a study is, of course, influenced by the availability of potential study subjects as well as by financial and other practical considerations. In addition, the relation between study size and precision should be considered carefully at the planning stage. A first step may be to estimate the expected number of cases in the different exposure categories (e.g., in the exposed and unexposed, respectively) with a certain study size. If it is possible to assess the occurrence of the exposure and the disease in the intended study base, then it is also possible to calculate 95 percent confidence intervals on the basis of various assumptions regarding the effect, for example, RR = 1, RR = 2, and RR = 4 (or RR = 0.5). How tight these intervals should be is naturally a matter of judgment. But there is usually reason to question whether the precision will be sufficient, if a strong or expected effect is accompanied by an interval that contains RR = 1, or if RR = 1 is accompanied by a confidence interval that contains marked effects. If so, one may decide to increase the planned size of the study, to improve its efficiency (see below), or to refrain from carrying out the study.

Efficiency

Precision can be improved by increasing the study size, but this as a rule also increases the costs. In any particular study, the precision may be low and the costs may be high. There are, however, several ways to improve *efficiency*, that is the relation between precision and study size or cost. *Size-efficiency* is the relation between precision and study size. *Cost-efficiency* (sometimes referred to simply as "efficiency") is the relation between precision and cost.

To illustrate the need for strategies to improve efficiency, consider a study of diet and colon cancer. Suppose that information on exposures (including potential confounders) is obtained at a cost of 100 USD per subject. The disease has an incidence rate of about $5*10^{-4}$ per year in men aged 40–74 years. Thus, during 5 years' follow-up of 20,000 men there would only be about 5 exposed cases (at RR = 1) if 10 percent were exposed. The cost for obtaining the exposure information was 20,000 * 100 = 2 million USD. In addition, there are other costs involved, including the cost for follow-up of disease occurrence. The relation between precision and cost would be even more unfavorable if the incidence rate was lower (colon cancer is one of the most common cancers), if less than 10 percent were exposed (which is true for several dietary factors), or if the cost for obtaining exposure information was higher.

Improving Efficiency

Precision increases with the occurrence of the exposure in the study population (up to 50 percent exposed at RR = 1). For example, consider a study of 10,000 subjects where IP = 0.02 regardless of exposure status (RR = 1). If the study population included 100 exposed subjects (2 cases) and 9,900 unexposed subjects (198 cases), precision would be low due to the small number of exposed cases. Precision would be higher if the study population included 5,000 exposed (100 cases) and 5,000 unexposed subjects (100 cases). With any particular study size, precision may be improved by selecting a study population where a high proportion (up to 50 percent at RR = 1) of the subjects are exposed. If the exposure is rare in the general population, the study population may be selected from a subgroup (e.g., occupational group) where a high proportion of the subjects are exposed. When the exposure has a strong effect, the optimal proportion of exposed may be above or below 50 percent. (The proportion of exposed that will give the highest cost-efficiency depends upon the relative risk and the cost of recruiting and examining exposed and unexposed subjects. Morgenstern, Winn 1983.) If there are different levels of exposure, and the effect is expected to increase with the level of exposure (so-called dose-response pattern), the study may be restricted to unexposed and highly exposed subjects, unless there is a wish to study the effect at different exposure levels.

Since precision is limited by a scarcity of cases, a high incidence may seem desirable. But if the absolute effect (e.g., the risk difference) is similar in two populations, the association will be most readily apparent in the population with the lowest disease incidence in the unexposed. On the other hand, if the relative effect (the relative risk) is similar in two populations, the one with the highest incidence in the unexposed will give the highest precision.

There are several ways of reducing the costs, and thus improving cost-efficiency, in a study. The costs may be reduced by using inexpensive methods for obtaining information on exposures (including potential confounders), and for follow-up of disease occurrence. Sometimes information on exposure or disease has been collected for other purposes and is available at a low cost. The gain in cost-efficiency should, of course, be weighed against any bias due to misclassification or lack of information.

The most powerful strategy for improving cost-efficiency is often to use exposure information only for the cases and, in addition, for a sample representing the study base or study population (so-called *referents* or "controls"). This is discussed in Chapter 6.

■■■ GENERALIZABILITY AND EFFECT MODIFICATION

Effect modification occurs when the effect of an exposure (as measured by, e.g., the relative risk or risk difference) is different in different subgroups of the population. For instance, the relative risk (reflecting the effect of a certain exposure on the risk of a certain disease) may be different in men and women. If so, sex is a *modifier* of the relative risk. The relative risk among men does not apply to women, and cannot be generalized to any population that includes women. Thus, the *generalizability* of the result is limited by effect modification. Effect modification is a natural phenomenon, and the object of investigation in some studies, rather than a source of error.

As an example of effect modification, consider a study of 800 tourists who visited a restaurant. Some of them ate a shrimp salad (exposed), others did not (unexposed). Some developed acute diarrhea within the next week (cases). But in addition, some subjects had and others had not received a vaccine that could protect against certain causes of acute diarrhea (Table 1–14).

Both the relative risk and risk difference are different in vaccinated and unvaccinated subjects; that is, both RR and RD are modified by vaccination status. When the disease occurrence in the unexposed is similar in each category (as in Table 1–14, where IP = 0.10 in both vaccinated and unvaccinated subjects), then both the relative and absolute effect, or neither, is modified. But if the disease occurrence in the

Table 1–14 Intake of shrimp salad and acute diarrhea—an illustration of effect modification (by vaccination status)

	Unvaccinated		Vaccinated	
	Exposed	Unexposed	Exposed	Unexposed
Cases	60	20	20	20
Subjects	200	200	200	200
Incidence proportion	0.30	0.10	0.10	0.10
Relative risk	RR = 3		RR = 1	
Risk difference	RD = 0.20		RD = 0	

unexposed is different in each category, then either the relative or absolute effect, or both, will be modified. For instance, suppose that (in Table 1–14) the incidence proportion in the unexposed would be 0.15 in unvaccinated and 0.05 in vaccinated. Then RR = 0.30/0.15 = 2 in unvaccinated and RR = 0.10/0.05 = 2 in vaccinated (i.e., no modification of the relative risk), but RD = 0.30 − 0.15 = 0.15 in unvaccinated and RD = 0.10 − 0.05 = 0.05 in vaccinated (i.e., modification of the risk difference). Thus, effect modification should always be specified as to what effect measure (e.g., RR or RD) is being modified.

If vaccinated and unvaccinated subjects in Table 1–14 were considered together, there would be 80 cases in 400 exposed (incidence proportion 0.20), and 40 cases in 400 unexposed subjects (incidence proportion 0.10): RR = 2, RD = 0.10. This represents the average effect in a mixed population with 50 percent vaccinated and 50 percent unvaccinated subjects, but no bias is introduced. (To introduce confounding, vaccination would have to be associated with the exposure and be a risk factor in the unexposed). But since the effect depends upon the vaccination status, there is an interest in the separate effects (i.e., the effect in unvaccinated subjects and the lack of effect in vaccinated subjects), rather than in the average effect in a mixed population (which will depend upon the proportion that is vaccinated). Information on such average effects are neither useful to vaccinated nor to unvaccinated subjects. In addition, the result would have very limited generalizability, since it would only apply (as an average) to populations with the same proportion of vaccinated. Thus, to the extent that an exposure has different effects in different subgroups of the population, there is an interest in the separate effects rather than in some weighted average (which will depend upon the occurrence of the modifier).

Effect modification may be dealt with by restriction when selecting the study population (e.g., including only unvaccinated subjects), or by restriction in the data analysis (e.g., estimating the effect in vaccinated and unvaccinated separately). To be able to estimate the separate effects with adequate precision, the study population should include a sufficient number of subjects in each category (e.g., vaccinated and unvaccinated). Otherwise, the study population should only include one category of the modifier (e.g., unvaccinated), and the results will apply to this category.

▄▄ STUDY DESIGN

Epidemiologic studies are designed with the overall objective of obtaining accurate results with limited resources. Decisions are based on considerations of possible sources of error, their impact on the results, and the strategies available to avoid or control the different errors. These strategies may be viewed as the building blocks used in the design of epidemiologic studies.

Asking the Questions

The design and accuracy of an epidemiologic study depend to a large extent on the question it is supposed to answer. To be able to obtain a useful answer, the question should be specific. Several questions can often be addressed in a single study. Each question should be specified with regard to exposure and disease, and the type of effect (effect measure) of interest. In addition, the effect of an exposure on the risk of developing a disease is likely to be different in different subgroups of the population (defined by effect modifiers), and during different periods of time (in relation to the time of exposure). Each question should be specified in these respects. This is discussed further in Chapter 2.

Selecting the Study Population and Follow-up Period

Accuracy (validity, precision) is influenced by the choice of study population and follow-up period. Confounding and misclassification bias may be reduced by restrictions with regard to confounders and factors that influence the accuracy of information. Selection bias may also be avoided by selecting a suitable study population and follow-up period. The induction time should be taken into account when selecting the follow-up period. Precision is influenced by study size, that is, the size of the study population and the duration of follow-up. The study population and follow-up period may be selected to improve efficiency, which depends upon the occurrence of the exposure, as well as the occurrence of the disease and the strength of the effect, in the study base. The cost and time necessary to conduct a study may be reduced by selecting a suitable study population and follow-up period, for example, by using register data or other available information. Finally, the generalizability and usefulness of the results may be improved by restrictions with regard to effect modifiers. This is discussed further in Chapter 3.

Obtaining Information on Exposures

The strategies used to obtain information on exposures (and potential confounders and modifiers) involve the definitions, the methods for measurement and classification of subjects, and the timing of the collection and handling of information. The concern is the accuracy of the study result, that is, the estimate of effect (rather than the accuracy of the exposure information itself). Thus, efforts should be made to avoid sources of differential exposure misclassification (e.g., recall bias and interviewer bias). This may influence the choice of definitions and methods, and the timing of the data collection. The possibility that an effect is underestimated or concealed by nondifferential exposure misclassification, will focus attention on any gap between the empirical and theoretical definition and on measurement errors that are independent of the disease. When subjects do not provide exposure information, the consequences may depend upon the timing of the data collection. This is discussed further in Chapter 4.

Follow-up of Disease Occurrence

The definitions and methods used in the follow-up of disease occurrence (or in the identification of prevalent cases) are important with regard to possible disease misclassification. Again, the concern is the accuracy of the study result, that is, the estimate of effect (rather than the accuracy of information on the disease under study). Thus, efforts should be made to avoid sources of differential disease misclassification, including any differences between the methods used in the follow-up of exposed and unexposed subjects. In some studies, it may be possible to use blinding with regard to exposure status. In order to avoid confounding by previous episodes of the same disease, a study is often limited to first cases of the disease. Sources of nondifferential disease misclassification may bias the result towards $RR = 1$ (specificity < 1), or reduce precision if fewer cases are identified (sensitivity < 1). Selection bias may be prevented by strategies used to avoid selective loss to follow-up. This is discussed further in Chapter 5.

Sampling from the Base (Case-Referent Strategies)

Low cost-efficiency is a major problem in many epidemiologic studies. Usually, precision is limited by the small number of cases, while the cost for obtaining exposure information is high due to the large number of subjects in the study population. The most powerful way to improve efficiency may be to select a sample, *referents* (also called *controls*), that reflects the occurrence of the exposure in the study base or study population (Miettinen 1985). The relative risk (RR = a∗D/b∗C, cf. Table 1–2A) is estimated as RR = a∗d/b∗c using exposure information only for the cases (a,b) and the referents (c,d). This is the basis for *case-referent studies* (also called *case-control studies*). If the referents reflect the occurrence of the exposure in the study base (i.e., if d/c = D/C), then a∗d/b∗c is an unbiased estimate of the relative risk. Otherwise a bias is introduced by the selection of referents. To avoid such *referent selection bias*, referents may be selected as a random sample of the study base or study population. But sometimes it may be preferable to select referents in some other way, for instance among other subjects admitted to the same hospital as the cases (so-called hospital referents). Case-referent strategies are discussed in Chapter 6.

Assignment of Exposure (Experimental Strategies)

The possibility of confounding by unidentified factors is a major concern in many epidemiologic studies. In *experimental studies*, the study subjects are assigned to receive or not to receive an intervention designed to change their exposure status (Meinert 1986). These assignments are, as a rule, made by *randomization* using a series of random numbers (randomized experiments). With an increasing number of subjects (or other units) involved in the randomization, the intervention and nonintervention group will tend to be similar with regard to other factors. In principle, this will prevent any confounding by unidentified as well as by identified factors present at the time of randomization. Sometimes it is also possible to avoid confounding that may be introduced by the intervention (or by awareness of the intervention), by using *placebo (sham treatment)* in the nonintervention group and *blinding*, that is keeping the study subjects, and perhaps also staff members, unaware of the assignments. High cost is a major limitation of experimental studies of disease causation and prevention. But sometimes the cost-efficiency may be improved, for example, by selecting a study population of subjects who are at high risk of the disease. Ethical and practical considerations may also introduce limitations in experimental studies. Experimental strategies are discussed in Chapter 7.

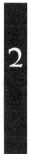

2 Asking the Right Questions

▬ INTRODUCTION

The General Question

"What are the causes of disease?" An obvious purpose of asking and trying to answer this question is to understand how disease arises (a scientific purpose). In addition, there are practical purposes: to prevent the occurrence of disease (a purpose of preventive medicine and public health) and to provide effective treatment of disease (a purpose of clinical medicine). An early example of the closeness between epidemiologic science, prevention, and treatment is found in Goldberger's studies of pellagra in 1914–1929 (Terris 1964).

There are, of course, different causes for different diseases. Thus, it makes sense to ask separate questions for each exposure (E) and disease (D): "Does E cause D?" But a single factor (E) is rarely, if ever, sufficient to bring about disease in all subjects. When we say that smoking causes lung cancer, we mean that smoking is a contributing cause that increases the risk of lung cancer. Thus, the question may be rephrased as follows: "Does E increase the risk of D?" In addition, there is an interest in the magnitude of an effect:

"Does E increase the risk of D—and if so, by how much?"

However, for those interested in the etiology, prevention, or treatment of disease, it may be just as important to learn about exposures that reduce the risk of disease (preventive factors):

"Does E reduce the risk of D—and if so, by how much?"

Sometimes the direction of the effect, if any, is not known in advance and the question may involve both possibilities:

> "Does E affect the risk of D—and if so, in what direction and by how much?"

These *general questions* should be specified in certain respects, as discussed in the following sections. *Specific questions* should be considered carefully in the planning of a study, since they are likely to influence the design and size of the study.

Effect Measures

The last part of the general question, ". . . by how much?", usually refers to the relative effect (relative risk). In addition, there may be an interest in the size of the public health problem involved, as reflected by the absolute effect and the attributable fraction.

Exposure

The question should be specific with regard to different aspects of the exposure. For example, consider the following question: "Does a high fat intake affect the risk of myocardial infarction—and if so, in what direction and by how much?" The effect may be of a different magnitude, and perhaps even different direction, depending upon the specific type of fat, for example, saturated, monounsaturated, or polyunsaturated fat. Thus, the question should be specific as to the type of fat or, in more general terms, the *type* of exposure. In addition, the question should be specific as to the *quantity* and *frequency* of exposure: what is meant by a "high" fat intake? If the level is defined in terms of an average daily (or weekly, monthly, etc.) intake, it may be worth considering whether the effect could depend upon the *patterns* of exposure, for example, a fairly constant daily intake close to the average versus a highly variable fat intake with levels sometimes much above the average. Sometimes the effect of an exposure may depend upon the *timing* of exposure in relation to other events. Finally, the *duration* of exposure usually has to be taken into account: a high fat intake during a short period of time may not have much impact on the risk of myocardial infarction.

Questions may be asked separately concerning the effects of the different aspects of an exposure mentioned above. But in practice, different aspects are often combined to define one or more *"exposed" categories*. Since the effect depends upon the alternative, the *"unexposed" category* should also be defined. This may be the absence of an exposure, such as smoking, or a low level of an exposure, such as fat intake. Usually unexposed means never exposed, since it may be difficult or impossible to rule out an effect of past exposure.

Induction Time

Following exposure, any effect on the risk of developing a disease is likely to vary over time. For example, the effect of current and past cigarette smoking on the risk of ulcerative colitis may be of different magnitude, and perhaps even different direction. Thus, it is appropriate to ask separate questions concerning the effect of current and past exposure. The time interval between exposure and effect varies considerably between different exposure-disease associations. Smoking may increase the risk of upper respiratory infections at once, but the risk of upper respiratory cancers only after several years. In many situations the induction time is not known in advance, and questions may be asked separately concerning the effect in different "time windows" following exposure. Sometimes there is an interest in estimating the length of the induction time, that is, to study the effect in different "time windows" following a *change* in exposure status (from unexposed to exposed, or vice versa).

Disease

The question should also be specific with regard to the disease (outcome) of interest. Consider the following example: "Does a high serum cholesterol affect the risk of stroke—and if so, in what direction and by how much?" The effect may be of a different magnitude, and perhaps even different direction, depending upon the specific type of stroke, for example, thrombotic or hemorrhagic stroke. Similarly, there are likely to be differences in the etiology of arthritis depending upon its type and localization, and differences in the causation of gallstones depending upon their chemical composition. The development of new diagnostic tools is likely to make it possible to separate an increasing number of disease entities that differ in their etiology. Sometimes there may be information from other sources, suggesting a subdivision of disease entities, for example, differences in the descriptive epidemiology of breast cancer in women occurring before and after menopause. Finally, there could be differences in the effect of an exposure between first and subsequent episodes of a disease, or between different degrees of severity of a disease. This is one reason for including these aspects in a definition of the disease.

Modifiers

A specific exposure may affect the risk of a specific disease differently in different subgroups of the population, so-called effect modification (see Chapter 1: Generalizability and Effect Modification). For example, a certain exposure may affect the risk of acute diarrhea differently in vaccinated and unvaccinated subjects. If so, there is effect modification by vaccination status, and an effect observed among unvaccinated subjects does not apply to vaccinated subjects or to any population that includes vaccinated subjects. There is not primarily an interest in the "average" effect in a population where a certain proportion is vaccinated. Instead, there is an interest in two separate questions: "What is the effect in unvaccinated subjects?" and "What is the effect in vaccinated subjects?". Thus, to put it in more general terms, potential modifiers should as far as possible be identified in advance and questions should be asked separately concerning the effect in each category of a modifier. The purpose of a study is often limited to address one of these questions. But sometimes a study is designed to address two or more of these questions, that is, to study effect modification.

Other Aspects

Potential confounders should, of course, be taken into account in a study. But when investigating the *effect* of an exposure, this is a methodologic issue rather than a part of the question addressed by the study. This also applies to other sources of error.

Sometimes, questions are rephrased in an attempt to overcome difficulties in the design or conduct of an investigation. For example, the purpose of a study of serum nutrients and cancer could be described as evaluating the effect of "nutrient levels in a serum sample" on the risk of cancer, because it may be difficult or impossible to measure nutrient levels over time. However, the risk of cancer is not likely to be affected by the nutrient level in a single serum sample but rather by nutrient levels over a period of time. The difference may be an important source of exposure misclassification (see Chapter 1: Misclassification). Questions should not be rephrased to avoid practical difficulties or sources of error. Thus, a question should be based on theoretical rather than empirical definitions.

Priorities

As the questions become more specific, the number of possible questions increases rapidly. This calls for priorities, although several questions may sometimes be addressed in a single study. Priority may be given to questions according to their scientific or practical importance. In addition, priorities may be based on the possibility of obtaining accurate results at a reasonable cost.

▬ EXERCISES

2:1 The effect of cigarette smoking on the risk of stroke in middle-aged women was investigated. What aspects of the exposure (cigarette smoking) should be considered? How should the exposed and unexposed categories be defined?

2:2 A study in Brazil showed that breast feeding reduced the risk of infant death due to diarrhea. What is the exposure of interest? What is the unexposed category?

2:3 A low level of occupational exercise was found to increase the risk of colon cancer. What is the exposure of interest? What subjects should be considered as highly exposed?

2:4 According to the findings of a study in New Zealand, a drug used in the treatment of asthma (fenoterol by MDI = metered dose inhaler) may increase mortality among subjects aged 5–45 under treatment for asthma.

A. What is the exposure of interest? What is the unexposed category?

In another study, it was found that a high dietary intake of protein increases the risk of rectal cancer.

B. What is the exposure of interest? What is the unexposed category?

2:5 According to the findings of an epidemiologic study, a family history of leukemia increases the risk of leukemia.

A. What is the exposure of interest?

Another study was planned to evaluate the effect of maternal smoking on infant mortality from respiratory and other diseases.

B. What is the exposure of interest?

2:6 A study in Japan showed that lung cancer mortality in nonsmoking wives of heavy smokers was twice that in nonsmoking wives of nonsmokers.

A. What is the exposure of interest?

B. How could the result of this study influence the definition of the unexposed category in a study where smoking is the exposure of interest?

Another study showed that blonde subjects have a higher risk of malignant melanoma of the skin than people with black hair.

C. What is the exposure of interest?

2:7   Vitamin E is known as an intracellular antioxidant that might protect against cancer, but studies on animals and humans have yielded somewhat conflicting results. An epidemiologic study focused on the effect of serum levels of vitamin E on the risk of cancer. Should serum levels, or dietary intake, of vitamin E be thought of as the exposure of interest?

2:8   In a randomized trial, the dietary intervention included advice on an increase in fatty fish intake. One of the questions at issue was if (and by how much) the exposure would reduce the risk of death from ischemic heart disease in men under 70 years of age who had recovered from a recent myocardial infarction. What is the exposure of interest?

2:9   In an outbreak of a severe infectious disease (listeriosis) in Los Angeles County, there were 142 cases, including 48 deaths. The specific bacterium responsible for listeriosis, Listeria monocytogenes, has been isolated from foods, water, sewage, and other environmental sources. An epidemiologic study was conducted with the purpose of identifying the sources of the outbreak. What was the exposure of interest?

2:10   The use of certain sedatives, such as benzodiazepines, may increase the risk of falls and other accidents. What aspects of the exposure (benzodiazepine use) should be considered when planning a study of its effect on the risk of hip fracture?

2:11   Pipe smoking has been found to increase the risk of cancer of the urinary bladder by about 20 percent in some American studies, and by about 200 percent in some European studies of men in similar age groups. If these results are accurate, what could explain the difference?

2:12 The effect of oral contraceptive use on the risk of breast cancer in premenopausal women was investigated. The study included women in two neighbor countries, and long-term (8+ years) use was associated with an excess risk in one of these countries but not in the other. What could explain this difference, if it was not due to random or systematic error?

2:13 It has been discussed, whether certain vitamins taken around the time of conception can reduce a woman's risk of having a child with a neural-tube defect. However, a study in California found no such effect and it was concluded that "the periconceptional use of multivitamins or folate-containing supplements by American women does not decrease the risk of having an infant with a neural-tube defect."

A. Why was the conclusion limited to apply to American women?
B. What was the exposure of interest?

2:14 Alcohol and aflatoxin (found in cassava, peanuts, and sometimes in corn) could each increase the risk of primary liver cancer. A study was planned to investigate this, as well as the joint effect of alcohol and aflatoxin. For each of these two exposures, subjects were considered to be either exposed or unexposed. Which were the "exposed" and "unexposed" categories? What were the general questions?

2:15 Tobacco and alcohol could each increase the risk of laryngeal cancer. There was an interest in studying the separate effects of tobacco and alcohol, as well as their joint effect, at three different levels of exposure: low, medium, and high. Which were the "exposed" and "unexposed" categories? What were the general questions?

2:16 The effect of smoking on all-cause mortality and mortality from some specific diseases was investigated in a study of male British doctors. To what extent should the general question, and thus the conclusions from the study, be restricted with regard to sex (men), nationality (British), occupation (doctors), and other factors such as age?

2:17 It has been suggested that large gallstones may increase the risk of gallbladder cancer. A study was conducted to investigate the effect of gallstone size, and growth, on the risk of gallbladder cancer. The study was planned as an interracial study. To what extent should questions be asked separately for different races? To what extent should different races be included in the study?

2:18 Occupational exposure to wood dust, and occupational exposure to textile dust, may each increase the risk of certain cancers of the nasal cavity and paranasal sinuses. When planning to study these effects, should questions be asked separately for men and women? Should both sexes be included in the study?

2:19 Cigarette smoking increases the risk of coronary heart disease (CHD). The magnitude of this effect was investigated, and there was an interest in the absolute as well as in the relative effect. Among nonsmokers, the incidence of CHD increases with age and is higher in men than in women. Should questions be asked separately for men and women? Should questions be asked separately for different age groups? Why/why not?

2:20 The effect of weight gain on mortality was investigated. Questions were specified with regard to effect measures, exposure, induction time, and potential modifiers. Should the questions be specified in some other respect? Which?

2:21 Surgical removal of a part of the stomach (partial gastrectomy), used in the treatment of benign ulcer disease, could increase the risk of gastric cancer. But when patients in Amsterdam were followed during 5 years after partial gastrectomy, there was no overall excess risk of gastric cancer. If this result is accurate, what additional questions should be considered before concluding that partial gastrectomy does not increase the risk of gastric cancer?

2:22 The possibility that pregnancy could increase the risk of gallstone disease has been discussed. But in a study of women aged 20–76 years, pregnancy had little or no overall effect on the risk of gallstone disease. What specific questions should be considered, before concluding that pregnancy does not increase the risk of gallstone disease?

2:23 Several studies have shown that oral contraceptive use reduces the risk of ovarian cancer. What are the appropriate questions to be addressed in a study aimed at investigating the length of the induction time?

2:24 Following surgery, limited mobility may lead to the formation of deep-vein thrombosis. Subcutaneous heparin is given with the purpose of preventing thrombosis formation, but may increase the risk of bleeding. A review of several randomized trials showed that subcutaneous heparin reduced the risk of deep-vein thrombosis by 2/3 (RR about 0.33), but increased the risk of excessive bleeding by 2/3 (RR about 1.67). What additional information would be useful, when comparing these effects?

2:25 "Does alcohol intake affect the risk of stroke in middle-aged women —and if so, in what direction and by how much?"

    A. Suppose the words "in middle-aged women" were left out in the above question. Would it make any difference? Why/why not?

    B. What aspects of alcohol intake should be considered? How should the exposed and unexposed categories be defined?

    C. Should the disease ("stroke") be further specified?

2:26 "Does vaccination with inactivated influenza virus vaccine reduce the risk of influenza in healthy subjects aged 30–60 years—and if so, by how much?"

    A. Suppose the words "in healthy subjects aged 30–60 years" were left out in the above question. Would it make any difference? Why/why not?

    B. What was the "exposure" of interest? What aspects of the exposure should be considered?

    C. What was the disease of interest? What aspects of the disease should be considered?

2:27 "Does coffee drinking increase the risk of myocardial infarction— and if so, by how much?" In what ways should this general question be specified?

2:28 In a study of high density lipoprotein (HDL) cholesterol and death from coronary heart disease (CHD), exposure information was obtained by determining the level of HDL cholesterol in a serum sample from each subject. Would it be appropriate to say that the purpose was to evaluate the effect of HDL cholesterol in a serum sample on the risk of death from CHD? Why/why not?

2:29 The purpose of a study was described as investigating the effects of grain farming and smoking on the prevalence of chronic bronchitis.

A. What determines the prevalence of chronic bronchitis, except its incidence?

B. There is likely to be an interest in the effects of the exposures on the incidence, rather than the prevalence, of chronic bronchitis. What is the difference?

2:30 The effect of X-ray exposure before puberty on the risk of breast cancer in women was investigated. Suppose that such exposure has different effects on the risk of breast cancer occurring before and after menopause. How could this be explained?

▬ GENERAL QUESTIONS

2:31 In studies of disease causation, what is the general question?

2:32 Two important aspects are the direction and magnitude of an effect. What effect measures may be used?

2:33 The questions should be specified with regard to exposure.

A. What different aspects of the exposure should be considered?

B. How should these aspects be used to define one or more exposed categories? Exemplify!

2:34 The effect of a certain exposure depends upon the alternative, that is, the unexposed category.

A. How should the unexposed category be defined? Exemplify!

B. When the joint effect of two or more exposures is being investigated, what is the unexposed category?

2:35 The questions should be specified with regard to the disease (outcome) of interest.

A. What different aspects of the disease should be considered?

B. How should these aspects be used to define the disease under study? Exemplify!

2:36 The questions should be specified with regard to modifiers, to identify one or more subgroups of the population where the effect is investigated.

A. What does this mean? Exemplify!

B. Why should the questions be specified in this respect?

2:37 The questions should be specified with regard to induction time, to identify one or more "time windows" where the effect is investigated.

A. What does this mean? Exemplify!

B. Why should the questions be specified in this respect?

2:38 Sometimes there is an interest in the effect of an exposure in different "time windows" following a *change* in exposure status, that is from unexposed to exposed or vice versa. Why?

2:39 Questions about disease causation may be considered from a theoretical (scientific) or practical (clinical or public health) point of view. What is the difference, if any? Exemplify!

2:40 Consider your own recent favorite study. What are the implications for that study of the general problems and possibilities exemplified in the different exercises in this chapter?

3 Selecting the Study Population and Follow-up Period

■■■ INTRODUCTION

General Aspects

The study population and follow-up period should be selected to achieve a high degree of accuracy (validity and precision) with limited resources. In principle, the study population could be selected from any part (defined by age, sex, residence, or other characteristics) of any source population. There are, however, considerable differences between populations in the occurrence of exposure, disease, confounders, and modifiers. In addition, there are differences between populations in the comparability, accuracy, and completeness of information that can be obtained. Conditions that should be taken into account when selecting a study population include the following:

A. The Occurrence of:

A:1. Exposure. Precision is improved by selecting a study population where a high proportion of the subjects are exposed (up to 50% at RR = 1). If the effect is expected to be stronger at higher exposure levels, the study may be restricted to unexposed and highly exposed subjects. The cost of recruiting and examining study subjects should also be taken into account. (See Chapter 1, Random Error: Improving Efficiency).

A:2. Disease. Precision is influenced by the occurrence of the disease and the strength of the effect, and the study population may be selected accordingly. If the relative effect is similar in two populations, the highest precision is obtained when using the population with the highest incidence in the unexposed. But if the absolute effect is similar in two populations, the effect will be most readily apparent in the one with the lowest incidence in the unexposed.

A:3. Confounders. Validity may be improved by restrictions with regard to potential confounders. For instance, confounding by sex is avoided if only women (or only men) are included in the study, and confounding by previous episodes of the disease is avoided by including only subjects who have not had the disease under study. Restrictions should be made according to strict criteria. Occasionally, matching of unexposed to exposed subjects is used to avoid confounding. (See Chapter 1, Confounding: Strategies in Dealing with Confounding).

A:4. Modifiers. The usefulness and generalizability of the results may be improved by restrictions with regard to modifiers. The category where the effect is most readily apparent should be selected (see A:2, above), unless there is an interest in the effect in some other category. When effect modification is investigated, each of the categories included in the study should be of sufficient size to permit assessment and comparison of effects. (See Chapter 1: Generalizability and Effect Modification).

B. The Comparability, Accuracy and Completeness of Information on:

B:1. Exposure. Although misclassification and failure to obtain information will not be apparent until the exposure information has been collected, the possibilities of avoiding these sources of bias are influenced by the choice of study population. Restriction may be used to improve the accuracy, comparability, and completeness of information, for example, by limiting the study to certain age groups or to people who speak the same language (using strict criteria).

B:2. Disease. The accuracy and completeness of information on disease may be improved by restricting the study to, for instance, certain age groups. Exposed and unexposed subjects should be selected to provide comparability with regard to follow-up and identification of cases. For instance, when exposed subjects are routinely offered a thorough follow-up of disease occurrence, this may suggest the choice of an unexposed group that is offered a similar follow-up.

B:3. Confounders. The possibility of controlling confounding in the data analysis (or avoiding confounding by restriction) depends upon the availability of accurate information on confounders. The information that can be obtained varies between population subgroups, and the study population may be selected accordingly.

B:4. Modifiers. The possibility of studying effect modification depends upon the information on modifiers that can be obtained for a selected study population.

Timing

Whenever possible, the study population should be defined prior to follow-up. When the study population is defined only after the cases have appeared, selection bias is introduced if the disease influences the selection of subjects for the study. Such definitions tend to conceal the sources and possible magnitude of a selection bias, and possibilities of avoiding selection bias may be overlooked. As an example, suppose that information on exposure to pesticides was obtained in a survey. Several years later an attempt was made to identify subjects who participated in the survey to see whether they had developed a neurologic disease. However, the possibility of identifying and examining subjects at that time may be influenced by the disease. For instance, subjects could be more interested in participating in the follow-up examination if they had developed the disease, particularly if they were exposed to pesticides. This would introduce selection bias. If the study population is defined as all subjects who participated in the follow-up examination, no information is provided on this bias. It would be preferable to define the study population prior to follow-up (from a list of participants in the population survey), and to provide information on the number of exposed and unexposed subjects lost to follow-up, on the reasons for loss to follow-up, and on the efforts that were made to avoid selective loss to follow-up.

Similar concerns apply to any restrictions that are made within a previously selected study population. When such restrictions (or divisions into subgroups) are made only after the cases have appeared, selection bias is introduced if the restrictions are influenced by the disease under study. This source of selection bias may be avoided if any restrictions are made "blind" (without knowledge of the disease) using strict criteria determined in advance.

In studies based on disease prevalence, the cases are usually present when the study population is selected. Selection bias may be avoided by selecting a study population that is likely to be defined independently of the disease (cf. Chapter 1), or by investigating asymptomatic disease. Any restriction to asymptomatic subjects should be made "blind" according to strict criteria.

Validity

Selection bias is introduced if the disease influences the selection of subjects for, or their participation in, a study (Chapter 1: Selection Bias). As mentioned above, selective entry into the study may be avoided by defining the study population prior to follow-up (before the cases appear). In addition, the study population and follow-up period should be selected in a way that is likely to minimize the possibility of selective loss to follow-up (cf. B:2, above) and selective lack of information (cf. B:1, above). In a study report, information should be provided on possible sources of selection bias.

Confounding may be avoided by restrictions with regard to potential confounders (cf. A:3, above). Sometimes these restrictions should be extensive and a study may include, for instance, only certain occupational groups or certain groups of patients (see Chapter 1, Confounding: Strategies in Dealing with Confounding). In addition, a study population should be selected that can provide accurate information on confounders to be controlled in the data analysis (Cf. B:3, above). As an example, consider a study of alcohol intake and myocardial infarction. Confounding by sex is avoided if the study is restricted to include only men or only women. Similarly, confounding by previous heart disease may be avoided by not including subjects with previous heart disease, and confounding by factors such as age and residence may be reduced by restrictions to a certain age interval and area of residence. But in addition, information is collected on confounders to be controlled in the data analysis, such as dietary habits including intake of fats and calories. The accuracy of information that can be obtained on such confounders may vary by age and sex and other characteristics, and this may be taken into account when selecting a study population.

Misclassification with regard to exposure and disease may be avoided by restrictions to improve the comparability and accuracy of information that can be obtained (cf. B:1 and B:2, above). When selecting a follow-up period, the induction time should be taken into account (Chapter 1). As an example, consider a study of the effects of certain dietary factors on the risk of gallstone disease. The accuracy of exposure information may be different in men and women. Since men and women also differ in their risk of gallstone disease, this would introduce a differential exposure misclassification. The comparability of exposure information may be improved by restriction to either men or women when selecting the study population (or in the data analysis), while the accuracy of exposure information may suggest restriction to women rather than men. To the extent that subjects change their dietary intake over time, the induction time should be taken into account. If the induction time is unknown, the effect may be studied in different "time windows" provided that the selected study population is large enough for adequate precision.

Precision and Cost

Precision, study size, and cost should be considered early in the planning of a study (see Chapter 1: Random Error). Precision may be improved by increasing the size of a study. But in addition, precision is influenced by the occurrence of the exposure (cf. A:1, above) as well as by the occurrence of the disease and the strength of the effect (cf. A:2, above). The study population and follow-up period should be selected to provide a high precision with the limited resources available. With the purpose of improving cost-efficiency, the cost of recruiting and examining study subjects should also be taken into account. As an example, consider a study to find out whether a drug, used in the treatment of arthritis, increases the risk of renal insufficiency. A high size-efficiency (and cost-efficiency) may be obtained by selecting a study population among people with arthritis where a high proportion (up to 50%) are exposed to the drug. A high cost-efficiency could also be obtained using a large subgroup of the general population, for example, people in a health surveillance program, for whom information on drug prescriptions is available from a computerized register at a low cost.

Generalizability and Effect Modification

The usefulness and generalizability of the results may be improved by restrictions when selecting the study population (see Chapter 1: Generalizability and Effect Modification). Sometimes there is an interest in studying the effect of an exposure in different subgroups of the population, that is to study effect modification (Chapter 2). If so, the study population should be selected to be of sufficient size in each category of a modifier (cf. A:4, above) and to provide adequate information on modifiers (cf. B:4, above). As an example, consider a study of the effect of an occupational exposure in an occupation where 90 percent are men and 10 percent women. The study population may be selected to include only men (or only women). If there would be an interest in studying the effect separately in men and women, the study population could be selected to include about 50 percent men and 50 percent women. But the study population should not be selected to reflect the sex distribution in the occupation: If the study population would include 90 percent men and 10 percent women, the number of women is likely to be insufficient to estimate the effect in women with adequate precision, whereas sex may still introduce bias (confounding; differential misclassification).

■■■ EXERCISES

3:1   The use of certain drugs during early pregnancy could increase the risk of cardiovascular malformations in the offspring. This was investigated among subjects born in Massachusetts during a 3-year period. The malformations develop during fetal life, but are usually identified only at birth. Thus, the study was based on prevalent cases among newborn babies. In what way could this have biased the relative risks, compared to a study based on incident cases during fetal life (if such a study could have been performed)?

3:2   Laboratory studies have shown that hair dye chemicals are genotoxic and may be carcinogenic when fed to rats and mice. But in a recent epidemiologic study of the effect of hair dye use on the risk of breast cancer in women, the relative risk was 0.8 (0.6–1.1, 95% confidence interval). The study population was women screened for breast cancer at the Guttman Breast Diagnostic Institute in New York City during a 5-year period.

A. The cases were primary breast cancers first detected at screening, including supplementary examinations such as aspiration or biopsy. Are these incident or prevalent cases?

B. Breast cancer screening is, of course, voluntary: "Certain women attend the screening center for yearly check-ups as a preventive measure. Others, however, seek screening only if they are experiencing symptoms which they fear may be breast cancer." How could this influence the validity of the study?

C. What are the advantages and disadvantages, respectively, of using screening participants and cases identified at screening?

3:3   The effect of certain behavioral factors (e.g., syringe sharing) and biologic factors (e.g., T4 lymphocytes) on the risk of HIV infection, was studied in intravenous drug abusers recruited from 15 drug treatment centers in northern Italy. A total of 933 HIV-negative subjects were enrolled, but 473 of these did not return for a second visit and were thus considered lost to follow-up. For the remaining 460 subjects, individual follow-up periods were defined on the basis of their returning for follow-up visits. (Participants were invited for follow-up visits every 3 months). Thus, 165 subjects had two visits, 195 had three visits, 75 had four visits, and 25 subjects were seen five times (mean duration of follow-up was 10.4 months). Could this way of defining the follow-up periods introduce, or conceal, a source of systematic error?

3:4   The effect of passive smoking on the risk of respiratory diseases in children was studied in Chang-Ning, a part of urban Shanghai in the People's Republic of China. Information on passive smoking, potential confounders, and respiratory diseases during the first 18 months of life, was collected by interview when the child was 18 months old. The study population included all babies born in Chang-Ning during a 3-month period, except babies who moved out of the area during their first 18 months of life. Babies born elewhere during the same period were included if they moved into the area during their first 18 months of life.

A. What is the main advantage and disadvantage, respectively, of not including babies who moved out of the area during their first 18 months of life?

B. What is the main possible advantage and disadvantage, respectively, of including babies who moved into the area during their first 18 months of life?

3:5   Of 6,403 women participating in a 5-day outdoor music festival in rural Michigan, nearly 50 percent developed gastroenteritis during, or within 7 days after, the festival. This outbreak was due to extensive transmission of a single strain of Shigella, isolated from cases. Transmission may be foodborne or person-to-person. All meals during the festival were included in the admission fee. After the festival, a study was conducted to identify food items or other sources of infection during the festival. Thus, the follow-up period had already elapsed when the study population was selected. In principle, the study population could include all festival participants. However, there was a large number of cases and the precision would still be acceptable with a smaller study population (which would reduce the cost of the study). How should the study population be selected, in order to avoid selection bias?

3:6   Physical exercise may reduce the risk of myocardial infarction. This was investigated in a 12-year follow-up of 7,644 men in the Honolulu Heart Program.

A. The study was restricted to men who, at the beginning of follow-up, were free from current and previous cardiac disease, including angina pectoris, coronary insufficiency, and myocardial infarction. Why?

B. Information was collected on several potential confounders (to be considered in the data analysis), including age, smoking, alcohol, serum cholesterol, systolic blood pressure, body mass index, resting ventricular rate, and left ventricular hypertrophy by ECG. What is required for one of these factors to introduce confounding?

c. Body mass may be associated with physical exercise, because exercise tends to reduce body mass. In addition, body mass (obesity) is a risk factor for myocardial infarction. Should body mass be considered as a confounder? Why/why not?

3:7 The effect of maternal smoking during pregnancy on infant (= first year of life) mortality was investigated. Previous studies had shown that smoking during pregnancy considerably increases the risk of low birth weight and preterm delivery. Low birth weight and preterm delivery are known risk factors for infant mortality. Should birth weight and gestation (preterm/fullterm delivery) be taken into account as potential confounders? Why/why not?

3:8 The effect of alcohol drinking on mortality among men was investigated in an American Cancer Society (ACS) study. In 1959, over one million men and women aged $\geq$ 30 years from 25 states in the United States were enrolled by the ACS, and provided information on alcohol drinking and potential confounders. All 276,802 white men aged 40–59 in 1959 were included in the present study. During a 12–year (1959–1971) follow-up, 42,756 deaths were identified. Compared to no alcohol intake, the relative risk (with 95% confidence interval) of death from all causes was 0.84 (0.81–0.87) at one drink/day, 1.08 (1.02–1.14) at four drinks/day, and 1.38 (1.32–1.45) at $\geq$ six drinks/day. Of all deaths, 44 percent were due to coronary heart disease (CHD). The relative risk of death from CHD was 0.79 (0.76–0.83) at one drink/day, 0.74 (0.68–0.82) at four drinks/day, and 0.92 (0.85–1.01) at $\geq$ six drinks/day.

A. Smoking is an important potential confounder, known to increase total mortality as well as CHD mortality. If smoking increases with the amount of alcohol consumed, in what direction would confounding by smoking bias the above relative risks?

About one-third of the subjects were classified as sick at enrollment, that is reporting a history of cancer, coronary heart disease, stroke, high blood pressure, cirrhosis of the liver, poor health, or current sickness.

B. Sickness may influence alcohol intake and increase the risk of death, and thus introduce confounding. In what direction would the relative risks be biased, if there was a tendency for sick people not to drink alcohol? How should this problem be dealt with?

3:9 It has been suggested that cervical cancer may be a sexually transmitted disease. Results from a study in Utah were considered to support this. The relative risk (with 95% confidence interval) was 8.99 (4.47–18.09) for women with ≥ 10 (compared to ≤ 1) sex partners, and 8.62 (4.04–18.42) for women having a current mate with ≥ 10 (compared to 1) sex partners. Women were included during any part of the study period (January 1, 1984–May 31, 1987) when they were aged 20–59 years and resided in any of four counties in Utah.

A. The above relative risks are adjusted for age, smoking, education, and church attendance. For each of the two relative risks, name one more potential confounder that could be important to take into account.

B. Women with a history of hysterectomy (surgical removal of the uterus) were not included in the study. Why?

c. Nonwhite women (less than 5% of the population) were not included in the study. Why?

3:10 In many countries, sudden infant death syndrome (SIDS) is one of the most common causes of death during the first year of life. Still, the causes of SIDS are unknown. The Collaborative Perinatal Project (CPP) followed the course of nearly 56,000 pregnancies at 12 medical-school-affiliated hospitals in the United States. Among 53,721 infants who were born alive and survived the neonatal period, 193 SIDS cases were identified.

A. The risk of SIDS was inversely related to maternal age: The relative risk for mothers aged 18–19, compared to mothers aged 35–41, was RR = 2.3. However, confounding by parity had not been taken into account. Mothers aged 35–41 had given birth to more children than women aged 18–19. In addition, the risk of SIDS increased with the number of previous children. Is the relative risk for women aged 18–19 higher or lower than 2.3, when confounding by parity is taken into account?

B. The risk of SIDS was found to be higher in infants of black mothers compared to nonblack mothers, RR = 1.4. Confounding by income and education was, however, not taken into account. Black mothers more often had a low income and education. Both income and education were inversely related to the risk of SIDS. Is the relative risk for black mothers higher or lower than 1.4, when confounding by income and education is taken into account?

c. Marital status was related to the risk of SIDS: The relative risk for single mothers compared to married mothers was RR = 1.4. But again, income was not taken into account as a potential confounder (see B, above). After adjustment for income, RR = 0.9 for single mothers. How was income related to marital status?

d. For mothers who had given birth to three or more children, compared to mothers with no previous children, the relative risk was 1.6. Confounding by maternal age was not taken into account (see A, above). Is the relative risk for mothers who had given birth to three or more children higher or lower than 1.6, when confounding by maternal age is taken into account?

3:11 Epidemiologic studies of coffee intake and the risk of coronary heart disease (CHD) have given apparently conflicting results. In one of these studies, the effect of coffee consumption on the risk of myocardial infarction and other CHD was investigated in about 100,000 subjects who received a multiphasic health examination in a prepaid health plan.

a. Age, total serum cholesterol, cigarettes/day, alcoholic drinks/day, blood glucose, systolic blood pressure, and body mass index all showed positive correlations with coffee consumption. In what direction is confounding by these factors likely to bias the relative risk?

b. Suppose that the average time of follow-up was 5 years, and that the incidence rate of myocardial infarction (MI) was 0.0015 per year. What is the expected number of cases of MI? What is the expected number of cases in the highly exposed, if 4 percent of all subjects were highly exposed (> 6 cups of coffee per day) and there was no effect (RR = 1)?

3:12 In a 17-year follow-up of 122,261 men and 142,857 women in Japan, there were 91 deaths (43 men, 48 women) from cancer of the sigmoid colon. The relative risk of death from such cancer for any versus no alcohol intake was 4.38 in men and 1.92 in women.

a. In addition to the information given above, what determines the precision of these results?

b. What could explain the difference in relative risk between men and women (if the results are accurate)?

c. The possibility of estimating the effect at different exposure levels was discussed. Available information allowed for a classification of subjects into four categories: high, medium, low, and no alcohol intake. These categories included 1.2, 5.5, 10.2, and 78.5 percent of all women, and 32.8, 27.9, 14.1, and 23.1 percent of all men in the study population. How do these distributions influence the possibility of estimating the effect at different exposure levels in women and men, respectively?

3:13 The effect of serum triglycerides on the risk of death from coronary heart disease (CHD) was investigated in Norway. During 1972–1977, 37,546 men aged 35–49 years were examined for serum triglycerides and potential confounders. Subjects were followed with respect to vital status and CHD deaths through December 31, 1983.

Consider the possibility of conducting a similar study, of the same size, among men aged 50–59 years. CHD mortality is considerably higher in that age group. Under what conditions would the precision be higher?

3:14 In a 6-year follow-up of 34,198 non-Hispanic white California Seventh-day Adventists, the effects of certain exposures on the risk of kidney cancer were investigated. Smoking and diet are likely to affect the risk of kidney cancer. The study population was described as follows: "The unique characteristics of this Seventh-day Adventist population include the fact that they are largely non-smoking and do not consume alcohol. Furthermore, about 58% are lacto-ovo vegetarians, and overall there is a large range of dietary habits."

A. How would these characteristics of the study population influence the accuracy (validity, precision), when studying the effects of certain dietary factors?

B. How would these characteristics of the study population influence the accuracy (validity, precision), when studying the effects of certain medications?

c. The incidence rate of kidney cancer was about $7*10^{-5}$ per year. What is the total number of cases that can be expected in the study? How could this influence the possibility of studying the effects of different exposures?

In another study of California Adventists, the effect of certain dietary exposures on mortality from prostate cancer was investigated. In addition, Adventists and non-Adventists were compared as regards the distribution of certain food frequencies. The frequency of intake of meat or poultry was reported as < 1 day/ week, 1–3 days/week, 4–6 days/week, or 7 days/week. Of 22,940 Adventists, the following percentage belonged to each of these categories: 54.8, 20.0, 13.4, and 5.8 percent, respectively. For non-Adventists, the corresponding percentage was 2.2, 9.0, 45.2, and 43.7 percent, respectively.

D. How are these distributions likely to influence the possibility of studying the effect of meat or poultry intake in Adventists and non-Adventists, respectively?

3:15 Does malnutrition increase the risk of childhood diarrhea? In an initial screening, children were enrolled for a study by a door-to-door survey in selected parts of the district of Tlalpan, Mexico City. A study population of 300 children under 2 years of age was selected. Information on nutritional status (weight for age, and other classifications of nutritional status) was obtained at the beginning of follow-up and every 3 months thereafter. During each 3-month period, the occurrence of diarrhea was recorded at weekly home visits. The study period was 1 year.

In the initial screening, 0.7 percent of all children under 2 years of age were found to have severe malnutrition, 5.3 percent moderate, 31.3 percent mild, and 62.8 percent no malnutrition (defined as <60%, 60–74%, 75–89%, and ≥90%, respectively, of weight for age of the National Center for Health Statistics reference tables).

A. Should the study population be selected to reflect the above distribution of the exposure (malnutrition) in the general population? Why/why not?

B. The relation between malnutrition and childhood diarrhea may be a complex one, since diarrhea is known to increase the risk of malnutrition. In what way could this affect the validity of the results?

c. The study was conducted in Tlalpan, a district of Mexico City described as the most heterogenous in terms of population and socioeconomic status. If this means a high variability of nutritional status, what are the consequences? If this means a high variability of potential confounders such as sanitation, hygiene, and socioeconomic status, what are the consequences?

3:16 Diabetes is among the 10 leading causes of death in the United States, and increases the risk of coronary heart disease and stroke. Non-insulin-dependent diabetes is by far the most common type of diabetes. Epidemiologic and metabolic data show that obesity is a cause of non-insulin-dependent diabetes. There is, however, uncertainty about the magnitude of the effect. The absolute and relative effect at different levels of obesity in women was investigated as part of the Nurses' Health Study. In 1976, a total of 121,700 female registered nurses, aged 30–55 years, living in 11 U.S. states, returned a mailed questionnaire that provided information on height, weight, and potential confounders. Those who were free from diagnosed diabetes, coronary heart disease, and cancer in 1976 were selected for the study. Follow-up was between the return of the 1976 questionnaire and June 1, 1984. Results showed a strong increase in the risk of diabetes with increasing body mass index (BMI = weight/height^2). Compared to BMI < 22 kg/m^2, the relative risk (with 95% confidence interval) was, for instance, 2.1 (1.4–3.3) at BMI = 22–22.9, 5.2 (3.7–7.5) at BMI = 25–26.9, and 58.2 (42.4–79.9 at BMI ≥ 35 kg/m^2). The absolute effect (IR difference) was, for instance, 72 cases per 100,000 person-years at BMI = 25–26.9 (compared to BMI < 22). It was estimated that about 90 percent of the cases of diabetes that occurred in these women were attributable to BMI ≥ 22 kg/m^2.

A. The study was restricted to female nurses aged 30–55 years in 1976 (30–63 years during follow-up). In what way could these restrictions have influenced the generalizability of the results?

B. In what ways could these restrictions have influenced the validity of the results?

C. Only nurses free from coronary heart disease and cancer in 1976 were included in the study. Why?

3:17 The effects of obesity and heredity on the risk of non-insulin-dependent diabetes in women was investigated among members of the Take Off Pounds Sensibly (TOPS) Club. In 1969, more than 83,000 members completed and returned a questionnaire providing information on the presence (at the time of the questionnaire) of diabetes, obesity (current weight and height), heredity (family history of diabetes), and other factors of interest. Since there was only a small proportion of men and blacks, these subjects were not included. After further restriction by age, the study included 32,662 white females aged 40–70 years, 1,744 (5.3%) of whom had non-insulin-dependent diabetes.

A. The study population was selected among members of the TOPS club in 1969. At that time the cases had already appeared. How could this influence the validity of the results?

B. The study population was selected among subjects who answered the 1969 questionnaire. At that time the cases had already appeared. How could this influence the validity of the results?

c. The study was based on prevalence, rather than incidence, of diabetes. How could this influence the validity of the results?

D. What are the advantages and disadvantages, respectively, of selecting the study population among TOPS members who answered the 1969 questionnaire?

3:18 The occurrence and etiology of "major depression" in subjects aged 18–44 was studied within the Epidemiologic Catchment Area Program. The study population was selected in 1980–1984 by drawing probability samples of adult residents from a combined total of 35,793 sampled households in five U.S. metropolitan areas. Information on current and past depression, as well as on exposures and potential confounders and modifiers, was collected soon after sampling. In 5,969 subjects aged 18–44, with no current or past depression, 194 cases were identified during one year's follow-up (incidence rate: 325 cases per 10,000 person-years). The relative risk (with 95% confidence interval) was 0.6 (0.4–0.8) for paid workers compared to those not working for pay, and 1.9 (1.2–3.1) for the separated and divorced compared to other marital groups.

The study population was selected for several purposes of the Epidemiologic Catchment Area Program. In what sense, if any, should the study population be representative of the general population when studying:

A. the current incidence (or prevalence) of major depression in the five U.S. metropolitan areas?

B. the incidence (or prevalence) of major depression in different subgroups of the population, for example in different ethnic groups?

c. the etiology of major depression?

3:19 Screening programs are available for the early detection of several diseases. In many countries, the frequency of routine screening examinations has increased rapidly during the past few decades. According to the 1982 U.S. National Health Interview Survey, the proportion of adults who ever had a routine screening examination was 81% for glaucoma test and 76% for electrocardiogram (both sexes, age ≥ 40 years), and 90% for breast examination and 89% for Pap smear (women, age ≥ 17 years).

People who have not experienced any symptoms of disease may attend a screening clinic or program for a health check. Cases identified among such screening participants are prevalent cases of asymptomatic disease. But in most screening programs there are also participants who have experienced symptoms of the disease when they attend the screening. These symptoms may have influenced their decision to attend the screening. In several epidemiologic studies, information has been collected on the presence of disease at screening and, at the same time, information on past exposure has been obtained by interview. Suppose that such a study was restricted to screening participants who had not experienced any symptoms or signs that could be related to the disease under study. How would this influence the possibility of:

A. selection bias?
B. differential exposure misclassification?

3:20 The effect of occupational exposure to amosite asbestos on cancer mortality was investigated among the workforce of a factory in London. Of all men ever employed at the plant, 4,820 were identified as exposed and 1,149 as unexposed. In addition, national cancer mortality rates for men by age and calendar period were used for comparison.

What are the advantages and disadvantages, respectively, of using national rates rather than rates in the 1,149 unexposed men for comparison?

3:21 Information on the effect of X-ray irradiation in childhood on cancer mortality was obtained in a study of children who had received radiotherapy for ringworm of the scalp. In Israel, nearly 20,000 children received such treatment between 1948 and 1960. The study was based on a follow-up of 10,834 of these exposed children and three different groups of unexposed children.

Exposed: Children born 1930–1960 who received their X-ray treatment before the age of 15, at four major Israeli treatment centers. Children were not included if they were of European-American origin, or if they had immigrated to Israel before 1948 or after 1960. Finally, restriction was made to those who could be identified in the Central Population Registry.

Unexposed (1): "For each irradiated subject, a nonirradiated, tinea-free comparison subject matched on sex, age, country of origin, and year of immigration was selected from the general population using the Central Population Registry."

Unexposed (2): "In addition, a nonirradiated, tinea-free sibling, also matched on age and with preference given to a sibling of the same sex, was chosen for approximately 50 percent of the irradiated subjects."

Unexposed (3): "Mortality rates specific for five-year age group, five-year calendar year, sex and ethnic origin . . . in the general population of Israel" were also used for comparison.

A. Unexposed children were selected to match the exposed children with regard to certain characteristics. Why?
B. For each of the three unexposed groups (1–3), to what extent could there be confounding by: Age and sex? Place of origin and time of immigration? Residential area and socioeconomic characteristics?
C. In general, what potential confounders should be considered when the exposure under study is a medical treatment?
D. Are any of the three unexposed groups likely to include exposed children? In what direction, if any, could this have biased the result?
E. Which of the three unexposed groups offered the highest and lowest precision, respectively?

3:22 When selecting a follow-up period, the induction time should be taken into account. Failure to do so will usually bias the result towards RR = 1 (like nondifferential exposure misclassification). This bias may be viewed as an instance of misclassification, where exposure information for an etiologically relevant time period is replaced by exposure information for some other time. However, as illustrated by the following study, the bias introduced by failure to take the induction time into account is not always towards RR = 1 (nondifferential).

It has been suggested that a low serum cholesterol might increase the risk of cancer. This was investigated in a study population where the cholesterol level was determined in a serum sample obtained from each subject at an examination in 1968–1972. Individual follow-up periods were from the date of examination until December 31, 1980. Low levels of serum cholesterol were found to be associated with a considerable increase in the risk of cancer diagnosed during this period. But the induction time, from exposure (serum cholesterol) until its effect in terms of symptomatic cancer, was not taken into account during the early parts of the follow-up period. (Slowly growing cancers may remain asymptomatic for several months or even years). In general, this would tend to bias the relative risk towards RR = 1. However, it was suggested that a cancer may lower the level of serum cholesterol even before the disease gives rise to symptoms and is diagnosed. In what direction would this bias the relative risk? If the induction time is unknown, how could this problem be handled?

3:23 A study of smoking and mortality was mentioned in Chapter 2 (exercise 2:16). A total of 34,440 subjects provided information on smoking habits, and were followed during 20 years with regard to all-cause mortality and mortality from specific diseases. When selecting the study population, restrictions were made with regard to nationality (British), sex (male), and occupation (doctors). In what ways, if any, could this have influenced the accuracy (validity, precision) of the results?

3:24 In many countries, mortality and morbidity from coronary heart disease (CHD) is reported to increase by 30–50 percent in winter compared to summer. This could be due to differences in environmental temperatures or in the occurrence of respiratory infections. It has also been suggested that exposure to sunlight in the summer might protect against CHD by increasing body levels of vitamin D. The effect of vitamin D on the risk of myocardial infarction (MI) was investigated in New Zealand. Subjects were included in the follow-up during any part of the study period (March 1986–February 1988) when they were aged 35–64 years and lived in the Central Auckland Statistical Area. One reason for selecting residents of this area for the study was the existence of a register that could be used to identify over 95 percent of all episodes of hospitalized and home-treated MI.

A. What characteristics of the study population, except for its size, will influence the precision of the results?
B. The study was restricted to subjects aged 35–64 years during follow-up. A lower age limit is justified since there are few cases of MI before the age of 35. But why was there an upper age limit at 64 years?

3:25 Several epidemiologic studies have shown that current use of oral contraceptives increases the risk of venous thrombosis. There are, however, considerable differences between different oral contraceptives in their hormone (estrogen and progestin) potencies. The effects of high and intermediate (compared to low) estrogen and progestin potency on the risk of deep venous thromboembolism was investigated. The study population was women aged 15–44 years who were Medicaid enrollees and had at least one prescription of an estrogen/progestin combination oral contraceptive (COC) during the study period (1980–1986). Individual follow-up periods were each 56-day period subsequent to a dispensed COC. Computerized Medicaid data were used to add such periods to a total of 244,071 women-years of follow-up, and to identify 141 cases of deep venous thromboembolism during follow-up (recurrent cases were not included). For estrogen potency, the results suggest a dose-response relationship with a relative risk (with 95% confidence interval) of 1.4 (0.8–2.3) for intermediate and 2.6 (1.2–5.5) for high estrogen potency (compared to low estrogen potency). For progestin potency there was no such increase in the risk of thromboembolism.

A. The definition of individual follow-up periods is based on certain assumptions. What assumptions?

Medicaid is a program for financing medical care for poor people in the United States. A computerized register provides information on Medicaid enrollees (personal identification number, demographic characteristics, periods of enrollment, etc.) and medical services paid for by Medicaid (pharmacy file: prescriptions filled, date and type of drug, etc.; inpatient file: hospital, diagnoses, admission and discharge dates, etc.).

B. What are the advantages and disadvantages, respectively, of selecting Medicaid enrollees as the study population for the present study?

In previous studies of oral contraceptives and venous thrombosis, the unexposed are usually women not using any oral contraceptives. Since the association between oral contraceptives and venous thrombosis has been widely recognized for many years, women considered to be at high risk of thrombosis are less likely to have a prescription for oral contraceptives. In addition, women could be more likely to have their thrombosis diagnosed if they use oral contraceptives.

C. Against this background, what are the advantages and disadvantages, respectively, of using women on low-estrogen/low-progestin oral contraceptives as "unexposed"?

3:26   The effect of dietary cholesterol intake on mortality from ischemic heart diease (IHD) was investigated among participants in the

Western Electric Study. In 1957, there were in all 5,397 men aged 40–55 years who had been working for at least 2 years at the Western Electric Company's Hawthorne Works near Chicago. Of these men, a random sample of 2,107 were examined with regard to dietary cholesterol intake and potential confounders and followed for 25 years with regard to death from IHD. Subjects were not included if, at the initial examination, they had ischemic heart disease, consumed ≥50 ml ethanol per day, or (in a separate analysis) reported that they were following diets.

A. The Western Electric Study was restricted to men aged 40–55 years in 1957, who had been working for 2 years or more at the Western Electric Company's Hawthorne Works near Chicago. How does this serve the purpose of the present study?

B. Participants were selected as a random sample of all men who fulfilled the above criteria. How does this serve the purpose of the present study?

C. Serum cholesterol is a risk factor for death from ischemic heart disease. Should serum cholesterol be taken into account as a potential confounder?

3:27 There is some evidence that certain vitamins may reduce the risk of cancer. The effect of serum vitamins A and E and carotenoids on the risk of cancer was studied among participants in the Hypertension Detection and Follow-up Program. This program enrolled 10,940 hypertensive men and women, aged 30–69 years, for a community-based trial of hypertension treatment. Before random allocation of participants to treatment groups, serum specimens were collected and stored at −70°C. For the study of serum vitamins and cancer, incident cases of cancer were identified during the subsequent 5 years. After this follow-up, vitamins were analyzed in the stored serum samples. But because of the breakdown of a large freezer, more than 50% of the serum samples were damaged, leaving specimens from 4,480 subjects available for analysis.

A. Why were subjects enrolled in a trial of hypertension treatment selected for a study of serum vitamins and cancer?

B. What were the disadvantages, if any, of selecting the study population from a trial of hypertension treatment?

C. What were the disadvantages, if any, of the breakdown of a large freezer resulting in loss of more than 50% of the serum samples?

3:28 The effect of HDL cholesterol on mortality from coronary heart disease (CHD) was investigated in a follow-up of participants in the Lipid Research Clinics Prevalence Study (cf. Exercise 2:28). The purpose of the initial study was to describe the distribution of serum lipids in an American population, and participants were selected from all ages and both sexes. After a first examination, all subjects with elevated serum lipids and a 15 percent random sample of all other subjects were invited to a second examination. People who were at least 30 years of age and participated in the second examination were selected for subsequent follow-up in the study of serum HDL cholesterol and CHD mortality.

    A. The study population was selected among participants in the Lipid Research Clinics Prevalence Study. Why?

    B. About 57 percent of the study population had been selected as a random sample of those who participated in the first examination. The distribution of HDL cholesterol in this sample reflects that of the source population. In addition, these subjects showed a wide age range and considerable geographic, socioeconomic, and occupational heterogeneity. How does this serve the purpose of the study of HDL cholesterol and CHD mortality?

    c. About 43 percent of the study population had been selected because they had elevated serum lipids at the first examination. How does this serve the purpose of the study of HDL cholesterol and CHD mortality?

    D. Among the 8,825 subjects originally included in the follow-up, there were 564 nonwhites and 688 subjects who had coronary heart disease at the time of the second examination (i.e., at the beginning of follow-up). Should these subjects be included in the study of HDL cholesterol and CHD mortality? Why/why not?

3:29 A study of smoking and mortality was based on subjects included in the Swedish Twin Registry (STR). In 1961, the STR enrolled nearly all like-sexed twins born in Sweden between 1886 and 1925. Of 12,889 twin pairs, approximately one-third were monozygotic, having all their genes in common, and two-thirds were dizygotic, sharing half their genes. Information on smoking and other characteristics was obtained in 1961. During follow-up (1961–1981), 6,447 of the subjects died. Within the study, two different study populations were selected as illustrated by the following results for any cigarette smoking (exposed) versus no smoking (unexposed) and all-cause mortality in men:

1. When all subjects were included, disregarding their twin status, there were 1,028 exposed cases (deaths) and RR = 1.4 (1.3–1.5, 90% confidence interval).

2. When comparing the twins within each pair, only those pairs were included where one twin was exposed and the other unexposed (smoking-discordant pairs). Among monozygotic twins, there were 35 exposed and 22 unexposed cases (first or only deaths within a pair), RR = 1.6. Among dizygotic twins, there were 102 exposed and 72 unexposed cases, RR = 1.4.

A. What is the principal advantage and disadvantage, respectively, of restricting the study to smoking-discordant twin pairs?

B. Suppose there was no twin registry and that, in 1981, an attempt was made to enroll smoking-discordant twin pairs for follow-up during the next 20 years (to use information on cases (deaths) occurring in 1981–2001). In what ways could failure to enroll all such twin pairs influence the accuracy of the results?

C. Suppose there was no twin registry and that, in 1981, an attempt was made to enroll smoking-discordant twin pairs where one twin had died since 1961 (to use information on cases (deaths) that occurred in 1961–1981). In what ways could failure to enroll all such twin pairs influence the accuracy of the results?

3:30 The effect of prenatal irradiation on the risk of cancer at age 4–39 years, was investigated in children exposed in utero by the A-bombs in Hiroshima and Nagasaki. Subjects selected for the study were born alive to A-bomb exposed mothers between August 6 (Hiroshima), or August 9 (Nagasaki), 1945, and May 31, 1946. Children who were still alive on October 1, 1950 were followed from that date. A supplementary survey of A-bomb survivors, conducted in 1960, identified additional children who had been exposed in utero. These children were followed from the time of the survey (1960). Follow-up was through December 31, 1984.

A. Could the choice of study population have influenced the estimate of the effect? Why/why not?

B. Among children identified in the 1960 survey, only cases that occurred after the time of that survey were included in the present study. Suppose there had been an attempt to identify cases of cancer that occurred in these children before 1960. How could this have influenced the validity of the results?

▅▅ GENERAL QUESTIONS

3:31 When selecting a study population, what strategies are available to improve the precision of the results? Exemplify!

3:32 When selecting a study population, what strategies are available to prevent confounding? Exemplify!

3:33 When selecting a study population, what strategies are available to prevent misclassification? Exemplify!

3:34 What are the principal reasons for making (or not making) restrictions with regard to age, sex, and other factors, when selecting a study population?

3:35 In what ways can selection bias be introduced (or avoided) by the choice of study population? Exemplify!

3:36 In what ways can validity and precision be influenced by the choice of study period, and individual follow-up periods? Exemplify!

3:37 How can the cost and time necessary to complete a study be reduced by the choice of study population? Exemplify!

3:38 Sometimes, findings from a follow-up of exposed subjects are compared to available information on morbidity or mortality in the general population. What are the possible advantages and disadvantages, respectively, of this approach?

3:39 In what ways, if any, should generalizability influence the choice of study population?

3:40 Consider your own recent favorite study. What are the implications for that study of the general problems and possibilities exemplified in the different exercises in this chapter?

4 | *Obtaining Information on Exposures*

■■■ INTRODUCTION

Definitions

Information should be obtained on exposures, including potential con-founders and factors that could influence misclassification or selection. Information should also be obtained on modifiers. As a first step, each exposure of interest is defined. Sometimes the theoretical definition should be supplemented by an empirical definition (or indicator), to be used as a basis for the collection of exposure information (cf. Chapter 1: Misclassification). For each exposure, at least two categories are defined: "exposed" and "unexposed." Different aspects of the exposure may have to be taken into account (cf. Chapter 2, Introduction: Exposure). There should be no overlapping between categories, and together they should cover all possible findings in the data collection. The unexposed category may include subjects free from the exposure under study or at the lowest levels of exposure. Only those who have never been exposed are in-cluded among the unexposed when there is uncertainty about the dura-tion of an effect. When the joint effect of two or more different exposures is being studied, the unexposed are those who belong to the unexposed category for both exposures.

Methods

A variety of methods are used to obtain exposure information in epide-miologic studies, and experts in the field should usually be involved at the planning stage. However, their main concern is likely to be the accuracy of measurements rather than the accuracy of the study results. For example, laboratory methods may be very accurate in determining blood nutrients or air pollutants at one point in time. But if the levels show considerable variation over time, there could be a large amount of misclassification in relation to the relevant exposure, which is likely to be the levels over a long period of time. Furthermore, and perhaps even more important, efforts to improve the accuracy of measurements may actually reduce the accuracy of the study results unless the comparability of exposure information is maintained (see Chapter 1, Misclassification: Differential Exposure Misclassification).

Questionnaires administered by mail, telephone, or face-to-face interview are used to obtain information on a wide range of exposures and potential confounders. Questioning has a strong advantage over other methods in that it can be used to obtain information on exposure at different times in the past and, in principle at least, to obtain a lifetime exposure history. However, the accuracy of information may sometimes be quite low due to poor or selective memory. Reporting of exposure may be influenced by "social desirability" (which could result in, for example, underreporting of the intake of candy, but overreporting of the use of a toothbrush), and recall of past exposure (e.g., past smoking) is likely to be influenced by current exposure (current smoking). The choice of method should be based on the comparability, accuracy, and completeness of information it yields, as well as its cost and feasibility. The objective is to obtain an accurate estimate of the effect of the exposure with the limited resources available.

Misclassification

Exposure misclassification may be introduced by measurement errors (including errors in the reporting of past exposure), and by the gap between an empirical (measured) and theoretical definition of the exposure. A similar error is introduced by failure to take the induction time into account (cf. Chapter 1: Misclassification).

Nondifferential exposure misclassification introduces a bias towards $RR = 1$ (Chapter 1, Misclassification: Nondifferential Exposure Misclassification). This general rule applies when there are only two exposure categories (exposed and unexposed), if the misclassification is independent of other errors and is not so extreme that the unexposed are more likely than the exposed to be classified as exposed (i.e., sensitivity + specificity ≥ 1). If the exposure does affect the risk of disease, nondifferential measurement errors may introduce some differential exposure misclassification when different levels of an exposure are included in a single category (Flegal et al. 1991). When there are three or more exposure categories, nondifferential exposure misclassification can sometimes result in an over- or underestimation of the relative risk if the misclassification involves a category other than the two being compared (Dosemeci et al. 1990). For example, when studying the effect of different levels of alcohol intake on the risk of liver cirrhosis, the relative risk associated with low levels of alcohol intake will be overestimated if there is a general tendency for exposed subjects to underreport their alcohol intake (but exposed subjects are not classified as unexposed). On the other hand, if people with a very high intake (alcoholics) would tend to deny any intake of alcohol, and thus be classified as unexposed, the relative risk associated with low levels of alcohol intake would be underestimated (biased towards RR = 0).

The "dilution" of the effect (bias towards RR = 1) introduced by nondifferential exposure misclassification also presupposes that there is a misclassification between "exposure" and "no exposure." But sometimes, one exposure may be misclassified as another. For example, when studying the effect of an analgesic drug on the risk of renal insufficiency, subjects may recall past intake of another drug as being the drug of interest. If so, the relative risk may reflect the effect of the other drug rather than that of the exposure of interest.

Regardless of whether the exposure information is collected before or after the cases appear, a differential exposure misclassification may be introduced if the accuracy of the exposure information is influenced by a risk indicator for the disease. But to the extent that such risk indicators are controlled in the data analysis, the remaining bias is towards RR = 1 (Chapter 1, Misclassification: Differential Exposure Misclassification).

Timing

In studies where the exposure information is collected (or handled) only after the cases have appeared, the disease may influence the accuracy and completeness of exposure information. This will introduce differential exposure misclassification and selection bias, respectively.

Differential Exposure Misclassification. When exposure information is collected (or handled) after the cases have appeared, the disease may influence the accuracy of the information, introducing differential exposure misclassification (bias towards RR = 0 or RR = ∞). For instance, when cases know that they are diseased, this may increase (or reduce) their tendency to recall and report past exposure ("recall bias"). In addition, the interviewer may be influenced by awareness of the disease status of a study subject ("interviewer bias"). Similarly, measurements and observations may (unintentionally) be influenced by awareness of the disease status of a study subject. In addition, measurements and observations reflect current rather than past exposure, and a differential misclassification is introduced if a subject's exposure status is influenced by the disease. Regardless of the methods and timing in the data collection, any handling (encoding, etc.) of exposure information after the cases have appeared may (unintentionally) be influenced by awareness of the disease status of a study subject. Finally, differential misclassification may be introduced when using different methods or different sources of exposure information for cases and noncases.

Differential exposure misclassification may be avoided by using the same examination methods and sources of information for cases and noncases. All handling of exposure information should be made "blind," that is, without knowledge of the disease status of the subjects. Sometimes, it may also be possible to use blinding of staff members collecting the exposure information. Whenever possible (in studies of asymptomatic disease), the study subjects should be kept unaware of their own disease status when the exposure information is collected. Indicators of an exposure may sometimes be used to improve the comparability of exposure information (but may increase nondifferential misclassification). When these measures are likely to be inadequate, it may be useful to consider the possibility of collecting exposure information prior to follow-up (before the cases appear).

Selection Bias. When exposure information is collected after the cases have appeared, the disease may influence the possibility of obtaining exposure information. Subjects may be lost because they have died, cannot be located or contacted, are disabled, or refuse to provide exposure information. Selection bias is introduced if the disease influences the extent to which exposure information is obtained (cf. Chapter 1: Selection Bias). The relative risk is overestimated (biased towards $RR = \infty$) or underestimated (biased towards $RR = 0$) if the disease influences the availability of information differently in the exposed and unexposed.

Selection bias may be avoided by selecting a study population that is likely to provide complete exposure information (Chapter 3), and by using suitable methods in the collection of exposure information. In addition, nonparticipation may be reduced by various techniques for tracing subjects and increasing their motivation to participate. When the exposure information is collected prior to follow-up (before the cases appear), the availability of exposure information is usually not influenced by the disease. But occasionally, a similar selection bias is introduced by selective loss of previously collected exposure information (cf. Chapter 1: Selection Bias). Information on subjects lost to the study because they did not provide exposure information should be presented together with the study results.

■ EXERCISES

4:1   Obesity may increase the risk of several diseases, including cardiovascular disease. But what is obesity, and how should it be measured? Several theoretical and empirical definitions have been proposed. The effects of three different aspects of obesity on the risk of developing essential hypertension was investigated in a study based on members of the Kaiser Permanente Medical Care Program in California. Centrally deposited fat (CDF) was estimated by measuring subscapular skinfold, peripherally deposited fat (PDF) was estimated by measuring triceps skinfold, and overall obesity was estimated by measuring body mass index (= weight/height^2). For each of these aspects of obesity, measured at baseline, the relative risk was 3.75, 2.29, and 3.85, respectively. After adjustment for confounding by the two other aspects, there was no association between PDF and hypertension, but CDF and overall obesity each increased the risk of hypertension. Three different aspects of obesity were investigated. How were they "defined":

    A. theoretically?
    B. empirically?
    C. What are the principal sources of exposure misclassification?

4:2   On November 6, 1985, a banquet was held for 1,362 employees at a factory in Connecticut. Within the next 48 hours, over 40 percent of those who ate the banquet foods developed acute gastroenteritis. Clostridium perfringens, a commonly identified cause of foodborne disease outbreaks, was identified in stool specimens from cases. On November 8, a questionnaire requesting information about food and beverage consumption at the banquet as well as subsequent illness (to identify incident cases of gastroenteritis that had occurred during the past 48 hours) was distributed to the factory employees. The purpose was to identify the food items responsible for the disease outbreak.

    Exposure information was collected only after the cases appeared (at the end of a 48-hour follow-up period). Suppose that the exposure information had been collected before the cases appeared (i.e., that subjects had been asked about their food intake during or immediately after the banquet). What difference would it make, in terms of possible differential exposure misclassification?

4:3   A study of physical exercise and coronary heart disease (CHD) in men was mentioned in Chapter 3 (Exercise 3:6). Inactive and moderately active men (here called "exposed") had a greater risk of CHD than physically active men (here called "unexposed"). In the age group 45–64 years, 406 cases were identified during 12 years' follow-up of 7,221 men:

	Exposed	Unexposed
Cases (CHD)	299	107
Noncases (no CHD)	4,503	2,312
All men	4,802	2,419
Incidence proportion (*1000)	62.27	44.23

$$RR = 62.27/44.23 = 1.41$$

Suppose there is no misclassification in these data. What would the results have been if there was:

A. a nondifferential exposure misclassification with sensitivity = 0.90 and specificity = 1.00?

B. a nondifferential exposure misclassification with sensitivity = 1.00 and specificity = 0.70?

C. a nondifferential exposure misclassification with sensitivity = 0.90 and specificity = 0.70?

D. a differential exposure misclassification with sensitivity = 0.90 and specificity = 1.00 among the noncases, but sensitivity = 1.00 and specificity = 1.00 among the cases?

E. a differential exposure misclassification with sensitivity = 1.00 and specificity = 0.70 among the noncases, but sensitivity = 1.00 and specificity = 1.00 among the cases?

F. a differential exposure misclassification with sensitivity = 0.90 and specificity = 0.70 among the noncases, but sensitivity = 1.00 and specificity = 1.00 among the cases?

4:4   A study on foods served at a banquet and acute gastroenteritis occurring during the next 48 hours was mentioned previously (Exercise 4:2). Gravy was considered as one possible source of infection. Exposure information was obtained by questionnaire after the cases appeared. Results were based on information from 671 subjects, including 294 cases. Suppose that, in the absence of any misclassification, the results would be as follows:

	Exposed	*Unexposed*	*Total*
Cases	41	253	294
Noncases	53	324	377
All subjects	94	577	671

$$RR = 41*577/253*94 = 0.99$$

The possibility of recall bias was discussed in exercise 4:2. Cases could be more likely than noncases to recall their exposure.

A. What would the relative risk have been, if 5 percent of the exposed noncases did not recall their exposure (i.e., sensitivity = 0.95; specificity = 1.00 among noncases, and sensitivity = 1.00; specificity = 1.00 among cases)?

In the above example (A), it was assumed that only 94/671 = 14 percent of the subjects were exposed. But in the present study, the vast majority of the subjects were exposed to gravy. Suppose that, in the absence of any misclassification, the results would be as follows:

	Exposed	*Unexposed*	*Total*
Cases	290	4	294
Noncases	372	5	377
All subjects	662	9	671

$$RR = 290*9/4*662 = 0.99$$

B. What would the relative risk have been, if the misclassification (sensitivity, specificity) was the same as above (A)?

4:5 Passive smoking may increase the risk of certain cancers and cardiovascular diseases. Some studies on the health effects of passive smoking in nonsmokers are based on questionnaires covering different sources of passive smoking at home, in the workplace, and in other environments. Empirical definitions of passive smoking are based on the different aspects of passive smoking covered by the questionnaire. However, another approach has been used in some studies of passive smoking in women: "marriage to a smoker" has been used as an indicator (empirical definition) of passive smoking.

A. Of the two approaches, which is likely to minimize the gap between the empirical and theoretical definition of passive smoking?

B. Of the two approaches, which is likely to minimize the measurement error when using a questionnaire?

C. In studies where exposure information is collected only after the cases have appeared, the disease could influence the accuracy of exposure information. Of the two approaches above, which is likely to minimize this source of differential exposure misclassification?

Two of the first studies of passive smoking and lung cancer in nonsmoking women were conducted in the 1960s–1970s, one in Japan (RR = 1.8) and the other in United States (RR = 1.2). In both studies, marriage to a smoker was used as an indicator of passive smoking.

D. Could the difference in result be explained by differences between the two countries in the degree to which the indicator reflects passive smoking? Why/why not?

4:6 Several studies suggest that passive smoking may increase the risk of respiratory diseases in children. Misclassification in respect of exposure is a potential problem in such studies. Different methods have been used to obtain information on passive smoking, including:

1. Questionnaires covering the smoking habits of each household member and exposure to passive smoking at home as well as in other environments.

2. Cotinine in serum, saliva, or urine. Cotinine is the major degradation product of nicotine metabolism and has a serum half-life of about 17 hours (i.e., about 17 hours after a maximum level due to exposure the serum cotinine is reduced to half).

A method used to determine serum cotinine (such as gas liquid chromatography) may be very accurate in measuring the true cotinine level in a single blood specimen.

A. When such a method is used, what is the most important source of exposure misclassification?

When exposure information is collected only after the cases have appeared, the disease could influence the accuracy of exposure information. This is a potential source of differential exposure misclassifcation in studies based on questionnaire data (recall bias).

B. Is this source of differential exposure misclassification avoided in studies based on serum cotinine? Why/why not?

4:7   It has been suggested that certain micronutrients, including retinol, beta-carotene, vitamin E, and selenium, may have an anticarcinogenic effect. Sera were available from 25,802 participants of a serum collection campaign in Maryland (autumn 1974). White participants born before 1950, with no history of cancer, were selected for a study. During the period January 1, 1975 through December 31, 1983, 72 study subjects were diagnosed with colon cancer. After follow-up, serum samples (stored at $-73°C$ since their collection in 1974) were analyzed to determine the levels of retinol, beta-carotene, vitamin E, and selenium. For each nutrient, serum values were categorized in quintiles, and the relative risk of colon cancer was estimated for each quintile compared with the highest quintile. With a possible exception for retinol, relative risks were only slightly elevated at the lowest nutrient level.

For each of the following problems related to the exposure information (1–6), in what direction are relative risks likely to be biased?

1. Errors arising from the collection and storage of sera. For instance, micronutrient levels are affected by recent intake: beta-carotene levels were higher in subjects who had eaten 2 to 5 hours before the time of blood donation.

2. Errors in the analysis of sera. For instance, serum samples run in duplicate showed some differences in results. In order to avoid any differences between cases and noncases, the serum samples were numbered randomly, handled "blind" by laboratory personnel, and analyzed in a sequence taking into account possible laboratory differences from day to day.

3. Duration (and other aspects) of exposure. The serum level at one point in time is not likely to have much impact on the risk of colon cancer. The exposure of interest is nutrient levels (or dietary intake) over a long period of time.

4. Induction time. The micronutrient levels were measured in serum collected shortly before a 9-year follow-up. However, the induction time (from exposure to clinically recognized colon cancer) could be several years.

5. Very few people in the rather well-nourished study population had deficient levels of micronutrients. Thus, when serum levels

are categorized in quintiles, even the lowest level (quintile) will contain few subjects with deficient levels of nutrients.

4:8   In environmental epidemiology, studies have dealt with exposures such as lead in the general environment or nitrogen dioxide in the indoor atmosphere. There may be large variations in the levels of these exposures, both in time and space. If so, a single measurement is not likely to reflect an individual's exposure over a longer, etiologically relevant, period of time. In what direction is this likely to bias relative risks, and what can be done to avoid such bias?

4:9   The effect of certain sedatives (benzodiazepines) on the risk of accidents resulting in hip fractures among elderly people was investigated (cf. Exercise 2:10). Information was available on whether or not a subject had been prescribed benzodiazepines. However, no information was available on whether or not the cases had actually taken the drug at the time of the accident. Thus, many of the cases that were classified as exposed on the basis of their prescriptions may not have been exposed to the drug at the time of the accident. But immediately after the accident, each case was examined at a hospital. Suppose that this examination of the cases could provide information on whether or not they had actually taken the drug at the time of the accident, and that only those cases who had actually taken the drug were considered as exposed. How would this affect the accuracy of the result (relative risk)?

4:10   Sometimes there is misclassification between different exposures, rather than between exposure and nonexposure. This is illustrated by the following study. A possible effect of sexually transmitted human papillomavirus (HPV) infection on the risk of cervical cancer was investigated in Sydney, Australia. In a screening program, 1,107 women (who fulfilled certain criteria) were found to have abnormal epithelial cells suggestive of HPV infection. During a 6-year follow-up, 30 cases of cervical cancer (carcinoma in situ) were identified among the exposed women. The relative risk was 15.6.

It was noticed, however, that the cytological findings considered typical for HPV infection were sometimes difficult to distinguish from mild dysplasia—which is known to increase the risk of carcinoma in situ. A supplementary study showed that of 86 women with mild dysplasia, 23 developed carcinoma in situ within 4 years. In the present study, a certain proportion of the 1,107 women classified as exposed to HPV may actually have had mild dysplasia. What proportion, approximately, would be required to explain the excess risk (RR = 15.6)?

4:11 Study subjects are often asked about their exposure in the past (retrospective exposure information). This possibility is a strong advantage of questioning over other methods (measurements, observations) which can usually provide information only on current exposure. However, several studies have shown that the recall of past exposure tends to be biased in the direction of current exposure. One of these studies was based on 9,394 middle-aged people who answered a detailed questionnaire on current and past smoking habits. Each subject answered the questionnaire twice, at 6-year intervals. Information on current smoking in the first questionnaire ("original information") was compared to information on smoking at the time of the first questionnaire, obtained in the second questionnaire ("retrospective information"). In relation to the original information on smoking, retrospective information showed a strong tendency to overestimate previous cigarette consumption among subjects who had increased their cigarette smoking, and to underestimate previous cigarette consumption among subjects who had reduced their cigarette smoking.

A study of the effects of current and past smoking on the risk of ulcerative colitis and Crohn's disease, was conducted in Stockholm, Sweden. Incident cases identified during follow-up (1984–1987) were approached up to 4 years after diagnosis to answer a questionnaire on their smoking habits at the time when the disease occurred (and before that time).

A. Symptoms of disease may influence peoples' smoking habits. In what direction could this have biased the relative risk, considering the findings of the study on retrospective smoking information mentioned above?

B. If the exposure information had been collected as the cases were identified, rather than up to 4 years later, what difference would it make?

4:12 Interview and questionnaire responses may, for certain kinds of questions, be biased in the direction of "social desirability." For example, people may tend to deny their drinking problems and taking certain drugs. On the other hand, people may tend to exaggerate their compliance with prescribed medications and programs aimed at quitting smoking or reducing the intake of calories. Sometimes, the tendency for such bias seems to be greater in face-to-face interviews than when answering a self-administered questionnaire.

A study of alcohol drinking and mortality was mentioned in Chapter 3 (Exercise 3:8). For total mortality, the results showed a J-shaped distribution with the lowest mortality at one drink/day, a somewhat higher mortality in men classified as nondrinkers, and the highest mortality at 6+ drinks/day. Exposure information was collected by questionnaire prior to follow-up.

A. Suppose that, due to social desirability, some subjects with drinking problems (highly exposed) would deny any intake of alcohol and thus be classified as nondrinkers. How would this bias the results?

In another study mentioned in Chapter 3, the possibility that cervical cancer is a sexually transmitted disease was investigated among young and middle-aged women in Utah (Exercise 3:9). A self-administered sexual history questionnaire was used to obtain information on certain exposures, such as the number of sex partners and history of genital infections. The information was collected only after the cases had been identified.

B. Suppose that the answers were influenced by social desirability. Could the resulting bias have been different because the exposure information was collected after (rather than before) the cases appeared? Why/why not?

4:13   The effect of vasectomy (surgical sterilization) on the risk of testicular cancer was investigated. Exposure information was obtained by telephone interview after the cases had been identified. The result showed a 50 percent excess risk associated with vasectomy: RR = 1.5 (1.0–2.2, 95% confidence interval). However, further analyses showed that the observed effect of vasectomy varied considerably by religious background: RR = 8.7 for Catholic, and RR = 1.0 for Protestant background. Could these results be explained on the basis of exposure misclassification? Why/why not?

4:14   Increases in asthma mortality during the past few decades have coincided with the introduction of certain drugs in the treatment of asthma. The possibility that such a drug (fenoterol by metered dose inhaler, MDI) increases the risk of death in asthma patients aged 5–45, was investigated in New Zealand (cf. Exercise 2:4).

Information on prescribed drug therapy for self-administration, including fenoterol, was obtained from hospital records. But for those who died during follow-up, information on prescribed drug therapy at the time of the fatal attack was obtained from a questionnaire answered by general practitioners for the National Asthma Mortality Survey. Fenoterol by MDI was found to be associated with a six-fold increase in mortality among patients on oral corticosteroids (RR = 6.5; 2.7–15.3, 95% confidence interval). Could this result be questioned on the basis of possible exposure misclassification? Why/why not?

4:15   Drugs used in the treatment of high blood pressure were among the exposures of interest in a study of kidney cancer mentioned previously (Exercise 3:14). A total of 34,198 subjects were followed during a 6-year period. Prior to follow-up, each subject answered a questionnaire that included questions on history of hypertension and use of antihypertensive medications. For those who had a kidney cancer diagnosed during follow-up, medical records were also available as a source of information. These records were used to obtain information on the diagnosis of kidney cancer, in order to reduce misclassification in respect of disease. In addition, the medical records of the cases could be used as a source of information on antihypertensive medications.

    A. Would this be likely to reduce the amount of exposure misclassification?

    B. Would this be likely to reduce bias due to exposure misclassification?

    c. How should the medical records of the cases be used as a source of information?

4:16   It was suggested that exposure to a drug (Bendectin, commonly used for nausea) during the first trimester of pregnancy could increase the risk of cardiovscular malformations in the offspring. A study was based on babies born in Massachusetts during a 3-year period (cf. Exercise 3:1). The same sources of exposure information were used for cases and noncases. Two separate sources of information were used:

1. A telephone interview with the biologic mother, using a detailed questionnaire, was conducted after the cases had been identified.

2. Information on drug use during pregnancy was abstracted from the obstetric record after the cases had been identified.

The two methods are different in that the interviews were conducted only after the cases had been identified, whereas the exposure information that was abstracted from the obstetric records had initially been collected before the cases had been identified (during pregnancy).

A. What is the principal advantage of using exposure information from the obstetric records rather than from the interviews?

B. What are the advantages of using information from the interviews rather than from the obstetric records?

4:17   Recall bias is due to the disease under study influencing the accuracy of exposure information obtained by interview or questionnaire. It has been suggested that the illness may act as a stimulus for people to report events that would otherwise be forgotten or unreported. Such recall bias would result in an overestimation of relative risks, and the results could show an excess risk even in the absence of an effect. (But sometimes the disease could reduce the tendency to report past exposure, resulting in underestimation of relative risks.) Although empirical data do not suggest that this is a frequent problem, it should be recognized as a possibility in any study where exposure information is collected only after the cases have appeared. In particular, the possibility of recall bias has been discussed for studies of congenital malformations and infant deaths. In some of these studies it has been possible to compare recalled exposure with information collected before the cases appeared.

In one study, exposure information obtained by interviewing 105 mothers of infants with major malformations and 165 mothers of nonmalformed infants was compared with data documented in obstetric records before the cases appeared. The number identified as exposed by both methods was divided by the number identified as exposed in the record (recall "sensitivity"). Of eight investigated exposures, five were reported "with little or no bias" and three were reported with a higher sensitivity by mothers of malformed infants.

A. Obstetric and other medical records often do not provide information on the presence (or absence) of an exposure for all subjects. Thus, many exposed subjects may not be classified as exposed due to lack of exposure information in the record. On what condition does the recall "sensitivity" reflect the true sensitivity?

B. Specificity (or recall "specificity") was not estimated. Suppose that mothers of malformed infants would be more likely than mothers of nonmalformed infants to report exposure even in the absence of exposure. In what direction would this bias the relative risk?

In another study, exposure information was obtained for 226 infants who died from Sudden Infant Death Syndrome (SIDS) and 226 living infants of the same age. Information on 25 exposures was available from interviews with the mothers (within 5 weeks after the cases occurred) and from medical records (recorded before the cases occurred). Recall "sensitivity" (defined as above) was higher in cases for 10 exposures, but higher in noncases for 14 exposures. Recall "specificity" was higher in cases for three exposures, but higher in noncases for 18 exposures. For 10 of the 25 exposures, the findings suggest that mothers of cases were more likely than mothers of noncases to report exposure. Relative risks were estimated using information from interviews and medical records, respectively. For 9 of the 10 exposures, the ratio of these two relative risks was between 0.9 and 1.5.

c. Recall "specificity" was calculated as the number not identified as exposed by any of the two methods divided by the number not identified as exposed in the medical record. The findings suggest that having a child die from SIDS tends to reduce recall "specificity." This may be due to an increased tendency to report exposure in the absence of exposure. But there could also be another explanation. Which?

D. If the outcome may act as a stimulus for people to report exposure, this effect is likely to depend upon the particular stimulus, that is, the disease (outcome) under study. What other factors are likely to influence this effect?

4:18 A possible effect of head trauma on the risk of Alzheimer's disease was investigated. Exposure information was collected by telephone interviews using a structured, standardized questionnaire. Information was obtained on whether a study subject had sustained "a head injury which 1) led him/her to visit a physician, 2) led him/her to seek hospital care, either in an emergency room (outpatient) or as an inpatient, or 3) resulted in a loss of consciousness, no matter how brief." Additional questions were asked concerning the duration of unconsciousness and other circumstances surrounding the injury. The interviews were conducted about 2 years after the cases had been identified (several years after a possible head trauma). Because of memory impairment and cognitive dysfunction in Alzheimer's disease, the cases were not able to answer the questionnaire themselves and relatives were used as surrogate respondents for all cases.

A. Should surrogate respondents be used for the noncases? Why/why not?

B. Surrogate respondents may not be available for all study subjects. How should this problem be dealt with?

C. The accuracy of exposure information provided by surrogate respondents is likely to be different for spouses, other relatives, and friends (depending upon how close they have been to the study subject). How should this problem be dealt with?

D. Suppose that, among the respondents, head trauma was perceived as a probable cause of dementia (Alzheimer's disease). How could this influence the accuracy of exposure information for cases and noncases, respectively?

E. For any head injury the relative risk was 3.5 (1.6–7.7, 95% confidence interval). Could a subdivision into severe and less severe head injury contribute information on the possibility of recall bias? Why/why not?

4:19   A study of the effect of using sunbeds and sunlamps on the risk of malignant melanoma of the skin was conducted in Ontario, Canada. Detailed interviews were made to obtain information on the use of sunbeds and sunlamps as well as on potential confounders. The interviews were conducted only after the cases had been identified, and the possibility of recall bias was discussed. In order to investigate this possibility, certain "distractor items" (microwave, personal computer, and video game usage) were included in the questionnaire. The reporting of these items was unrelated to melanoma. On what conditions does this show that the excess risks that were found in the present study (RR = 1.88 in men, RR = 1.45 in women) could not be explained by recall bias?

4:20   Differential exposure misclassification may be introduced if the exposure information is influenced by the disease under study. In principle, this could happen when exposure information is collected or handled after the cases have appeared. This is illustrated by the following four studies, all based on prevalent cases.

Study 1. The effects of sexual habits and contraceptive use on the risk of cervical human papillomavirus (HPV) and herpes simplex virus (HSV-2) infections in women aged 20–39 years was studied in Greenland and Denmark. The study included 1,247 subjects who participated in an interview on exposure history (sexual habits, oral contraceptives) and, at the same time, a physical examination to obtain biologic samples (blood, cervical cells) used to identify cases. Subsequent laboratory analyses identified 159 prevalent cases of HPV, and 386 prevalent cases of HSV-2.

A. On what conditions could the diseases under study have influenced the exposure information?

Study 2. It has been suggested that serum cholesterol might affect the risk of colorectal cancer. Colorectal polyps increase the risk of such cancer. Against this background, a possible effect of serum cholesterol on the risk of colorectal polyps was investigated in Michigan. Among 1,380 men who participated in a screening program, 246 were found to have at least one colorectal polyp. At the same time, blood samples were drawn and analyzed for serum cholesterol.

B. On what conditions could the disease under study have influenced the exposure information?

Study 3. The effect of alcohol intake, body mass, and serum cholesterol on the risk of gallstones in Mexican Americans aged 20–74 was studied in the Hispanic Health and Nutrition Examination Survey. Ultrasonography of the gallbladder of 2,293 study subjects identified 169 subjects with gallstones, and an additional 137 subjects who had their gallbladder removed due to previous gallstone disease. Exposure information was collected (interviews, examinations, blood specimens) at the time of the screening.

C. On what conditions could the disease under study have influenced the exposure information?

Study 4. Hypertension, obesity, and family history have been found to increase the risk of cardiovascular disease. A study of the effect of obesity and family history of hypertension on the risk of hypertension was conducted in Ottawa, Canada. Of 2,479 subjects screened for high blood pressure, 193 were identified as hypertensive. While waiting to be tested, each subject answered a one-page self-administered questionnaire on height and weight (used to calculate body mass index), family history of hypertension, and their own history of hypertension. Of the 193 cases identified at screening, 89 indicated that they had a previously known hypertension.

D. On what conditions could the disease under study have influenced the exposure information?

4:21 The effect of current exposure to certain analgesic drugs on the risk of bleeding gastric ulcer was investigated. As the cases appeared, information on the intake of analgesics on the day of the gastric bleeding was obtained from the cases. Similarly, noncases were interviewed about their intake of analgesics on the day of the interview. Suppose that noncases were contacted by mail or telephone to select a day for the interview at their convenience. Could this introduce a bias? Why/why not?

4:22 The collection of exposure information usually includes several steps. In a study of sexually transmitted disease in U.S. women aged 18–28, information on contraception, sexual history, and personal behaviors was collected only after the cases appeared. In addition, the study included comparisons between different methods of data collection (mail questionnaires and in-person interviews):

Subjects selected for the mail protocols were sent a packet on April 10, 1986 containing an introductory letter, a survey (color coded by case-control status), a stamped, addressed return envelope, and a postcard which the subject could use to request study results. Two weeks following the initial mailing, a postcard reminder was mailed. Three weeks after the initial mailing, a replacement survey was sent. A different stamp was placed on the return envelope in order to determine the response rate to the second mailing. Subjects assigned to the in-person interview were mailed an introductory letter on April 10, 1986. Callers began to follow up the letters on April 14, 1986. Interviewers sheduled appointments at the subjects' convenience. Interviews occurred during April 15–June 30, 1986. (Am. J. Epidemiol. 1989; 129:1052–1061).

A. Questionnaires were color coded by disease ("case-control") status. Could this be a source of bias? Why/why not?
B. Interviewers scheduled appointments at the subjects' convenience. Could this be a source of bias? Why/why not?

4:23   The interviewer may sometimes be a source of differential exposure misclassification in studies where interviews are conducted only after the cases have appeared. If the interviewer knows whether or not a subject has the disease under study, questions could (unintentionally) be asked in slightly different ways when cases and noncases are interviewed. In addition, the interviewer may be aware of the expected findings of the study and thus pay more attention to certain questionnaire items when the cases are interviewed. To avoid this source of differential exposure misclassification, all study subjects should be asked the same questions in the same way. This may be achieved by interviewers trained to approach all study subjects in a similar fashion using carefully structured questionnaires. Efforts are sometimes made to keep interviewers unaware of the subjects' disease status, or of the expected findings, or both. But such "blinding" is not always feasible. This is illustrated by the following studies.

Study 1. A structured questionnaire covering the use of specific drugs for over 40 indications, was used in a methodologic study. The interviewers were "nurses trained to administer the interview in a standard manner". They were "not informed of particular hypotheses under investigation."

Study 2. Two different sources of exposure information were used in a study of drug exposure during pregnancy and cardiovascular malformations in the offspring (cf. Exercise 4:16). One of these sources was "a detailed telephone questionnaire administered by one interviewer throughout the study. . . Although the interviewer was aware, by necessity, of the pregnancy outcome, she had no knowledge of the hypotheses under investigation or of the specific diagnosis of congenital heart disease."

Study 3. In a study of hair dye use and breast cancer among screening participants (cf. Exercise 3:2), standardized telephone interviews were conducted. "The interviewing was carried out by three trained interviewers who were kept 'blinded' as to the case or control status of the respondents until after the questions concerning hair dyes had been asked."

Study 4. When investigating periconceptional vitamin use and neural-tube defects (cf. Exercise 2:13), each mother was interviewed by telephone by two different interviewers. The first interviewer "obtained details about neural-tube defects. . . The mothers were then instructed not to discuss neural-tube defects or the presence or absence of other defects in their children with the second interviewer." The second interviewer, who was kept unaware of the infant's disease status, collected information on exposure and potential confounders using a standard questionnaire.

A. In these studies, attempts were made to keep the interviewer unaware of the subjects' disease status or of the expected findings of the study. Which is more important?

B. When the interviews are conducted only after the cases have been identified, the study subjects are usually aware of their own disease status. Give an example of a study where this is not the case.

c. When collecting the exposure information, it may be difficult to keep the investigator (interviewer) unaware of the subjects' disease status. There is another situation where it may be both feasible and important to keep an investigator unaware of the subjects' disease status. Which?

4:24 The effect of cigarette smoking on the risk of coronary heart disease was investigated (cf. Exercise 2:19). Smoking status was defined as current, past, or never (= unexposed), and current cigarette smokers were classified according to the number of cigarettes smoked per day. Consider two alternatives for a classification into three categories (with different cut-off points):

1. 1–14; 15–24; $\geq$ 25 cigarettes/day,
2. 1–9; 10–19; $\geq$ 20 cigarettes/day.

Could the choice between these two alternatives affect the amount of exposure misclassification?

4:25 Intake of saturated fat was one of several exposures of interest in a study of diet and kidney cancer. Dietary fat is an important source of energy, and intake of saturated fat means intake of calories. How should the calories contributed by saturated fat be regarded when defining exposure to saturated fat?

4:26 The costs for obtaining information on exposure and potential confounders should be considered in any study. A small difference in cost per subject may translate into a large difference in total cost when a large number of subjects are examined. With limited financial resources, any savings could be used for other purposes such as increasing the size of the study and thus its precision. Priorities should be made with the purpose of obtaining results that are as accurate as possible with the resources available.

Information on occupational exposures can be obtained in different ways. A study in Montreal, Canada included comparisons of five possible methods of data collection: 1) job titles abstracted from routine records, 2) job titles abstracted from routine records and processed through a job exposure matrix to derive exposure data, 3) job titles obtained by interview, 4) job titles obtained by interview and processed through a job exposure matrix to derive exposure data, and 5) job descriptions obtained by interview and processed by a team of experts to derive exposure data. Of the total estimated costs for data collection in 1988, some costs were strongly related to the number of subjects examined, while others were independent of the number of subjects examined (e.g., $20,000 for buying and implementing a job exposure matrix). The total cost was lowest for alternative (1): $13.75–125 per subject, and highest for alternative (5): $325–600 per subject, depending upon the number of subjects examined. The different methods should be compared, not only with regard to costs, but also with regard to the comparability, accuracy, and completeness of exposure information that can be obtained. In general, what sources of bias may be reduced (avoided) by the choice of method for obtaining exposure information? What are the priorities?

4:27 Of 11,136 men selected for the Honolulu Heart Program, 8,006 (72%) participated and 3,130 (28%) did not participate in the baseline examination, which was completed at the end of 1968. During a 14-year follow-up (January 1969 through December 1982), nonparticipants had a higher mortality than participants. This applies to total mortality as well as to mortality from cancer and from coronary heart disease (CHD).

Most results are based on participants only. How could the above nonparticipation be expected to bias the results of a study aimed at estimating:

A. the mortality (total, cancer, or CHD) in the study population that was originally selected for the program?
B. the effect of a certain exposure on mortality (total, cancer, or CHD)?

4:28 As part of the collaborative Lipid Research Program, a study of cardiovascular disease was conducted to investigate the effects of several exposures. Of 2,854 men selected for the study, 532 (19%) did not provide information on exposures and potential confounders. But telephone interviews were conducted with a sample of the nonrespondents, and it was found that certain exposures and potential confounders were more common among respondents than among nonrespondents. How could the results have been biased by this nonresponse, if the exposure information was collected:

A. before the cases appeared?

B. only after the cases appeared?

4:29 A possible preventive effect of vitamin intake around the time of conception on a woman's risk of having a child with a neural-tube defect was investigated (cf. Exercise 4:23). Exposure information was obtained by interviewing the mothers after the cases had been identified. Of the cases, 351 were identified as exposed (any vitamin supplements or cereals) and 214 as unexposed (no vitamin supplements or cereals).

A. If 62% of the study population was exposed and 38% was unexposed, what was the estimated relative risk?

In the study population, a total of 831 cases were identified. But only $351 + 214 = 565$ of these cases agreed to participate in the interview. For the remaining 266 cases, no exposure information was available.

B. Mothers who had given birth to a child with a neural-tube defect could be more willing to participate in the interview if they had used vitamins during pregnancy. If so, in what direction would the lack of exposure information bias the relative risk?

C. Suppose that, of the 266 cases lost to interviews, 50% were exposed and 50% were unexposed. What would the relative risk have been, if exposure information had been obtained for all cases?

D. As the most extreme outcome of B (above), suppose that exposure information was obtained for all cases that were exposed (i.e., that the 266 cases who did not provide exposure information were all unexposed). What would the relative risk have been, if exposure information had been obtained for all cases?

4:30 Failure to obtain exposure information is influenced by the methods used to collect the information as well as by the choice of study population (Chapter 3). The response may be different for different methods such as mail questionnaires, telephone interviews, and face-to-face interviews. The content, wording, and sequence of questions and the length of the questionnaire may also influence nonresponse. Study subjects may perceive a questionnaire or examination as trying, boring, interesting, or helpful, and this may influence their willingness to participate. In a study of sexually transmitted disease (cf. Exercise 4:22), exposure information was collected only after the cases appeared. The women were randomly assigned to one of three data collection strategies: 1) an in-person interview, 2) a self-administered mail survey (equivalent to the interview), and 3) a modified mail questionnaire.

A. For each of the three methods, 82–85 percent of the noncases returned the questionnaire (or participated in the interview). In what other respects should the three methods be compared?

B. Compared to the women responding to mail questionnaires, those interviewed in person were less likely to report yeast infections (24% vs. 44%), and more likely to state that one-time relationships were "not applicable" to them (69% vs. 31%). How could this be explained, and what are the possible consequences in terms of exposure misclassification?

GENERAL QUESTIONS

4:31 A gap between the theoretical and empirical definition of an exposure should be considered as a source of exposure misclassification. Why? Exemplify!

4:32 What are the advantages and disadvantages, respectively, of questioning as compared with other methods used to obtain exposure information? Exemplify!

4:33 Reporting of exposure may be influenced by social desirability, and recall of past exposure may be influenced by current exposure. How could this bias the results of a study? Exemplify!

4:34 The possibility of bias due to exposure misclassification is influenced by the timing of the collection and handling of exposure information. How? Exemplify!

4:35 Differential exposure misclassification may be introduced by respondents (recall bias). What different strategies have been proposed to avoid, assess, or control recall bias? Exemplify!

4:36 Differential exposure misclassification may be introduced by the interviewer or examiner. How can this be avoided? Exemplify!

4:37 Differential exposure misclassification may be introduced in the handling (e.g., encoding) of exposure information. How can this be avoided? Exemplify!

4:38 Some study subjects may not provide exposure information. In what ways could this bias the results of a study? Exemplify!

4:39 What could be done, and what should be done, to reduce non-response in the collection of exposure information? Exemplify!

4:40 Consider your own recent favorite study. What are the implications for that study of the general problems and possibilities exemplified in the different exercises in this chapter?

5 *Follow-up of Disease Occurrence*

■■ INTRODUCTION

Definitions

Information on disease occurrence is obtained by follow-up during a certain period of time (in studies based on incidence), or by examining each subject at one point in time (in studies based on prevalence). As a first step, the disease or diseases (outcomes) of interest are defined. In clinical medicine, disease entities are more or less clearly separated by clinical and laboratory findings, as well as the patient's history, with a view toward treatment and prognosis. In both epidemiologic and clinical research there is often a need for more explicit definitions, and for criteria that are uniformly applied. In epidemiology, there is an interest in the etiology (causation) of disease. Thus, a disease should be defined with regard to its localization, macroscopic and microscopic appearance and so forth, to the extent that such aspects could be related to causation. Symptoms (e.g., chest pain), signs (e.g., in electrocardiograms), and tests (e.g., serum enzyme levels) may suggest the presence of a disease (e.g., myocardial infarction). A set of *diagnostic criteria* based on such indicators may be viewed as an empirical definition of the disease. These criteria are more or less accurate in reflecting a theoretical definition of the disease. An International Classification of Diseases (ICD) is available, and revised periodically (World Health Organization 1992–1993), but for many diseases there are no well-defined and generally accepted diagnostic criteria. As new diagnostic tools become available, this is likely to make it possible to separate an increasing number of disease entities which differ in their etiology.

The development of a disease episode is usually a gradual process that may reach different degrees of severity. As a basis for making the distinction between the disease-free and the diseased state, a definition should specify the stage at which the disease is considered to occur (cf. Chapter 1: Measures of Disease Occurrence, and Figure 1–1). Among people who have had the disease previously, the risk of developing the same disease again may be much increased (e.g., myocardial infarction) or reduced (e.g., specific infectious diseases). Thus, to avoid confounding by previous episodes of the disease under investigation, a study is often limited to first cases of the disease (cf. Chapter 1: Confounding). Finally, the exposure under study should never be included in a definition of the disease or among the diagnostic criteria. For example, when studying the effect of obesity on the risk of diabetes, obesity (or body mass) should not be included among the diagnostic criteria for diabetes.

Methods

In principle, follow-up of disease occurrence means continuous surveil-lance (examinations) of each study subject to determine if, and when, there is an incident case, that is a transit from the disease-free to the diseased state according to the definition. In most studies, however, cases are identified as individuals go to visit a doctor because of symptoms of disease. These are incident cases when the disease is defined on the basis of "symptoms severe enough to see a physician" (incident cases of symptomatic disease). There may, however, be considerable differences between individuals in their tendency to seek medical advice. Screening programs are sometimes available for the detection (and treatment) of early, asymptomatic disease. In addition, patients who seek medical advice or treatment for one condition are subjected to routine examinations that may identify other diseases at an early, asymptomatic stage. These are prevalent cases of asymptomatic disease (some of which would progress further to become incident cases of symptomatic disease). Incident cases may, under certain conditions, be identified indirectly by repeated screening examinations of subjects initially free from screening detectable disease (incident cases of screening detectable disease). Studies are sometimes based on mortality, and deaths caused by the disease may be considered as incident cases of disease severe enough to be fatal (incident cases of fatal disease). However, when the disease is merely present at the time of death, it is not an incident case (but rather a prevalent case of nonfatal disease) although the distinction is occasionally difficult to make.

In practice, a variety of methods may be used to identify incident (or prevalent) cases of disease. The choice of methods depends upon the particular disease under study and on the avaliable sources of information. Questioning or close surveillance of study subjects may be necessary to identify cases that would not come to the attention of the medical services. Study subjects may have to be examined repeatedly. Questionnaires may provide information on symptoms, episodes of illness, physician-diagnosed disease, and hospitalizations. Reviews of medical records, death certificates, and other sources of data will often provide additional useful information. The accuracy of the information varies considerably depending upon the particular disease (outcome) of interest and the methods used for examination (e.g., autopsy). Register data are sometimes available as a source of information on morbidity or mortality. This is likely to save cost and time. But it may also conceal sources of bias unless attention is paid to the comparability, accuracy, and completeness of the original information. In addition, reporting and registration may be incomplete or incorrect with regard to the outcome of interest or the information necessary to identify study subjects (e.g., personal identification numbers).

Misclassification

Disease misclassification may be introduced by the definition (diagnostic criteria), follow-up or examination, diagnosis, reporting, and recording of disease. Nondifferential disease misclassification introduces no bias (sensitivity < 1), or a bias towards RR $= 1$ (specificity < 1). Stringent diagnostic criteria tend to reduce the probability that people who do not have the disease are classified as having it, that is, increase specificity and thus prevent a bias towards RR $= 1$. But stringent criteria are also likely to increase the probability that people who have the disease are classified as not having it, that is, reduce sensitivity. This will not introduce any bias due to misclassification—but reduces the number of cases, and thus precision. Differential disease misclassification introduced by a factor associated with the exposure is nondifferential within strata and may result in a bias towards RR $= 1$ when the factor is controlled in the data analysis (cf. Chapter 1, Misclassification: Differential Disease Misclassification).

Since the cases occur only after an exposure of interest, there is always the possibility that the exposure could influence disease misclassification. But steps can often be taken to avoid this source of differential misclassification. As mentioned previously, diagnostic criteria should be independent of the exposure. In addition, the exposed and unexposed should be examined for disease in a similar way using the same methods and sources of information. Thus, if exposed subjects are offered frequent medical examinations, the unexposed should be provided with a similar intense follow-up in order to avoid "detection bias" (differential misclassification). This may influence the selection of exposed and unexposed subjects for the study (cf. Chapter 3). Sometimes, exposed subjects may have concerns about the possible health effects of the exposure, and this may influence their tendency to seek medical advice and to report symptoms of illness. This source of differential misclassification can sometimes be avoided by selecting a study population where the unexposed have similar concerns, by close surveillance (frequent examinations) of all study subjects, or, in experimental studies, by the use of placebo and blinding. Similarly, physicians who know that the exposure may affect the risk of disease could tend to examine a patient more thoroughly, or use a certain diagnosis more frequently, when the subject is exposed. This source of differential misclassification may be avoided by the use of standardized criteria and examination methods, and sometimes by blinding with regard to exposure status, that is, keeping the examiner unaware of whether a subject is exposed or unexposed. Finally, exposed subjects may be more likely than the unexposed to participate in screening examinations for the detection and treatment of early, asymptomatic disease. This could introduce a bias towards $RR = \infty$ (by screening during follow-up, if prevalent cases of screening-detectable disease are included among the cases) or towards $RR = 0$ (by screening prior to follow-up, resulting in a depletion of cases-to-be in studies of symptomatic disease).

Selective Loss to Follow-up

Individual follow-up periods may be defined to cover the entire study period, or parts thereof (cf. Chapter 1: Study Population and Follow-up Period). Selection bias is introduced if the disease under study influences the termination of follow-up (Chapter 1: Selection Bias). Subjects may be lost to follow-up because they have died or can no longer be followed, perhaps after moving abroad or refusing further participation in the study. The loss to follow-up may be selective. For example, subjects may be more inclined to return for a follow-up examination if they have developed symptoms of the disease. This tendency may be different in the exposed and unexposed, resulting in overestimation (or underestimation) of the relative risk. Definitions of individual follow-up periods may sometimes conceal this source of bias. For example, if subjects with a certain occupational exposure would tend to leave their job when they develop symptoms of disease, exposed cases may not be identified if follow-up periods are defined to last only as long as the employment.

In order to avoid selection bias, follow-up periods should be independent of the disease, and efforts should be made to avoid selective loss to follow-up. Loss to follow-up may be avoided by the choice of study population and follow-up period (Chapter 3), and by using suitable methods for follow-up. In addition, various techniques have been used to trace and motivate subjects for continued follow-up. Attention should be paid to the possibility of selective withdrawals, and it may sometimes be possible to examine subjects for the presence of disease at the time of withdrawal. In experimental studies, randomization, placebo, and blinding may be used to avoid any differences between the exposed and unexposed with regard to selective loss to follow-up. Information about subjects lost to follow-up should be presented together with the study results.

■■■■ EXERCISES

5:1   The disease or outcome of interest should be specified. The extent to which this is done is likely to influence the results, as illustrated by the following studies:

Study 1. The effect of physical activity on total mortality (death rate) was investigated among 16,936 Harvard alumni during 12–16 years of follow-up.

A. Death is a rather unspecific outcome. In what ways, if any, does this influence the interpretation of the results?

Study 2. The effect of dietary vitamin A intake on the risk of lung cancer in men aged 35–79 years was investigated.

B. The outcome of interest was primary lung cancer. Would it be useful to specify the outcome further? Why/why not?

Study 3. The effect of serum cholesterol on mortality from stroke was investigated in a follow-up of 350,977 men screened for the Multiple Risk Factor Intervention Trial. Even at the highest level of serum cholesterol there was little or no effect.

C. Could an effect have been concealed by defining the outcome as death from stroke? Why/why not?

Study 4. The etiology of gallstone disease in middle-aged women was investigated. The outcome under study was symptomatic gallstones in women with no previous symptoms of gallstone disease.

D. Should the outcome be specified further? Why/why not?

5:2 The effect of alcohol drinking on the risk of diabetes in women was investigated among participants in the Nurses' Health Study. Women with any alcohol intake (here called "exposed") had a lower risk of diabetes than women with no alcohol intake (here called "unexposed"). In the age group 50–59 years, 281 cases were identified during 4 years' follow-up of 30,297 women:

	Exposed	*Unexposed*
Cases (diabetes)	156	125
Noncases (no diabetes)	20,271	9,745
All women	20,427	9,870
Incidence proportion ($*10^4$)	76.37	126.65

$$RR = 76.37/126.65 = 0.60$$

Suppose there is no misclassification in these data. What would the results have been if there was:

A. a nondifferential disease misclassification with sensitivity = 0.90 and specificity = 1.00?

B. a nondifferential disease misclassification with sensitivity = 1.00 and specificity = 0.99?

C. a nondifferential disease misclassification with sensitivity = 0.90 and specificity = 0.99?

D. a differential disease misclassification with sensitivity = 0.90 and specificity = 1.00 among the exposed, but sensitivity = 1.00 and specificity = 1.00 among the unexposed?

E. a differential disease misclassification with sensitivity = 1.00 and specificity = 0.99 among the exposed, but sensitivity = 1.00 and specificity = 1.00 among the unexposed?

F. a differential disease misclassification with sensitivity = 0.90 and specificity = 0.99 among the exposed, but sensitivity = 1.00 and specificity = 1.00 among the unexposed?

5:3 An outbreak of gastroenteritis at an outdoor music festival was investigated in a study mentioned in Chapter 3 (Exercise 3:5). For exposure to a tofu salad served at the festival the results were approximately as follows:

	Exposed	*Unexposed*
Cases	120	40
Noncases	32	183
All subjects	152	223

$$RR = 4.40$$

Suppose there was no misclassification in these data.

A. What would the result (RR) have been, with an overreporting of the disease among the exposed (sensitivity = 1.00; specificity = 0.95) but not among the unexposed (sensitivity = 1.00; specificity = 1.00)?

The proportion of subjects who fell ill was quite high in this study. In another study, the number of cases may only have been 10% of that in the table above:

	Exposed	*Unexposed*
Cases	12	4
Noncases	140	219
All subjects	152	223

$$RR = 4.40$$

Suppose there was no misclassification in these data.

B. What would the result (RR) have been, if the misclassification (sensitivity, specificity) was the same as above (A)?

5:4   Acute lower respiratory infections (LRI) are a common cause of illness and death among children in the developing countries. The World Health Organization (WHO) has recommended that children with certain signs of severe LRI should be referred for inpatient treatment. In addition, certain signs have been used to identify cases of severe LRI in epidemiologic studies. In rural Gambia, children under 5 years of age were surveyed for 1 year by trained field workers. They identified 222 children with symptoms of respiratory infection. Of these children, 216 were examined by chest radiography: severe LRI (lobar consolidation) was present in 25 (cases) and absent in 191 (noncases). The possibility of identifying cases in the absence of radiography was investigated. Three different signs were evaluated: bronchial breath sounds or decreased air entry on auscultation (BB or RAE), respiratory rate above 60 per minute (RespR > 60), and axillary temperature above 38.5°C (T > 38.5). The findings were as follows:

Lobar consolidation:	BB or RAE:		RespR > 60:		T > 38.5:	
	yes	no	yes	no	yes	no
yes	8	17	15	10	15	10
no	6	185	52	139	35	156

A. For each of the three signs, calculate the sensitivity and specificity in identifying cases with lobar consolidation.

B. The sensitivity and specificity of each sign depend upon the equipment and method used for examination as well as on the skills of the examiner. When using similar equipment, methods, and examiners, would the findings (sensitivity, specificity) apply to any population of children of the same age? Why/why not?

c. None of the three signs had a sensitivity greater than 60 percent. However, information on two signs may be combined: the presence of both may be required to identify a case, or the presence of either one may be sufficient to identify a case. Which should be preferred in order to improve the sensitivity?

D. The signs that are most useful in epidemiologic studies are likely to be different from those that should be used to identify cases for inpatient treatment. Why?

5:5 In a review of methods used to identify cases of atherosclerotic peripheral arterial disease, it was concluded that "the intermittent claudication questionnaire lacks sensitivity, but is highly specific; palpation of pulses is more sensitive, but less specific."

A. Suppose that a "positive" result by either one of the two methods (questionnaire or palpation of pulses) would be sufficient for diagnosis. How would this affect the sensitivity and specificity, respectively?

B. Suppose that a "positive" result by both methods (questionnaire and palpation of pulses) would be required for diagnosis. How would this affect the sensitivity and specificity, respectively?

5:6 In the Framingham Study, a follow-up of 459 subjects who had experienced an initial myocardial infarction (MI) identified 275 cases of MI (reinfarction) and 344 deaths from coronary heart disease (CHD). Systolic blood pressure, serum cholesterol, and diabetes were found to increase the risk of MI and death from CHD.

Most other studies are based on "clinically recognized" cases of MI—that is, subjects who had symptoms (such as chest pain) severe enough to seek medical care and where an examination showed findings (electrocardiograms, serum enzymes, etc.) indicating MI. But in the Framingham Study, clinically unrecognized cases of MI were identified by routine biennial examinations, including electrocardiograms. About one third of all cases of MI identified in the Framingham Study were not clinically recognized (but had a similar long-term prognosis).

A. How could the results (RR) be biased if, as an outcome, only clinically recognized cases of MI were identified?

B. How could the results (RR) be biased if, as an outcome, only nonfatal cases of MI were included?

5:7 The World Health Organization (WHO) criteria for "definite myocardial infarction" are as follows:

1. a definite ECG abnormality, or

2. typical or atypical symptoms together with a probable ECG abnormality and abnormal enzymes, or

3. typical symptoms together with abnormal enzymes with an absent, non-codable or non-evolving ECG;

4. fatal cases, whether sudden or not, with naked-eye appearances of fresh myocardial infarction and/or recent coronary occlusion found at necropsy.

Of 905 cases of definite myocardial infarction according to the previous WHO criteria, 739 (82 percent) also fulfilled the above, new WHO criteria for definite myocardial infarction. There is, in addition, always a discrepancy between an empirical definition (based on criteria like those above) and a theoretical definition of myocardial infarction. Even in the absence of any measurement error, this is likely to introduce some misclassification in relation to the theoretical definition.

A. How could this bias relative risks?

Despite guidelines for "definite" and "probable" abnormality of an electrocardiogram (ECG), there is likely to be some misclassification due to differences between hospitals, and between individual physicians, in the interpretation and recording of ECGs. Enzymes are considered "abnormal" when a value is more than twice the laboratory "normal," but variations between laboratories, and even within the same laboratory, are likely to introduce some misclassification. The description and evaluation of "typical" and "atypical" symptoms (although specified further) rests with the individual patient and physician. Thus, measurement errors are likely to introduce some misclassification in relation to the WHO criteria, even among subjects who are thoroughly examined.

B. How could this bias relative risks?

The identification of nonfatal cases of MI depends heavily on the availability of ECG and enzyme data. Many cases, for example those with mild symptoms, are not examined routinely (cf. Exercise 5:6). Fatal cases among sudden deaths and out-of-hospital deaths may not be identified. Autopsy rates vary considerably, and fatal cases may never be examined according to (4).

C. How could this bias relative risks?

5:8 Some studies are based on incidence, others on prevalence. But incident and prevalent cases should not be mixed. The difference between incident and prevalent cases is illustrated by the following studies.

Study 1. An outbreak of meningococcal disease occurred in 1986 in Gloucestershire, England. Symptom-free carriers are a major source of meningococcal infection. Thus, a population survey was conducted to identify meningococcal carriers. Each symptom-free subject was examined once for the presence of meningococci. During one month (November 1986), 69 carriers of outbreak strains were identified.

A. Are these incident or prevalent cases?

Study 2. The effect of maternal smoking during pregnancy on the risk of oral clefts in the offspring was investigated. During one year, 28 infants were born with cleft lip with or without cleft palate.

B. Are these incident or prevalent cases?

Study 3. A study of dietary vitamin C and uterine cervical dysplasia was based on women attending two screening clinics in Bronx, New York. During the study period, 87 cases of cervical dysplasia were identified by Pap smears.

C. Are these incident or prevalent cases?

Study 4. An examination of 15,812 necropsy reports identified 33 cases of gastric cancer that had not been diagnosed during life.

D. Are these incident or prevalent cases?

5:9 The effect of oral contraceptive use on the risk of cervical cancer was investigated in the Royal College of General Practitioners' Oral Contraception Study in England. The development of a cancer of the uterine cervix is a gradual process. A transition, as seen in the microscope, from normal cells to dysplasia and further to carcinoma in situ and eventually invasive cancer, may take one or more decades. However, the rate of progression—and possible spontaneous regression—is not well known, since identification is nearly always followed by treatment. The early stages may be asymptomatic, but sometimes there are vaginal bleedings. Later there may be vaginal discharge, profuse bleeding, and pain. Tumor dissemination by regional and distant metastases is followed by general manifestations. Death from cervical cancer is reported in 10–90 percent of patients with invasive cervical cancer, depending upon the stage at diagnosis.

What is an incident case of cervical cancer?

5:10 Like cervical cancer, endometrial cancer has a gradual onset and its first manifestation is often vaginal bleeding. The findings of several studies suggest that postmenopausal estrogen use increases the risk of endometrial cancer. However, estrogen use may induce vaginal bleeding. Such bleedings may prompt a gynecologic examination, which is likely to identify a prevalent case of asymptomatic endometrial cancer, if present. In practice it may be difficult or impossible to know whether the bleeding was induced by estrogen or was a first manifestation of an incident case of symptomatic cancer. This is a possible source of differential disease misclassification ("detection bias").

A. When all cases are considered as incident cases, in what direction is this likely to bias the relative risk?

In order to estimate the possible magnitude of such detection bias, a study was conducted to identify cases of endometrial cancer that remain undetected during life. A review of over 50,000 necropsy reports showed that, among deceased women aged $\geq$ 45 years, about 30/10,000 had a previously undetected endometrial cancer at the time of death. If these were prevalent cases at the time of death, the prevalence proportion of undetected endometrial cancer was 30/10,000 in women aged ≥ 45 years. (If these were incident cases, the appropriate denominator would include all living women rather than those who died.) According to data from the State Tumor Registry, the incidence rate of endometrial cancer diagnosed during life in women aged ≥ 45 years was about 5/10,000 per year.

    B. How many cases of endometrial cancer would be diagnosed during life in 10,000 women aged 45 years? (Suppose that, on average, they live until age 75).

    c. How many cases would be added, if all cases detected at necropsy would have been diagnosed during life?

    D. Estrogens should not be prescribed for women with endometrial cancer, and women asking for a prescription of estrogen are usually examined with regard to possible endometrial cancer. In what direction is this likely to bias the relative risk?

    E. An effect of estrogen use on the risk of endometrial cancer is likely to occur only after several months of use. But vaginal bleedings due to estrogen tend to occur early during estrogen treatment. In what direction is this likely to bias the relative risk?

5:11 The effect of tubal sterilization and hysterectomy on the risk of epithelial ovarian cancer in women aged 20–54 years was investigated in the Cancer and Steroid Hormone Study. Allowing for an induction time of 6 months, the relative risk (with 95% confidence interval) was 0.69 (0.50–0.95) for tubal sterilization, 0.55 (0.38–0.81) for hysterectomy only, and 0.60 (0.31–1.17) for hysterectomy with unilateral oophorectomy.

    A. A detection bias could be introduced if women who had a tubal sterilization or hysterectomy were subjected to examinations during follow-up that could identify an early asymptomatic ovarian cancer. Could this explain the findings of the present study? Why/why not?

    B. Another possibility is that women were examined during (or before, or within 6 months after) surgery for the presence of an early asymptomatic ovarian cancer or premalignant condition. Could this explain the findings of the present study? Why/why not?

5:12 In a study of prostate cancer, the most common cancer in men, subjects with heart disease had an increased risk of having a prostate cancer diagnosed during follow-up. One possible interpretation of this finding would be that heart disease, or a risk factor or treatment for heart disease, increases the risk of prostate cancer. Another possibility, that was discussed, is that the association was due to detection bias. Like cervical cancer in women (cf. Exercise 5:9), prostate cancer develops gradually over an extended period of time. In medical care, patients are being examined for the presence of prostate cancer—and of other diseases—on different grounds:

1. *General examination.* Patients admitted for other diseases are routinely subjected to physical examination as well as to certain blood tests, and perhaps also X-rays, electrocardiograms, and other examinations. Questioning about symptoms, and sometimes also palpation of the prostate gland, are included in such routine examinations.

2. *Differential diagnosis.* Patients admitted for diseases that give rise to symptoms similar to those seen in prostate cancer are examined more carefully for the presence of a prostate cancer. For instance, benign enlargement of the prostate gland is a common condition in elderly men. Patients admitted for this condition are also examined for the presence of prostate cancer.

   A. If the association between heart disease and prostate cancer was due to detection bias, what is the likely explanation and how should this problem be handled?
   B. What is the main difficulty in identifying incident cases of symptomatic prostate cancer?

5:13   Non-insulin-dependent diabetes is another disease that may be asymptomatic and remain undetected for a long period of time. But subjects who are being examined and treated for other diseases are often subjected to blood and urine tests that are likely to detect an early diabetes.
   A. On what condition could this introduce a detection bias resulting in overestimation of the relative risk?
   B. How should this problem be handled?
   C. According to definitions proposed by the National Diabetes Data Group, weight is used as a criterion in the diagnosis of non-insulin-dependent diabetes. How would this bias the results when studying the effect of obesity on the risk of diabetes?

5:14 In July 1980, a Canadian newspaper reported that four employees of Toronto Star (another newspaper firm) who had worked with video display terminals (VDTs) during pregnancy had subsequently given birth to malformed infants. In addition, some clusters of spontaneous abortions were reported during the next few years and the possibility of an association with VDT use was discussed in the media. Against this background, an epidemiologic study of VDT use and the risk of spontaneous abortion was conducted in Calgary, Canada.

    A. Suppose that information on spontaneous abortions was obtained by interview at the end of the follow-up period. How could the events mentioned above have influenced the possibility of misclassification in respect of spontaneous abortion? (In a previous study on the accuracy of spontaneous abortion recall, 75 percent of previously recorded abortions were recalled under relatively favorable conditions).

    B. In the present study, cases were identified as they were admitted to the gynecological units of hospitals, and spontaneous abortion was defined as "the unintentional cessation of pregnancy before 20 weeks of gestation." Compared with A, above, how does this alter the possibility of differential misclassification?

5:15 The association between smoking and the prevalence of chronic bronchitis was investigated (cf. Exercise 2:29). Smoking has long been the single most prominent, known cause of chronic bronchitis. Mild forms of the disease may exist for years with only slight cough, such as the morning "cigarette" cough, getting worse after acute upper respiratory infections. The condition may progress to severe chronic cough with mucoid or purulent sputum, and eventually irreversible impairment of pulmonary function.

    A. In the absence of other signs of the disease, the clinical diagnosis of chronic bronchitis is often based on an evaluation of the symptoms mentioned above. Attention is usually paid to the smoking habits of the patient. How could this influence the possibility of bias due to disease misclassification?

    B. In the present study, cases were not identified by clinical diagnosis. Instead, information on respiratory symptoms was obtained by questionnaire and chronic bronchitis was defined as "cough productive of sputum for at least three months per year for the previous two consecutive years." How could this influence the possibility of bias due to disease misclassification?

5:16 Injuries among inner-city women were studied in an urban black community in Pennsylvania. A case was "defined as any injury event . . . which led to care or evaluation at a hospital surveillance site or resulted in death . . ."

A. What is the main advantage and disadvantage, respectively, of defining a case in this way?

During one year, nearly 10 percent of women aged $\geq$ 15 years suffered at least one injury event resulting in an emergency room visit. Injury rates were found to be highest for women aged 25–34 years (157.1 per 1,000 woman-years at risk) and lowest for women aged $\geq$ 65 years (48.5 per 1,000 woman-years at risk). Injury events were classified according to the International Classification of Diseases, Injuries, and Causes of Death, Clinical Modification (ICD-9-CM). The most frequent type of injury (E-code) was falls (25.1 cases per 1,000 woman-years at risk), followed by violence (20.8 cases per 1,000 woman-years at risk).

B. Suppose that there was a tendency for certain kinds of injuries by violence to be misclassified as falls or other types of injuries (E-codes). Under what circumstances would this bias relative risks of injury by violence?

5:17 A study of the effect of passive smoking on the risk of respiratory diseases in children was mentioned in Chapter 3 (Exercise 3:4). Information on passive smoking, potential confounders, and respiratory diseases during the child's first 18 months of life was collected by interview when the child was 18 months old. In principle, it would be possible to ask the parents of each child about: 1) signs of respiratory disease, 2) respiratory disease diagnosed by a doctor, or 3) hospitalizations for respiratory disease. What are the advantages and disadvantages, respectively, of each of these three approaches?

5:18 In rural Bangladesh, a study was conducted of diarrhea in children under 5 years of age. Follow-up was made by health assistants who, accompanied by a local female worker, visited each home and interviewed the mother or any adult present to record the diarrhea episodes experienced by children during the preceding week. Diarrhea was defined as "three or more loose motions in a 24-hour period with or without the presence of blood and mucus. An episode was considered new if there was an interval of at least 48 hours between symptoms."

Each home was visited once a week. Of 7,380 reported diarrheal episodes, 43 percent started during the 2 days prior to the day of visit. The number of episodes reported on each day fell gradually from 2 to 6 days prior to the day of visit. This drop was more pronounced for episodes without fever than for episodes with fever, and more pronounced for episodes with a low (3–4/24 hours) than for episodes with a high ($\geq 7/24$ hours) frequency of motions. It was assumed that a diarrheal episode was equally likely to start on any day of the week. Thus, the observed differences between days in reported onsets of diarrhea were interpreted as reporting errors. Compared to the 2 days prior to the visit, the underreporting of diarrheal episodes on day 3–6 before the visit day was estimated at 42 percent for episodes without fever.

How would an underreporting of this magnitude bias the relative risks when studying the effects of exposures such as feeding, malnutrition, and hygiene on the risk of diarrhea?

5:19   In many epidemiologic studies, computerized registers are used to identify cases. The accuracy of such register data depends not only on the extent to which disease episodes are identified and correctly diagnosed, but also on the completeness and accuracy of reporting and registration. The world's oldest population-based cancer registry, operating on a national scale, is the Danish Cancer Registry (DCR). The completeness of registration of cases of invasive cervical cancer in the DCR, from its start 1943 until 1966, was evaluated by linkage to a complementary data file with information on 5,674 cases of invasive cervical cancer enrolled in a clinical study. The purpose was to find out to what extent these cases could be identified in the DCR.

A. What information, except diagnosis and date, is needed for a record linkage?

B. In the record linkage, 80 percent of the cases in the clinical study were identified in the DCR. What could explain the 20 percent deficit?

5:20   Death is the outcome of interest in many epidemiologic studies, and death certificates are a common source of information on the causes of death. A single death may be due to several diseases (e.g., pneumonia, coronary heart disease, and diabetes). But in studies of mortality, each death is often considered as being due to only one disease, usually the so-called underlying cause of death on the death certificate.

Mortality from different diseases was investigated in a 25-year follow-up of 2,046 men in the Chicago Western Electric Study. Of all 766 death certificates, 45.7 percent listed a single cause of death, 33.9 percent two causes, 14.9 percent three, and 5.5 percent four or more causes of death. The number of death certificates with a certain cause of death mentioned as the underlying cause (and other mentions) was 452 (61) for cardiovascular disease, 202 (20) for cancer, 16 (43) for influenza-pneumonia-bronchitis, and 3 (44) for diabetes.

A. No less than 34 of the 47 decedents with any mention of diabetes had cardiovascular disease as the underlying cause of death. Could this bias the relative risks in a study of death from diabetes, including cases with any mention of diabetes on the death certificate? Why/why not?

B. The association between diabetes and cardiovascular disease is well-known among physicians, and they could be more likely to mention diabetes on the death certificate when the underlying cause of death is cardiovascular disease. Could this bias the relative risks in a study of death from diabetes, including cases with any mention of diabetes on the death certificate? Why/why not?

C. Would it be preferable to include only cases where diabetes is mentioned as the underlying cause of death? Why/why not?

5:21 The diagnoses that are mentioned on death certificates reflect, to some extent, physician terminology preferences. This is illustrated by the findings in a study of 2,268 deaths in Maryland, using the ninth revision of the International Classification of Diseases (ICD-9). For instance, the choice between chronic heart disease (ICD–9:414) and chronic cardiovascular disease (ICD–9:429.2 or 402.9) as an underlying cause of death was related to the availability of advanced diagnostic methods, length of patient care, medical school of the certifier and, in addition, to the race and sex of the decedent.

A. When could this bias the relative risk of chronic heart disease (ICD–9:414) towards RR = ∞ (or RR = 0)?

B. When could this bias the relative risk of chronic heart disease (ICD-9:414) towards RR = 1?

C. What should be done to avoid these sources of bias?

5:22 In elderly people, osteoarthritis of the hip is a common cause of chronic pain and disability. In epidemiologic studies, the diagnosis is often based on X-ray findings such as osteophytes, joint space narrowing, and subchondral sclerosis. Diagnostic criteria and classification schemes have been based on different combinations of such radiologic features. But the findings in a study of men aged 60–75 years suggested that a single X-ray feature (minimal joint space) could be "the best radiologic criterion of the disease for epidemiologic studies." It is easy to use, and covaries with other X-ray findings. In addition, minimal joint space compared well with many other radiologic indexes as regards the agreement between classifications of the same X-rays made by different observers (between-observer variation) and by the same observer on different occasions (within-observer variation).

A. Between- and within-observer variation in the interpretation of X-rays are likely to bias relative risks towards RR = 1, unless there are observer differences between the exposed and unexposed. Such differences may introduce differential disease misclassification. How can this be avoided?

An important question is, of course, to what extent a certain radiologic criterion, or combination of criteria, identifies subjects who actually have the disease. There is, however, some uncertainty about how osteoarthritis of the hip should be defined in epidemiologic studies. To the extent that there is an interest in the etiology of a disease that causes human suffering, pain and disability are characteristics of osteoarthritis of the hip.

B. How could this be used in the evaluation of criteria such as minimal joint space?

As for many other diseases, it remains uncertain whether the concept "osteoarthritis of the hip" could include two or more conditions with differences in their etiology. If so, it would be useful to try to separate these conditions in epidemiologic studies.

C. How should this influence the choice of radiologic features to be examined in an epidemiologic study?

5:23 Common cold may be prevented by using an intranasal spray with alpha$_2$-interferon, as suggested by a study in Adelaide, Australia. The study subjects were kept unaware of whether they were exposed (using interferon spray) or unexposed (using placebo spray). During follow-up, they used a daily symptom diary to record any symptoms (runny nose; stopped-up nose; sore, scratchy throat; cough; hoarseness; chills; fever; muscle ache). Respiratory episodes were defined on the basis of these symptoms. The diaries were analyzed and computer-coded by staff members who were kept unaware of the subjects' exposure status (interferon or placebo spray). When respiratory symptoms developed, study subjects called a study nurse, who made a home visit to collect specimens for viral cultures and serologic analyses.

A. The study subjects were kept unaware of their own exposure status (interferon or placebo spray). In what way could this influence disease misclassification?

B. Staff members were kept unaware of the subjects' exposure status (interferon or placebo spray) when they analyzed and computer-coded the diaries. In what way could this influence disease misclassification?

5:24 The possibility that symptoms of heart disease could increase the risk of panic attacks was investigated as part of the National Institute of Mental Health Epidemiologic Catchment Area Program. An initial interview provided information on exposure (cardiac symptoms) and panic attacks, and 12,823 people who reported that they had never experienced a panic attack completed a follow-up interview 12 months later. According to the second interview, 383 subjects had experienced panic attacks since the time of first interview. Symptoms of heart disease were found to increase the risk of panic disorder, severe panic attacks, and other panic attacks. A subdivision was also made into panic attacks with cardiovascular symptoms (such as heart pounding, breathing difficulty, and chest pain) and panic attacks with psychologic symptoms. Although these categories were not mutually exclusive, the effect of cardiac symptoms appeared to be much stronger for panic attacks with cardiovascular symptoms (RR = 8.36; 3.70–18.89, 95% confidence interval) than for panic attacks with psychologic symptoms (RR = 2.23; 1.02–4.89). In what ways, if any, could these results be explained on the basis of misclassification?

5:25 A study on the occurrence and etiology of depression in subjects aged 18–44 was discussed in Chapter 3 (Exercise 3:18). In order to obtain information on exposures, as well as on current and past depression, all subjects selected for the study were invited to a first (baseline) interview. But 24 percent did not participate in this interview. One year later, the subjects were invited to a second (follow-up) interview, to obtain information on incident cases of depression since the time of the first interview. But 20 percent did not participate in the second interview.

When investigating the effects of certain exposures on the risk of first-time depression, all subjects originally selected for the study were eligible except those with a history of depression at the time of the first interview. But some of these subjects were lost to the study, because they did not participate in the first interview. In addition, some subjects were lost to follow-up because they did not participate in the second interview. As a possible source of bias, what is the principal difference between nonparticipation in the first (baseline) and second (follow-up) interview, respectively?

5:26 The possibility that a high alcohol intake could increase the risk of non-insulin-dependent diabetes, has been discussed. As part of a survey in California, subjects aged 40–79 years were examined with regard to diabetes, alcohol intake, and potential confounders (baseline examination). Those who did not have diabetes (by history or fasting hyperglycemia) at baseline were followed for more than 10 years to identify cases of non-insulin-dependent diabetes. The results could be presented as follows:

	Alcohol intake:	
	Exposed	*Unexposed*
Cases (Diabetes)	a	b
Person-years	C	D
Incidence rate (IR)	a/C	b/D

IR ratio $= a*D/b*C$

IR difference $= a/C - b/D$

In the present study, a considerable proportion of the subjects did not participate in the follow-up examinations. Loss to follow-up could bias the relative effect (IR ratio) and the absolute effect (IR difference).

A. If alcohol intake (but not diabetes) influenced the loss to follow-up, would this introduce a bias? (For example, suppose that 40% of the exposed and 10% of the unexposed were lost, regardless of whether or not they developed diabetes).

B. If diabetes (but not alcohol intake) influenced the loss to follow-up, would this introduce a bias? (For example, suppose that 40% of the cases and 10% of the person-years were lost, regardless of whether or not the subjects were exposed).

c. If diabetes and alcohol intake jointly influenced the loss to follow-up, would this introduce a bias? (For example, suppose that 40% of the exposed cases and 10% of the others were lost).

5:27   The effect of sexually transmitted human papillomavirus (HPV) infection on the risk of cervical cancer was investigated in a study dicussed in Chapter 4 (Exercise 4:10). A gynecological screening program in Sydney, Australia, identifed 1,107 women free from cervical cancer who had abnormal epithelial cells suggestive of HPV infection. These exposed women were asked to return repeatedly for follow-up examinations (Pap smears) to identify cases of cervical cancer (carcinoma in situ) during a 6-year period following the initial examination. However, 261 women did not return for any follow-up visits despite reminders. The remaining 846 women, returning for one or more follow-up visits, contributed a total of 3,448 women-years among the exposed. A total of 30 cases were identified in the exposed.

A. Among the exposed, how many woman-years were lost to follow-up?

B. Women could be more likely to return for follow-up visits if they developed minor bleedings from a cervical cancer. If so, in what direction would the relative risk be biased by the loss of exposed women to follow-up?

c. By how much could the loss of exposed women to follow-up, according to B (above), have biased the relative risk? (With the extreme assumption that the 30 identified cases were all cases that occurred in the 1,107 exposed women during the 6 years).

5:28   Selection bias may be present even if the observed occurrence of the exposure and disease are accurate, as illustrated by the following example. As part of the Framingham study, the effect of alcohol consumption on the risk of hip fracture was investigated. The 5,209 study subjects aged 28–62 years in 1948 were examined biennially. During the study period 1952–1985, information on alcohol intake from the most recent examination was used for exposure classification, and the follow-up of hip fractures was based on several sources (chart reviews, hospital record reviews, face-to-face interviews, and telephone interviews). For women aged < 65 years, the findings were as follows:

	Exposed (> 1 oz/week)	Unexposed (≤ 1 oz/week)	Total
Hip fractures	17	13	30
Person-years	11,565	26,000	37,565

Among these women in Framingham, the incidence rate of hip fracture was $30/37,565 = 8.0 * 10^{-4}$ per year, and the occurrence of the exposure was $11,565/37,565 = 30.8\%$. The relative risk was RR $= 17*26,000/13*11,565 = 2.94$

Suppose that no person-years (or hip fractures) were lost in this study. In another study, however, there could be a substantial loss to follow-up, for example, among alcohol-exposed subjects who suffered hip fractures. Imagine a study (with the same study population and study period) where 4,626 person-years including 11 cases among the exposed, and 10,400 person-years including one case among the unexposed, were lost to follow-up. What would the results of such a study have been, when estimating:

A. the incidence rate of hip fracture (true value: $8.0 * 10^{-4}$ per year)?

B. the occurrence of the exposure (true value: 30.8%)?

C. the relative risk of hip fracture (true value: 2.94)?

5:29 The follow-up of migrating study subjects may be both expensive and time consuming. In a community, 622 subjects were examined with regard to exposures of interest for a study of cardiovascular disease (baseline examination). In a follow-up four years later, 142 (23%) of these subjects could not be located at their original addresses. A standard tracing protocol was used, according to which the investigators "first attempted to trace participants through a contact person provided by the participant at baseline examination. Afterward, the names of participants who could not be found were sought through the state driver's license bureau. If this information was inadequate, calls were made to the last known place of employment and/or visits made to the participant's original home address." Current addresses were obtained through the contact person for 81 percent, and by adding the other steps of the protocol for a total of 96 percent of those who had moved.

A. For comparison, a commercial firm was used to trace the same 142 subjects. In what respects should comparisons be made between different strategies used to trace subjects?

B. The commercial firm provided current addresses for 58 percent of those who had moved within the same area, but only for 10 percent of those who had moved outside the initial study area. What is the principal advantage and disadvantage, respectively, of restricting the study to subjects who had not moved outside this area?

5:30   A total of 51,672 male health professionals aged 40–75 years answered a six-page questionnaire regarding their medical history, current diet, and life-style habits. Two years later, a mail questionnaire was used for a first follow-up of disease occurrence. After up to three mailings by nonprofit bulk mail, there were still 12,233 nonrespondents. These were included in an experimental study, designed to evaluate six different mailing methods aimed at reducing nonresponse to follow-up. Certified mail gave the highest response among initial nonrespondents, 63.2 percent after one and 79.5 percent after two mailings. Questionnaires sent by certified mail were more than twice as likely to be completed and returned as questionnaires in standard window envelopes sent first class mail. In addition, hand-addressed envelopes were found to increase response. After a third mailing, the final overall follow-up was 95.7 percent. What factors, other than the questionnaire and mailing strategies, may have contributed to the high response?

■■■ **GENERAL QUESTIONS**

5:31   What aspects should be considered when defining the disease under study? Exemplify!

5:32   What is the difference between incident and prevalent cases of disease? Exemplify!

5:33   Among people with mild or moderate symptoms of disease, some may and others may not seek medical advice. In what circumstances could this introduce a bias? Exemplify!

5:34   Differential disease misclassification may be due to differences between the exposed and unexposed in the frequency of medical examinations. What can be done to avoid or assess this source of bias? Exemplify!

5:35 Differential disease misclassification may be introduced if the physician (examiner) tends to examine or diagnose exposed and unexposed subjects differently. In what ways can this source of bias be avoided? Exemplify!

5:36 Differential disease misclassification may be introduced if exposed and unexposed subjects differ in their reporting of symptoms or disease. In what ways can this source of bias be avoided? Exemplify!

5:37 In screening programs, and at routine examinations in medical care, cases of many diseases are being detected (and subsequently treated) at an early asymptomatic stage. What problems and possibilities does this introduce with regard to study design and validity? Exemplify!

5:38 What are the possible advantages and disadvantages, respectively, of using morbidity and mortality registers to identify cases? Exemplify!

5:39 How can the study results be biased by loss to follow-up of disease occurrence? Exemplify!

5:40 Consider your own recent favorite study. What are the implications for that study of the general problems and possibilities exemplified in the different exercises in this chapter?

6 Sampling from the Base (Case-Referent Strategies)

INTRODUCTION

Purpose and Principles

Usually a large study population has to be followed over a considerable period of time in order to obtain the number of cases required for acceptable precision. It may be very costly to obtain information on exposures (including potential confounders) from all subjects in a large study population. But if the study size is reduced, in order to reduce the costs, precision may not be sufficient. The relation between precision and cost, that is, the *cost-efficiency* of a study, may be improved considerably by using a sample that reflects the occurrence of the exposure in the study base or study population.

In a study where the comparison is based on incidence rates, the results may be presented as in Table 6–1A (cf. Table 1–2A). The relative risk (IR ratio) is calculated using exposure information for the cases (a, b) and the person-time in the study base (C, D). The information needed for the study base is the relative size of the unexposed and exposed part, that is D/C. But D/C may be estimated using a representative sample of the study base. This sample should be representative in the sense that it should reflect the occurrence of the exposure in the study base, that is $d/c = D/C$, where c is the size of the exposed part of the sample, and d is the size of the unexposed part of the sample. If so, *RR = a∗d/b∗c using information only from the cases and the base sample*. The subjects in the base sample are referred to as *referents* (or *controls*), and the study is called a *case-referent study* (or *case-control study*). The results from a case-referent study may be presented as in Table 6–1B.

Table 6–1   Tables of results (incidence rate).

A. Not using referents (cf. Table 1–2A):

	Exposed	Unexposed
Cases	a	b
Person-time	C	D

$$RR = \frac{a*D}{b*C}$$

B. Using referents ("case-referent study"):

	Exposed	Unexposed
Cases	a	b
Referents	c	d

$$RR = \frac{a*d}{b*c}$$ (provided that $d/c = D/C$, i.e. that the referents reflect the occurence of the exposure in the study base).

In studies based on *incidence rates*, the referents should reflect the occurrence of the exposure in the *study base*, that is, the total person-time experience that generated the cases (as above). In studies based on *incidence proportions*, the referents should reflect the occurrence of the exposure in the *study population* (i.e., all subjects at risk at the beginning of follow-up). Similarly, when the comparison is based on *prevalence proportions*, the referents should reflect the occurrence of the exposure in the *study population* (i.e., all subjects examined for the presence of disease). Thus, the referents should be representative of the study population in the sense that $d'/c' = D'/C'$ where c' and d' are the numbers of exposed and unexposed referents, and C' and D' are the numbers of exposed and unexposed subjects in the study population (cf. Table 1–2B). If so, $RR = a'*d'/b'*c'$ using exposure information for the cases and referents. Sometimes the referents are selected as a representative sample of the *noncases* that is, $d'/c' = (D'-b')/(C'-a')$, and the *odds ratio* is $OR = a'*d'/b'*c'$. When the study population is large in relation to the number of cases ("rare disease assumption"), that is, when $(D'-b')$ is approximately equal to D' and $(C'-a')$ is approximately equal to C', the odds ratio may be used as an estimate of the relative risk.

Sampling

The referents should reflect the occurrence of the exposure in the study base or study population (i.e., the appropriate denominator for all cases in a study, referred to here simply as the *"base"*). Referents may be selected as a *random sample* of the base. The principal advantage of this approach is that the sample will give an unbiased estimate of the occurrence of the exposure in the base. Thus, no *sampling bias (referent selection bias)* is introduced. A necessary prerequisite is, of course, that the base is available for random sampling.

Referents are sometimes selected as a *non-random sample* of the base. The purpose may be to improve the comparability of exposure information between cases and referents, that is, to reduce differential exposure misclassification. For example, in studies of specific congenital malformations, infants with other malformations have sometimes been used as referents in an effort to avoid a possible recall bias. Another purpose may be to make the collection of exposure information from the referents more convenient, and perhaps also to reduce nonresponse among the referents. Potential advantages of this approach must, however, be weighed against the possibility of a referent selection bias that is introduced if the sample does not reflect the occurrence of the exposure in the base.

Many case-referent studies are initiated by a defined case-series, such as all subjects diagnosed with the disease under study at a certain hospital during the study period. This is often convenient and reduces the cost of follow-up of disease occurrence. But the cases may or may not represent all cases of the disease that occurred during the study period in a certain population, for example, among people living in the catchment area of the hospital. The hospital may not even serve a well-defined population. Still, the study population is the population that generated the cases (cf. Chapter 1). In principle, the study base may be defined secondary to the cases as "the person-time experience of people who would have been diagnosed at the hospital during the study period if they had developed the disease under study." In order to avoid a referent selection bias, the referents should reflect the occurrence of the exposure in the base. Referents may be selected among other subjects admitted to the same hospital during the study period (hospital referents). This approach is convenient and reduces the cost of identifying and examining referents. Several strategies may be used to avoid a referent selection bias when selecting hospital referents.

Sample Size and Sampling Fraction

Precision increases with the *sample size*, that is, the number of referents. But as the number of referents becomes large in relation to the number of cases, precision is limited by the number of cases rather than by the number of referents. With a certain number of cases, a *maximum precision* is approached by increasing the number of referents. The proportion of the maximum precision that is reached in any particular study is approximately $r/(r + 1)$, where r is the number of referents divided by the number of cases. Thus, if the number of referents is equal to the number of cases ($r = 1$), precision will be about $1/(1 + 1) = 0.50$, or 50 percent of the highest possible (with that number of cases). If the number of referents is four times the number of cases ($r = 4$), the study will yield about $4/(4 + 1) = 0.80$ or 80 percent of the maximum precision. As the number of referents is further increased, the additional gain in precision becomes increasingly marginal. But the total cost for obtaining exposure information usually continues to rise with an increasing number of referents. Depending upon the costs involved, the highest *cost-efficiency* is often obtained when the number of referents is one to four times the number of cases. (This applies within each stratum in a stratified data analysis. Thus, overall there should sometimes be more than four times as many referents as cases).

The *sampling fraction* is the number of referents (the sample size) divided by the number of person-years in the study base, or the number of subjects in the study population, that is represented by the referents. When the sampling fraction is known, not only the relative effect (relative risk) but also the *absolute effect* (e.g., rate difference) can be estimated in a case-referent study.

Matching Referents to the Cases

Sometimes referents are matched to the cases with regard to one or more potential confounders. One possibility is *individual matching*: For each case, a referent is selected as the subject most similar to the case in respect of one or more potential confounders (e.g., age). Individual matching may include one referent for each case (matched pairs), or two or more referents for each case. Another possibility is *frequency matching*: The study base (or study population) is divided into strata of one or more potential confounders, for example, different age groups. In each stratum (age group) a number of referents is selected in relation to the (expected) number of cases, in order to obtain a similar proportion of the referents and cases in each stratum.

The purpose of matching is to improve *efficiency*, rather than to control confounding (which may be achieved in the data analysis regardless of matching). Efficiency may be improved if there is a strong association between the matching factor (e.g., age) and the disease under study. Otherwise matching may reduce efficiency (so called overmatching).

Matching introduces some potential problems and limitations in a study. A bias is introduced because matched referents do not reflect the occurrence of the exposure in the study base (or study population), but rather a distortion according to the distribution of the cases. In principle, this bias may be removed in a matched data analysis. But in practice, individual matching may virtually double the number of subjects lost due to nonresponse (since pairs are analyzed together), or introduce bias because pairs are not analyzed together or because referents that have been lost are replaced by others (who may be different with regard to exposure). Whenever matching is used, the study cannot be utilized to investigate how the risk of disease is influenced by a factor on which subjects have been matched. When two or more diseases are being studied, individual matching means that new referents have to be matched to the cases of each disease, whereas the same unmatched referents may be used for cases of different diseases. Thus, there are several reasons for showing restraint with matching in the selection of referents.

Other Aspects

Referents are selected with the purpose of reducing the number of subjects that have to be examined in respect of exposures, and thus reduce costs and improve cost-efficiency. Exposure information is obtained by collecting primary information (e.g., blood specimens, questionnaire responses), and processing this information (e.g., by analyzing blood specimens or questionnaire responses and transferring the information to a medium suitable for data analysis). In many studies, both steps are limited to cases and referents. But in some case-referent studies, the primary information is obtained for all subjects in the study population (prior to follow-up) but the information is processed only for the cases and referents (after the cases have been identified). The purpose is to avoid differential exposure misclassification in the first step (cf. Chapter 4), and to reduce the costs in the second step (where differential exposure misclassification may be avoided, e.g., by blinding).

In some studies, more detailed and costly exposure information is collected only for the cases and referents (after the cases have been identified), while less detailed and costly information on the same exposure is obtained for all subjects in the study population (prior to follow-up). Sometimes, information on certain exposures (confounders, modifiers) is collected only for the cases and referents (after the cases have been identified) while information on others is obtained for all study subjects (prior to follow-up).

The gain in cost-efficiency by using exposure information from the cases and referents, rather than from all subjects in the study population, increases when the occurrence of the disease is low and when the cost for obtaining exposure information is high. When the cost is low or negligible, or when a large proportion of the study population are cases, there may be no point in selecting referents, since this may not improve cost-efficiency. However, referents are useful in obtaining information on current exposure in the study base, and in obtaining exposure information for a study base where people enter and leave during the study period (such as the person-time experience of the population in a town with people moving in and out, sometimes referred to as an "open" or "dynamic" population). The cost-efficiency of a study can sometimes be further increased by utilizing the same referents when studying two or more diseases within the same study base.

▬ EXERCISES

6:1 The effect of cigarette smoking on the risk of breast cancer in women aged 40–59 years was investigated in the Canadian National Breast Screening Study. When attending the screening, each woman completed a self-administered questionnaire on smoking and potential confounders. Of 59,781 women who underwent their initial screening between September, 1982 and March, 1985, 254 were found to have breast cancer at the first visit ("prevalent cases"). Among women who did not have breast cancer at their first visit, 317 developed a breast cancer that was identified at a subsequent screening visit ("incident cases"). The effect of cigarette smoking was investigated separately in one study based on prevalent cases, and another study based on incident cases of breast cancer.

A. What is the appropriate denominator for the prevalent and incident cases, respectively?

Two series of referents were selected, one in the study based on prevalent cases and another in the study based on incident cases.

B. How should the referents be selected in each of the two studies?

In the present study the number of selected referents was three times the number of identified cases ($r = 3$). Results were based on exposure information from cases and referents only. Consider the alternative of using exposure information from the entire study population.

C. What is the purpose of selecting referents, rather than using information from the entire study population?

D. How is precision influenced by selecting referents, rather than using information from the entire study population?

E. What sources of bias are introduced by selecting referents, rather than using information from the entire study population?

6:2 The possibility that low serum vitamin E levels could increase the risk of certain cancers was investigated in Finland, among 15,093 women initially free from cancer. A blood sample was drawn from each woman and serum was kept frozen at $-20°C$. Cancers diagnosed among these women during follow-up were identified by record linkage to a national cancer register. A total of 356 cases were identified, and twice as many referents were selected. For each case and each referent, a serum sample was thawed and analyzed for vitamin E. Relative risks were estimated, using exposure information from the cases and referents.

A. Consider possible sources of bias. In what ways, if any, does the present study differ from a study where the serum samples of all 15,093 women are analyzed for vitamin E?

B. Consider precision and cost. How does the present study differ from a study where the serum samples of all 15,093 women are analyzed for vitamin E? (Suppose that the analysis of each serum sample cost 50 USD).

C. In the present study, twice as many referents as cases were selected, that is $r = 2$. However, it may be useful to consider precision and cost for different sample sizes. Calculate the percentage of the maximum precision, and the total cost for analyzing vitamin E, for the following alternatives: $r = 1$, $r = 2$, $r = 4$, $r = 8$, and $r = 16$. Present the results in a table.

6:3 Five different methods for obtaining information on occupational exposures were compared in a study mentioned in Chapter 4 (Exercise 4:26). Costs were lowest for method 1 (job titles abstracted from routine records), and highest for method 5 (job descriptions obtained by interview and processed by a team of experts to derive exposure data). The cost per subject was $13.75–125 for method 1, and $325–600 for method 5, depending upon the number of subjects examined. Suppose that one of these two methods was to be selected for use in a study with 16,000 study subjects. The cost of obtaining exposure information for all study subjects would be $13.75 * 16,000 = 220,000$ using method 1, and $325 * 16,000 = 5,200,000$ using method 5. In order to improve cost-efficiency, consider the possibility of collecting exposure information only for the cases and a similar number of referents ($r = 1$) using either method 1 (at a cost of $125 per subject) or method 5 (at a cost of $600 per subject).

A. Suppose that, when studying a disease with low incidence, 80 cases would occur in the study population during follow-up. What is the total cost of obtaining exposure information in the case-referent study when using method 1 and 5, respectively?

B. Suppose that, when studying a disease with high incidence, 800 cases would occur in the study population during follow-up. What is the total cost of obtaining exposure information in the case-referent study when using method 1 and 5, respectively?

C. For each alternative (in A and B, above), how much is the cost of obtaining exposure information reduced by using referents? How much is the precision reduced, in relation to the maximum precision in a study with that number of cases?

D. How is the gain in cost-efficiency (by using referents) influenced by the occurrence of the disease?

E. How is the gain in cost-efficiency (by using referents) influenced by the cost per subject for obtaining exposure information?

6:4 When studying the effect of short-acting sedatives on the risk of accidents resulting in hip fractures among elderly people (cf. Exercise 4:9), subjects may be classified as exposed or unexposed depending upon whether or not they have a prescription. But since these drugs are often used occasionally and the exposure of interest is recent intake, this is likely to introduce considerable non-differential exposure misclassification. Many cases classified as exposed because they had a prescription may not have taken the drug at the time of the accident. But information on recent drug intake at the time of the accident, obtained from the cases when they enter the hospital, cannot be used unless similar information is available for the study base (since this is likely to bias the relative risk towards $RR = 0$ due to differential exposure misclassification, cf. Exercise 4:9). How should information on recent drug intake be obtained for the study base? In what way, if any, could referents be used to provide this information?

6:5 A study of diet and colon cancer was conducted in an adult population of about 1 million residents in Stockholm, Sweden. During the study period, people were moving into and out of the Stockholm area. People were included in the study (follow-up) during any part of the study period when they lived in Stockholm. (Such populations, with people entering and leaving during the study period, are sometimes referred to as "open" or "dynamic" populations.) Efforts were made to identify all cases of colon cancer that occurred in this population during follow-up.

A. As the cases were identified, they were interviewed about their dietary habits in the past. Similar information is required for the study base. How could referents be used to provide this information?

B. The relative effect (IR ratio) is estimated using exposure information for cases and referents. What additional information is needed to estimate the absolute effect (IR difference)?

6:6   The effect of oral contraceptive use on the risk of breast, endometrial, and ovarian cancer was investigated in the Cancer and Steroid Hormone Study. The study population was women aged 20–54 who resided in eight geographic locations in the United States during the study period. Attempts were made to identify all incident cases of breast, ovarian, and endometrial cancer that occurred in the study population during the study period. Referents were selected by random digit dialing of households in the eight geographic locations during the study period. A random sample of household telephone numbers were called, information on household members was requested, and referents were selected among women aged 20–54 according to strict rules. Are there any potential sources of referent selection bias and if so, how could these sources of bias be avoided?

6:7   A study of the effect of using sunbeds and sunlamps on the risk of malignant melanoma of the skin was mentioned in Chapter 4 (Exercise 4:19). The study population was subjects aged 20–69 years (with no history of melanoma) living in six counties in Southertn Ontario, Canada. Efforts were made to identify all cases of malignant melanoma of the skin that occurred in the study population during the study period. Referents were selected from the study population during the study period, as a random sample of people listed in the property tax assessment rolls for the 39 municipalities in the study area.

A. Could there be a referent selection bias and if so, what can be done to avoid such bias?

Exposure information was obtained by interviewing cases and referents. The possibility of recall bias was discussed, since the interviews were conducted only after the cases had been identified and the cases could be aware of a possible association between the use of sunbeds and sunlamps and their own disease. In the interviews, efforts were made to avoid and assess any recall bias (cf. Exercise 4:19). In addition, another series of referents was selected from the study population during the study period: patients who for the first time attended the clinic where the cases were identified, "having a suspicious pigmented lesion needing a skin biopsy" but who were found not to have melanoma.

B. How is the possibility of recall bias influenced by using these referents?

C. How is the possibility of referent selection bias influenced by using these referents?

6:8   The possibility that a high vitamin intake around the time of conception could reduce a woman's risk of having a child with a neural-tube defect was investigated (cf. Exercise 4:29). The cases were infants born with a neural-tube defect in a study population of newborn infants. Two series of referents were selected: one among nonmalformed infants, and the other among infants born with other major malformations, in the study population. Exposure information was obtained by telephone interviews with case and referent mothers. The exposed were babies to mothers who reported a high vitamin intake around the time of conception.

A. What is the difference between the two series of referents, with regard to possible referent selection bias?

B. What is the difference between the two series of referents, with regard to possible recall bias?

C. Suppose that a high vitamin intake was found to reduce the risk of having a child with a neural-tube defect when using the nonmalformed referents, but not when using the malformed referents. How would you interpret these results? (For simplicity, consider only two potentially important sources of error: referent selection bias and recall bias.)

D. Suppose that a high vitamin intake was found to reduce the risk of having a child with a neural-tube defect when using the malformed referents, but not when using the nonmalformed referents. How would you interpret these results? (For simplicity, consider only two potentially important sources of error: referent selection bias and recall bias.)

6:9 A study was done to evaluate the effects of several exposures, including naevi (pigment patches in the skin), on the risk of malignant melanoma of the skin. During a 3-year period, efforts were made to identify all cases of malignant melanoma of the skin that occurred among subjects aged 20–79 years living in a defined area in England. During the same period, referents were selected as a random sample of subjects of the same ages living in the same area, who had "any inpatient or outpatient attendance at any of the hospitals used by the cases, and who were therefore recorded on the Patient Master Index of the hospital."

A. Could there be any referent selection bias? Why/why not?

B. Suppose that the referents had been sampled from a list of hospital attendances (rather than from a list of subjects with any hospital attendance). How would this influence the possibility of referent selection bias?

6:10 The possibility that a drug used in the treatment of asthma increases the risk of death in asthma patients aged 5–45 was investigated in two studies mentioned in Chapter 4 (Exercise 4:14). In the second of these studies, the cases were "all patients aged 5–45 years who died from asthma in New Zealand during the period January, 1977—July, 1981, and who had been admitted for athma to a major hospital during the 12 months before death." Referents were selected at random among patients discharged from these hospitals during the study period who "had a previous hospital admission for asthma during the 12 months before the admission under consideration." For both cases and referents, exposure was assessed on the basis of the drug prescriptions documented in the hospital record relating to the previous admission.

A. Could there be any referent selection bias? Why/why not?

B. Assessment of exposure was done only after the cases had been identified. Could this introduce a differential exposure misclassification? Why/why not?

6:11 Tobacco, alcohol, and dietary factors were among the exposures of interest in a study of kidney cancer. The study population was subjects aged 30–85 years who resided in the Minneapolis—St. Paul Standard Metropolitan Statistical Area during the study period. Efforts were made to identify all cases that occurred in the study population during the study period. Exposure information for cases and referents was obtained by interview. However, many cases had died before they could be interviewed and exposure information for dead cases was obtained from surrogate respondents.

A. Should dead referents be selected for dead cases? Why/ why not?

In the study, a series of living referents were selected from the study base and a series of dead referents were selected at random from all deaths (except kidney cancers) that occurred in the study base. Several exposures, including smoking, intake of certain drugs and alcoholic beverages, and adulthood diseases, were reported more frequently for dead referents than for living referents.

B. What conclusions can be drawn from this?

Consider the possibility of conducting a study where only the living cases (and living referents) are included.

C. Would this improve the validity of the results? Why/why not?

6:12 A study of alcohol consumption and cancer of the sigmoid colon included about 122,000 men and 143,000 women (cf. Exercise 3:12). A total of 91 cases (43 men, 48 women) were identified during follow-up. In the study population, about 61 percent of the men and 7 percent of the women had a high or moderate intake of alcohol. When these subjects were considered as exposed, and those with little or no alcohol intake as unexposed, the relative risk was approximately RR = 4. Suppose that this effect was similar among men and women:

Men:

	Exposed	*Unexposed*	*Total*
Cases	37	6	43
Study population	74,000	48,000	122,000
	RR = 4.0		

Women:

	Exposed	*Unexposed*	*Total*
Cases	11	37	48
Study population	9,893	133,107	143,000
	RR = 4.0		

Sex is a confounder, since sex is associated with the exposure (almost 61% of the men, but only 7% of the women, are exposed) and with the risk of disease among the unexposed (incidence proportion: $6/48,000 = 13*10^{-5}$ in men, and $37/133,107 = 28*10^{-5}$ in women). When the relative risk is calculated separately for men and women (as above) there is, of course, no confounding by sex. But the confounding effect would be obvious, if the relative risk was calculated for men and women together.

A. Calculate the relative risk for men and women together (without adjustment for sex).

The study population is large in relation to the number of cases. Suppose that referents were selected, matched to the cases by sex. Selecting three times as many referents as cases ($r = 3$), would give $3*43 = 129$ male, and $3*48 = 144$ female, referents. These referents should reflect the occurrence of the exposure in the study population, among men (almost 61% exposed of $129 = 78$ exposed referents) and women (7% exposed of $144 = 10$ exposed referents):

Men:

	Exposed	Unexposed	Total
Cases	37	6	43
Referents	78	51	129

$$RR = 4.0$$

Women:

	Exposed	Unexposed	Total
Cases	11	37	48
Referents	10	134	144

$$RR = 4.0$$

When the relative risk is calculated separately for men and women (as above) there is, of course, no confounding by sex. The referents are matched to the cases by sex, and reflect the occurrence of the exposure among men and women, respectively, in the study population.

B. Calculate the relative risk for men and women together (without adjustment for sex), using the data for cases and matched referents.

C. Is confounding by sex controlled by matching referents to the cases on sex?

D. What is the purpose of matching referents to the cases on a confounder like sex, age, or residence? In what circumstances can this purpose be achieved?

6:13   In the previous study (Exercise 6:12), the occurrence of the disease was different in unexposed men and women. Suppose that the study was done in another population where the occurrence of the disease is similar in unexposed men and women:

Men:

	Exposed	Unexposed	Total
Cases	81	13	94
Study population	74,000	48,000	122,000

RR = 4.0

Women:

	Exposed	Unexposed	Total
Cases	11	37	48
Study population	9,893	133,107	143,000

RR = 4.0

These tables are identical to the first two tables in Exercise 6:12, except that the number of cases is increased among men (so that the occurrence of the disease is similar in unexposed men and women).

A. Calculate the relative risk for men and women together (without adjustment for sex).

As in the previous exercise suppose that, for every case, three sex-matched referents were selected to reflect the occurrence of the exposure among men and women, respectively, in the study population:

Men:

	Exposed	Unexposed	Total
Cases	81	13	94
Referents	171	111	282

RR = 4.0

Women:

	Exposed	*Unexposed*	*Total*
Cases	11	37	48
Referents	10	134	144

$$RR = 4.0$$

B. Calculate the relative risk for men and women together (without adjustment for sex), using the data for cases and matched referents.

C. What conclusion can be drawn, when comparing the answers to (A) and (B)?

6:14 The effect of alcohol intake on the risk of hip fracture was investigated (cf. Exercise 5:28). During 117,224 person-years of follow-up, a total of 217 cases were identified. Their age distribution is shown in the table. Suppose that 200 cases were anticipated and that an equal number of referents were selected as a random sample of the study base. These unmatched referents would have an age distribution similar to that of the study base:

	Age (years):			
	<65	65–74	≥75	Total
Cases	41	62	114	217
Referents:				
unmatched	140	48	12	200
age-matched	38	57	105	200

If there is confounding by age, cases and referents in each age group are analyzed together to control confounding. In the age group ≥ 75 years, there are 114 cases but only 12 referents and precision is limited by the small number of referents. With a further subdivision according to sex or other confounders, there may be some strata with no exposed (or no unexposed) referents, resulting in loss of information in the data analysis.

One way of handling this problem is to increase the number of unmatched referents, selected at random from the study base. In order to obtain a similar number of referents as cases ($r = 1$) in the age group ≥ 75 years, the total number of referents would have to be increased about ten times (from 200 to about 2,000) in the present study.

Another way of handling the problem is to select age-matched referents, for example, as a random sample of the study base within each age group (frequency matching by age). A total of 200 referents selected in this way would have an age distribution similar to that of the cases (see table). This would increase the number of referents in the age group $\geq$ 75 years without increasing the total number of referents. (In addition, precision could be further improved by increasing the number of referents to, e.g., 400.)

How is the choice between these two alternatives influenced by:

A. the strength of the association between age and hip fracture?
B. the cost of identifying additional referents and obtaining information on their exposure and potential confounders?

6:15 In a study of sudden infant death syndrome (SIDS), 193 cases were identified among 53,721 infants who were born alive and survived the neonatal period (cf. Exercise 3:10). The exposures of interest included previous pregnancies and certain gestational factors. In addition, several sociodemographic variables were expected to be associated with SIDS, including maternal age, race, income, education, and marital status. In order to improve efficiency, referents were selected to provide information on the occurrence of exposures in the study population. Referents may be selected as a random sample of the study population. Another possibility is individual matching where, for each SIDS case, a referent is selected with the same maternal age, race, income, and so on, as the case. What potential problems and limitations are introduced by individual matching (except for any overmatching)?

6:16 Some epidemiological findings suggest that alcohol consumption might increase the risk of breast cancer in women. In addition, descriptive epidemiological data indicate that there are differences in etiology between pre- and postmenopausal breast cancer. The effect of alcohol intake on the risk of breast cancer was investigated in The Netherlands. Caucasian women of Dutch nationality were included in the study during any part of the study period when they were aged 25–44 or 55–64 years and lived in the catchment areas of 17 hospitals. During the study period, 168 cases of breast cancer in women of these ages were diagnosed at these hospitals. In addition, 548 referents were sampled from the municipal population register for the catchment area of the hospitals.

The study base may be defined as the person-time experience of caucasian women of Dutch nationality aged 25–44 or 55–64 years, included in the municipal population register for the catchment area of the 17 hospitals, during the study period. If the referents were selected as a random sample of this study base, no referent selection bias is introduced.

A. Suppose that some of the women identified as cases were not listed in the municipal population register. Should these cases be included in the study?

B. Suppose that some cases of breast cancer that occurred in women living in the catchment area of the 17 hospitals were diagnosed at a private clinic outside these hospitals. Should these cases be included in the study?

6:17 Certain anti-inflammatory drugs (NSAID) may increase the risk of perforated peptic ulcer. This was investigated in England, at a hospital that "provides all the acute services for a population of 300,000." During the study period, a total of 269 patients were admitted with perforated peptic ulcers. Suppose that these were all incident cases of perforated peptic ulcer that occurred in the 300,000 population during the study period.

A. Define the study base.

B. Referents were selected at random from among patients admitted as surgical emergencies to the same hospital during the same period. Could there be a referent selection bias? Why/why not?

6:18 Age-related cataract is a common cause of visual loss in elderly people. A study of its etiology was conducted in Parma, Italy. The cases were all subjects aged 45–79 years who, during a 2-year period, had an age-related cataract in at least one eye diagnosed at three ophthalmic clinics providing "outpatient care for nearly the entire population of the metropolitan Parma area." Suppose that these clinics identified all cases that were diagnosed in this population during the study period. But all incident cases of cataract may not have been diagnosed. Age-related cataract has a gradual onset and may only cause slight or moderate visual loss in one eye, symptoms for which elderly people may or may not see an ophthalmologist. The relative risk is biased if the exposure is associated with people's tendency to see an ophthalmologist and have their cataract diagnosed (cf. Chapter 5). Against this background, consider the following two alternatives:

1. The study base is defined as the person-time experience of subjects aged 45–79 years and living in Parma during the study period. Referents are selected as a random sample of the study base, for example, from a continuously updated population register.

2. The study base is defined as the person-time experience of subjects (aged 45–79 years and living in Parma during the study period), who would see an ophthalmologist if they experienced symptoms like those of cataract. Referents are selected among subjects who seek advice for other conditions giving rise to similar symptoms.

A. Could any bias introduced by failure to identify all incident cases of cataract (in alternative 1), be avoided by defining the study base, and selecting the referents, according to alternative 2?

B. What other consequences should be taken into account before deciding whether to select referents according to alternative 1 or 2?

6:19   Hip fractures will almost invariably come to medical attention and diagnosis. The effect of estrogen replacement therapy on the risk of hip fracture in postmenopausal women was investigated at four hospitals in Connecticut. The cases were all women aged 45–74 years who, during the study period, were admitted to these hospitals for hip fracture.

A. How should the study base be defined? (Suppose that the hospitals did not serve a geographically or otherwise defined population, but rather admitted patients on the basis of complex preferences and socioeconomic factors).

The referents were women aged 45–74 years who, during the study period, were admitted for trauma to the inpatient surgical services of the same hospitals as the cases.

B. What are the potential sources of referent selection bias?

6:20   A classic study of cigarette smoking and lung cancer was conducted in England in 1948–1952. The cases were 1,488 patients admitted for lung cancer to the participating hospitals. A similar number of referents were selected among patients who, during the study period, were admitted to the same hospitals for other diseases (except diseases suggested to be related to smoking). About 70 percent of the cases were identified at hospitals in London, and over 90 percent were men. In London, the smoking habits of the hospital referents were compared with those of people in a random sample of all residents. These comparisons showed that, among men of similar ages, smoking was more common in the hospital referents than in the population sample. As suggested by the investigators, this could be explained by previously unknown associations between smoking and several diseases.

A. Suggest another possible explanation for a difference in smoking habits between patients admitted to a hospital and the residents of the catchment area.

Among men of similar ages, the percentage of nonsmokers was 7.0 percent in the hospital referents and 12.1 percent in the population sample. The percentage smoking at least 25 cigarettes per day was 13.4 percent in the hospital referents and 8.5 percent in the population sample.

B. For a disease that appears to be unrelated to smoking (RR = 1) when using the hospital referents, what would the relative risk be when using the population sample?

A similar study of cigarette smoking and lung cancer in women was conducted in the United States in 1955–1957. Hospital referents were selected among patients admitted for a variety of diseases "reflecting the experience encountered in surgical and medical services." The proportion of smokers among these referents was found to be similar to that of female hospital referents in other studies, but higher than among women in a general population sample. This difference persisted when patients with coronary and respiratory diseases were excluded. Among women aged 45–54 years, for example, the percentage who never smoked was 57 percent in the hospital referents and 69 percent in the population sample. The percent "current, regular cigarette smokers" was 35 percent in the hospital referents and 23 percent in the population sample.

C. For a disease that appears to be unrelated to smoking (RR = 1) when using the hospital referents, what would the relative risk be when using the population sample?

6:21 Possible effects of drinking water composition on the risk of myocardial infarction (MI) in middle-aged men were investigated in Finland. The cases were "all male patients aged 30–64 years who were discharged (alive or dead) from Kotka Central Hospital after their first myocardial infarction." Hospital referents were selected "among male patients discharged with a surgical diagnosis" from the same hospital during the same period. In addition, another series of referents were selected "from the population register for persons living in Kotka Central Hospital district." Samples of drinking water were collected from the homes of cases and referents, and analyzed in the laboratory.

Very low fluoride concentration in drinking water (< 0.1 ppm) was found to increase the risk of MI considerably when using the referents selected from the population register (RR = 4), but to a lesser degree when using the hospital referents (RR = 2). Name two possible explanations for a difference in exposure (fluoride in drinking water) between patients hospitalized for surgical conditions (the source of the hospital referents) and subjects living in the catchment area of the hospital.

6:22 In a study of the effect of coffee consumption on the risk of myocardial infarction in women aged 30–49 years, referents were selected among patients who, during the study period, were admitted to the same hospitals as the cases. Of 6,815 women hospitalized for "conditions not known to be caused or prevented by coffee use," 980 were admitted for "conditions that usually have a rapid onset and require urgent admission to hospital" (acute condition referents). Most of the remaining 5,835 women "had been hospitalized, often electively, for chronic illnesses" (chronic condition referents).

Coffee intake was less common in the chronic condition referents than in the acute condition referents. As suggested by the investigators, long-standing illness may reduce the intake of coffee. The proportion of coffee drinkers was found to decrease with increasing number of reported visits to a physician or clinic within the preceding year, both among the chronic condition referents (who had more visits) and among the acute condition referents.

A. Which referents would give the highest relative risk?

Among the chronic condition referents, 42 percent did not drink coffee and 15 percent consumed ≥ 5 cups of caffeine-containing coffee per day. Among the acute condition referents, the corresponding percentages were 35 percent and 19 percent, respectively.

    B. Suppose that no effect was found when using the acute condition referents (RR = 1). What would the relative risk be, when using the chronic condition referents?

    C. Should hospital referents be selected among patients admitted for chronic conditions, among patients admitted for acute conditions, or as a representative sample of all patients admitted to the same hospitals as the cases during the study period?

6:23   Several exposures were investigated in a study of cervical cancer in women aged 20–79 in Utah. During the study period, cases were identified through a population-based cancer incidence registry covering the state, and referents were selected as a random sample of residents of the state.

    In addition, a separate analysis was based on a subset of the cases: those diagnosed at two large metropolitan hospitals. For this analysis, hospital referents were selected at random among patients admitted to the gynecological services of the same hospitals as the cases (except for gynecological cancers and elective abortions).

    For 10 out of 11 studied exposures, a higher proportion was exposed in the hospital referents than in referents selected among residents. Adjusted relative risks in the analysis based on all cases and referents selected among residents (and the corresponding result based on the cases and referents identified at the two hospitals) were as follows: age ≤ 16 at first intercourse RR = 2.3 (RR = 1.1), age ≤ 17 at first marriage RR = 1.6 (RR = 1.0), age ≤ 17 at first pregnancy RR = 2.8 (RR = 1.1), number (≥ 2) of sexual partners RR = 4.8 (RR = 1.8), number (≥ 2) of marriages RR = 4.1 (RR = 1.4), marital status (separated or divorced) RR = 3.8 (RR = 1.2), current smoking RR = 4.8 (RR = 2.4), treated for venereal disease RR = 1.9 (RR = 1.3), husband treated for venereal disease RR = 3.0 (RR = 2.7), previous vaginal infections RR = 1.6 (RR = 0.5), birth control pills (ever used) RR = 1.3 (RR = 1.3).

    A. How could the differences in results be explained?

    B. Which results should be considered more valid?

6:24   Oral contraceptive use was found to reduce the risk of epithelial ovarian cancer by about 25 percent (RR = 0.75) in a WHO collaborative study. Cases were included if they had been identified at one of the participating hospitals during the study period, were of certain ages and had been residents of the area served by the hospital for at least 1 year. Referents were selected among women admitted to the same hospitals during the same period, with the same restrictions on age and residence.

A. What is the purpose of the referents?

B. Women admitted to obstetric or gynecological wards were not selected as referents. Why?

C. When selecting hospital referents, should other restrictions be made because of possible associations between oral contraceptive use and referent diseases—and if so, what kind of restrictions?

D. Among patients admitted to a hospital there are likely to be women with a history of disease that is not related to their current hospitalization. If such disease, like diabetes or cardiovascular disease, is associated with oral contraceptive use, should these women be included among the referents?

E. When selecting hospital referents, should restrictions be made for reasons other than possible associations between oral contraceptive use and referent diseases—and if so, what kind of restrictions?

6:25 The extent to which BCG vaccination prevents meningitis tuberculosis (MT) in children aged 0–12 years was evaluated in a study in Brazil. MT is a severe disease, requiring hospitalization. Cases and referents, identified among children admitted to the same hospital during the study period, were examined with regard to BCG vaccination status. The cases were children admitted for MT. The referents were children admitted for acute diarrhea (AD referents), or acute nontuberculous bacterial pneumonia (BP referents).

A. Would it be preferable to select referents among all children admitted to the hospital during the study period? Why/why not?

The hospital was "considered one of the most important reference centres for MT" in the state, and a larger proportion of the cases than of the referents lived outside the metropolitan region where the hospital was located.

B. Does this indicate a possible referent selection bias and if so, how could this problem be dealt with?

6:26 The effect of alcohol intake on the risk of primary liver cancer was investigated (cf. Exercise 2:14). Information on alcohol intake was obtained from cases and referents identified at certain hospitals. Among all patients that could be selected as hospital referents, many are unlikely to reflect the alcohol intake of people in the study base: 1) patients admitted for diseases that are caused (or prevented) by alcohol; 2) patients admitted for chronic or recurrent diseases that may have influenced their alcohol intake in the past; 3) patients admitted electively for any condition, since alcohol consumption may be related to the probability of being admitted electively. Most patients admitted to a hospital are likely to belong to one (or more) of these categories, and thus contribute to a referent selection bias.

    A. In order to avoid a referent selection bias, referents should be selected among patients admitted for diseases that are not caused (or prevented) by alcohol, that could not have influenced past alcohol intake, and that require hospitalization (like liver cancer). Patients admitted for lung cancer are likely to fulfill these requirements. Would patients admitted for lung cancer be suitable as referents? Why/why not?

    B. In the present study, referents were selected among "patients from the surgical and medical wards, such as accident victims or those with myocardial infarction, etc, who showed normal livers after liver function tests." Could these patients have introduced a referent selection bias? Why/why not?

6:27 Convenience and low cost are among the main advantages of selecting hospital referents, which are readily available at the hospital where the cases are identified. A possible referent selection bias is the main concern. Referents have been selected in different ways in efforts to avoid bias while maintaining convenience and low cost. One approach is to select referents among friends of the cases, or among those accompanying patients to the hospital.

    A possible effect of sunlight exposure on the risk of senile cataract was investigated at a university hospital. The cases were patients admitted for cataract surgery during the study period. The referents "were selected from among those waiting for a friend or relative who was attending one of the ophthalmology clinics" at the same hospital during the study period. Subjects were accepted as referents only if they had never had a cataract, were found to be free of cataract at examination, and were not currently under treatment in any of the eye clinics.

  A. Was referent selection bias avoided by selecting referents among those waiting for a friend or relative attending one of the clinics? Why/why not?

  B. Suppose that referents were selected by asking each case to select his best friend. Would referent selection bias be avoided by selecting referents in this way? Why/why not?

6:28   The effect of oral contraceptive use on the risk of cerebral ischemia or thrombosis in young women was investigated. The study included women aged 15–44 years, with some additional restrictions. The cases were women who, during the study period, were admitted to certain hospitals for stroke (cerebral ischemia or thrombosis). For each case, a referent was selected from among women living in the same neighborhood. These neighbor referents were identified using a strict scheme, that involved "listing household units by number and working counterclockwise from the residence of the patient with stroke until arrival at a randomly designated household. From this point on, all members of households were identified and listed until the first woman meeting all the requirements was located. All efforts were to be made to interview this woman, and replacement was not permitted for any reason."

  A. Suppose that the participating hospitals served a geographically defined population, and that the cases of stroke occurring in this population were identified at these hospitals. Was a referent selection bias avoided by selecting neighbor referents? Why/why not?

  B. Suppose that the participating hospitals did not serve a geographically defined population, but rather admitted patients on the basis of complex preferences and socioeconomic factors. Was a referent selection bias avoided by selecting neighbor referents? Why/why not?

  C. All efforts were made to interview a woman selected as referent, and no replacements were permitted. Why?

6:29   Studies in occupational epidemiology suggest that electrical workers are at increased risk of certain cancers, especially leukemia. One of these studies was based on information from the New Zealand Cancer Registry. This registry "obtains data from public and private hospitals throughout the country as well as from death certificates and incidental autopsy findings, and registration was virtually complete for the study period." The registry also includes information on each patient's most recent occupation at the time of registration. The study was restricted to men aged 20 years or more, and used information on cancers that occurred during the study period. In a series of analyses, the cases were men with one type of cancer (e.g., leukemia) and the referents were men with all other types of cancer. Relative risks were estimated for electrical workers (exposed) compared to men in all other occupations (unexposed).

A. Define the study base.

B. Could a referent selection bias have been introduced by using men with all other cancers as referents? Why/why not?

c. What are the advantages of using men with other types of cancer as referents?

6:30 Excess risks of certain cancers have been found in pulp and paper production workers exposed to toxic chemicals. A study used information from death certificates for all pulp and paper mill workers in New Hampshire, who died during an 11-year period. The deaths were classified by underlying cause of death according to the eighth revision of the International Classification of Diseases (ICD-8). As an estimate of the relative risk, a proportionate mortality ratio (PMR) was calculated by dividing the proportion of all deaths that occurred in a specific cause of death category with the corresponding proportion of all deaths in the United States population. The study was restricted to white males aged ≥ 20 years.

A. Define the study base.

B. Who were the exposed and unexposed, respectively?

c. The PMRs were adjusted for age and year of death. Suggest some other potential confounders.

D. The PMR was used as an estimate of the relative risk. PMR = a:c/b:d = a*d/b*c, where a and b are the number of cases (cancer deaths), and c and d are the total number of deaths, in the exposed and unexposed, respectively. On what condition is PMR = RR?

GENERAL QUESTIONS

6:31 What is the purpose of selecting referents, and what conditions influence the extent to which this purpose is achieved?

6:32 What potential sources of bias are introduced by using referents, and how can such bias be avoided?

6:33 In many studies, referents are not selected as a random sample of the study base or study population. Why?

6:34 Precision is influenced by the number of referents selected. How?

6:35 What information is needed to estimate the absolute effect (e.g., the rate difference) in a case-referent study?

6:36 Sometimes, referents are matched to the cases. What is meant by matching? What is the purpose of matching, and in what situations could this purpose be achieved?

6:37 What limitations and potential problems are introduced by matching referents to the cases?

6:38 What are the advantages and disadvantages, respectively, of using the cases diagnosed at a certain hospital and selecting the referents among other patients admitted to the same hospital during the study period?

6:39 When hospital referents are selected, patients are sometimes not accepted as referents if they have been admitted electively or for chronic or recurrent conditions. Why?

6:40 Consider your own recent favorite study. What are the implications for that study of the general problems and possibilities exemplified in the different exercises in this chapter?

7 Assignment of Exposure (Experimental Strategies)

■■■ **INTRODUCTION**

Purpose and Principles

The possibility of confounding by unidentified (unknown) risk factors is a major concern in many epidemiologic studies. Such confounding may be avoided in studies where the subjects are assigned to receive or not to receive an intervention to alter their exposure status. In *experimental studies (trials)* the intervention is assigned with the purpose of improving validity, usually by randomization (randomized experiments, randomized trials).

The purpose of random assignment of exposure is to avoid bias due to differences between the exposed and unexposed (subjects assigned to receive and not to receive the intervention). With a very large number of subjects involved in the randomization, the groups will tend to be equal with regard to other factors prior to the intervention. Thus any confounding (and differences with regard to misclassification and selection) due to such factors will be avoided. With a limited number of subjects involved in the randomization there may still be confounding due to chance differences between the groups, but this becomes increasingly unlikely with an increasing number of subjects (or other units) involved in the randomization.

Random assignments are made using a table of random numbers, or a series of computer-generated random numbers. A table of random digits 0–9 (occurring on average the same number of times, but with no discernible pattern) may be used to assign the intervention for certain digits but not for others (simple randomization). Usually, the digits are selected to obtain a similar number of subjects in each group, for example, 0–4 for intervention and 5–9 for no intervention (equal randomization). A chance difference in group size may be avoided by restricted randomization (e.g., blocked randomization). A chance difference between the groups with regard to a known potential confounder may be avoided by stratification prior to randomization (stratified randomization). When studying the effects of two different exposures (interventions A and B), subjects may be randomly allocated to three groups: A, B, and no intervention. But precision may be improved by random allocation to four groups: A, B, A+B, and no intervention (factorial design).

The randomization is usually based on individual study subjects. But sometimes the unit of randomization is families, wards, or even communities, rather than individual subjects. This may offer advantages with regard to cost and convenience, and may reduce the likelihood of the intervention influencing subjects assigned not to receive the intervention ("spill-over effect"). On the other hand, it will reduce the number of randomized units and thus the possibility of achieving the purpose of randomization.

The major advantage of experimental over nonexperimental studies is the possibility of avoiding confounding by unidentified factors. In some experimental studies, the use of placebo and blinding may offer additional advantages (see below). The major disadvantage is a low cost-efficiency, due to a high cost per subject and the large number of subjects usually required to obtain adequate precision in studies of disease causation and prevention. In addition, there may be limitations due to ethical concerns or practical problems such as noncompliance with the intervention.

Procedures

A study population is selected according to the principles described in Chapter 3. But since the exposure status is to be altered by intervention, all study subjects should be unexposed if the intervention is designed to induce the exposure (and vice versa). In addition, participation presupposes ability and willingness to comply with the intervention and with other procedures of an experimental study. Subjects are included only if they are considered to be able to participate in the trial, as judged from an informal evaluation or from their compliance during a formal run-in period prior to randomization. Subjects should not be included unless they are expected to tolerate the intervention (no contraindications), and respond to the intervention by a change in exposure status.

Subjects may enter a trial only if they fulfill specified *eligibility criteria*, based on restrictions with regard to potential confounders and modifiers and ability to provide accurate information (see Chapter 3), and on their exposure status and expected ability to participate in the trial (see above). Before subjects enter a trial they should also give their *informed consent*—that is, they should be informed about the trial and give their consent to participate (written consent may be required). In addition it may be necessary to obtain approval from their physicians. Subjects who fulfill the eligibility criteria and give their informed consent should formally *enter the trial* and receive a unique number (001 for the first subject, etc.) on a list of participants. In a *baseline examination* (before the intervention), each subject is examined with regard to potential confounders and modifiers (cf. Chapter 4). A *randomization list* is usually prepared in advance, and gives the consecutive assignments based on random numbers (see above). Subject registration and randomization should be handled by an independent person (e.g., a statistician) who is not involved in the enrollment, examination, treatment, or follow-up of study subjects. It is essential that staff members are not informed about, and cannot predict, the next assignment before the subject has formally entered the trial (otherwise the assignments could be influenced by the staff, e.g., by order of enrollment).

Placebo and Blinding

Sometimes it is possible to use *placebo (sham) treatment* for the subjects in the nonintervention group. Placebo treatment should be identical to the "active" treatment given to subjects in the intervention group, except for the specific component designed to alter the subjects' exposure status. In addition, placebo treatment should be perceived as being identical to the active treatment in order to make blinding possible. In *single-blind* trials, the study subjects are kept unaware of their own assignment (active or placebo treatment) during the study. In *double-blind* trials, both the study subjects and the staff involved in the treatment and follow-up are kept unaware of the assignments during the study.

The purpose of placebo and blinding is to avoid bias due to differences between the groups with regard to factors that are introduced or influenced by the intervention (placebo), or by awareness of the intervention (blinding). Thus, placebo and blinding are used to avoid that the intervention introduces the following:

1. Confounding. For example, in a study of hypertension and cardiovascular disease, treatment of hypertension could make people

aware of other risk factors and thus introduce changes in their diet and smoking habits. In addition, treatment of hypertension includes medical surveillance that may result in other treatments. Placebo and blinding are used to avoid confounding, by making the intervention and nonintervention group similar in these respects.

2.   Differences in disease misclassification. For example, treatment of hypertension includes medical surveillance that may influence the identification of cases. In addition, awareness of the treatment could influence the study subjects in their perception and reporting of symptoms. Placebo and blinding are used to avoid differential misclassification, by making the intervention and nonintervention group similar in these respects.

3.   Differences in selective loss to follow-up (or selective loss of information). For example, symptoms of disease may influence the loss to follow-up differently in subjects who are, and subjects who are not, under treatment for hypertension. Placebo and blinding are used to avoid differential selection, by making the intervention and nonintervention group similar in these respects.

When placebo and blinding are used, any differences between the groups in compliance or in loss to follow-up may be due to chance—or signal that the blinding has been broken. Any differences in side effects between active and placebo treatment may also interfere with the possibility of achieving the purposes of blinding. In many trials, the study subjects are followed with regard to factors that may be introduced or influenced by the intervention (or by awareness of the intervention).

Sources of Bias

To achieve the purpose of randomization, the results of a trial should be based on all subjects involved in the randomization, considering those assigned to receive the intervention as exposed and those assigned not to receive the intervention as unexposed (or vice versa). Thus, exposure classification is based on assignment rather than on actual intervention or (change in) exposure status. *Exposure misclassification* is introduced if subjects allocated to the intervention group would not receive the intervention (e.g., due to noncompliance), or if the intervention would fail to bring about the intended change in exposure status in all subjects. In addition, exposure misclassification is introduced if subjects allocated to the nonintervention group would have (or develop) the exposure status induced by the intervention. The exposure misclassification tends to bias the result towards RR = 1, and may explain "negative results" in several randomized trials. This bias may be reduced if the results are based only on subjects who received the intended intervention ("on-treatment" analysis). However, the purpose of randomization may not be achieved unless the results are based on all randomized subjects according to their assignments ("intention-to-treat" analysis).

Randomization is used to prevent *confounding*. But confounding could still be present due to chance differences between the groups or improper randomization procedures. Confounding introduced by the intervention (or by awareness of the intervention) is not avoided by randomization, but may be prevented by the use of placebo and blinding in some experimental studies. However, such confounding may be introduced if the blinding is broken or if there are differences in side effects. As in nonexperimental studies, information on potential confounders (obtained at baseline and during follow-up) may be used to control confounding in the data analysis.

A specific intervention could, in principle at least, affect the risk of developing the disease (outcome) under study by changing the exposure status—or by other pathways. The latter possibility would introduce confounding when studying the effect of a change in exposure status. For example, nonexperimental data suggest that a high serum cholesterol increases the risk of cardiovascular disease. When studying this effect in a randomized trial using a drug to lower serum cholesterol, confounding is introduced if the drug would affect the risk of cardiovascular disease by other pathways.

Differential *disease misclassification* may be avoided by the use of placebo and blinding (and to some extent also by randomization), but could be introduced by broken blinding or by differences in side effects. Nondifferential disease misclassification is not influenced by randomization, placebo, or blinding.

Selection bias is introduced if loss to follow-up (or loss of information) is influenced by the disease (outcome) under study (see Chapter 1: Selection Bias). Differential selection may be avoided by placebo and blinding (and to some extent also by randomization), but could be introduced by broken blinding or by differences in side effects. Nondifferential selection (resulting in overestimation or underestimation of the absolute effect) is not influenced by randomization, placebo, or blinding.

▬ EXERCISES

7:1   A randomized trial was conducted to study the effects of certain dietary factors on the risk of myocardial infarction (MI) in men under 70 years of age who had recovered from a previous MI. Patients admitted to certain hospitals for MI were recruited when they had recovered. Each subject was checked with regard to eligibility criteria: MI diagnosis, age (under 70 years), sex (male), and restrictions with regard to other potential confounders and modifiers (as discussed in Chapter 3). In addition, to be eligible for a trial, subjects should: a) not be exposed regardless of the intervention, and b) be able and willing to participate in the intervention. Eligible subjects, and their physicians, were informed about the trial and asked to give their approval (informed consent). Thus, the following three steps determined whether or not a subject could enter the trial:

1. Subject recruitment

2. Eligibility check

3. Informed consent

Each subject entering a trial (after 1–3) is given a unique trial number (e.g., 001 for the first subject entering the trial, and so on). This number is recorded on a list of participants together with the subject's name and other identifications (e.g., date of birth, hospital) and the date of entry on the trial. Only after this formal entry should a subject be randomly assigned to receive or not to receive the intervention (e.g., diet). The random assignment is usually made from a randomization list that has been prepared in advance.

A. Confounding is introduced by risk factors associated with the exposure (Chapter 1). In the assignment of exposure, randomization is used with the purpose of avoiding confounding by making the exposed and unexposed (those assigned to receive and not to receive the intervention) equal with regard to other risk factors. How does the number of subjects (or other units) involved in the randomization influence the possibility of achieving this purpose?

B. Confounding may also be dealt with by restrictions when selecting the study population and by methods used to control confounding in the data analysis (Chapter 1). Compared with these startegies, what is the principal advantage of random assignment of exposure?

C. Does random assignment of exposure prevent all sources of confounding? Why/why not? Exemplify!

D. To be eligible for a trial, subjects should not be exposed regardless of the intervention. Thus, men who already intended to eat the intervention diet were not included in the present study. If they had been included, what difference would it make?

E. Staff members involved in the recruitment of subjects for a trial, or in the decision about formal entry on the trial, should be kept unaware of the next assignment on the randomization list until the subject has formally entered the trial. If they were aware of the next assignment, what difference would it make?

7:2   Nonexperimental epidemiologic findings suggest that vegetables rich in beta carotene may reduce the risk of certain cancers. Against this background, a randomized double-blind trial was done to study the effect of beta carotene supplements on the risk of skin cancer (basal-cell or squamous-cell carcinoma) in people at high risk of such cancers. Subjects who fulfilled certain eligibility criteria, and who gave their informed consent to participate in the trial, were assigned by computer-generated random numbers to receive capsules containing either 50 mg of beta carotene or placebo identical in appearance.

A. Prior to randomization, information was obtained on age, sex, skin type, smoking habits, and other potential confounders. The final report provided information on the occurrence of these factors in subjects assigned to receive beta carotene and placebo, respectively. In addition, adjustment for such factors was made when calculating the relative risk. Why?

B. Is it possible to check whether the randomization was "successful" in achieving the purpose to avoid confounding? Why/why not?

7:3   The effects of certain vitamin supplements, taken around the time of conception, on the risk of neural tube defects in the offspring was investigated in a randomized double-blind trial. Only women at high risk, due to a previous pregnancy affected by a neural tube defect, were eligible for the study. In addition, only women who were willing and able to participate were included: "Women invited to join the trial were given a week to decide if they wished to take part, so that they could consider the matter at leisure and discuss the matter further with others if they wished. All patients were given a printed information leaflet about the trial."

In another randomized double-blind trial, the effect of beta carotene supplements on the risk of skin cancer was investigated (cf.

Exercise 7:2). Study subjects were recruited among people who were at high risk of skin cancer because they had had a skin cancer previously. Subjects who fulfilled specified criteria (e.g., restrictions with regard to age, pregnancy, and medical history), and gave their informed consent to participate, were included in a test: "A total of 1,968 persons (38 percent of all those initially identified) began a one-month placebo run-in period to assess their willingness and ability to comply with the study protocol." Subjects found to be willing and able to participate entered the trial and were randomly assigned to receive either beta carotene or placebo.

A. In both trials, actions were taken that could actually increase the loss of otherwise eligible subjects prior to randomization. Why?

B. In both trials, study subjects were selected among people at high risk because they had previously had the outcome of interest. Why?

7:4   The possibility of using a drug (allopurinol) to prevent renal calculi (calcium oxalate calculi) in people previously affected by such calculi was investigated in a randomized double-blind trial. A total of 72 subjects were randomly assigned to receive either drug or placebo of identical appearance.

Simple randomization is done by preparing a randomization list from a table (or computer-generated list) of random numbers (0 to 9) where the drug may be assigned for digits 0–4 and placebo for digits 5–9.

A. The following series is obtained from a table of random numbers: 6,8,1,5,6,7,7,5,7,5,3,4 . . . (where the first digit is used for assignment of subject no 1, and so on). Which of the first 12 study subjects are assigned to receive the drug?

In the present study, the total number of subjects involved in the randomization was relatively small. Thus, there may by chance be an imbalance between the number of subjects assigned to receive drug and placebo, respectively, when using simple randomization. Restricted randomization is sometimes used to ensure that there will be a similar number of subjects in each group. One way to restrict randomization is to use blocked randomization (random permutated blocks). In the present study "(a) block size of six was used, allowing placement of equal numbers of subjects receiving placebo and allopurinol in each multiple of six patients." A table of random permutations of numbers is used for random assignment of three subjects to receive the drug and three subjects to receive placebo, with a different sequence within each block of six subjects, when drug treatment is assigned for digits 0–2 and placebo for digits 3–5.

   B. The following series is obtained from a table of random permutations of numbers 0 to 5 (= six numbers for a block size of six): 0,1,4,5,3,2,3,5,4,2,1,0 . . . Which of the first 12 study subjects are assigned to receive the drug?

   c. What is the purpose of blocked randomization, and in what situations would it be a useful alternative to simple randomization?

7:5 The effect of dietary intake of protein on the risk of renal failure in subjects with chronic renal insufficiency was investigated. Study subjects were randomly assigned to receive either a protein-restricted or a regular diet. Suppose that blocked randomization was used, with a block size of two, and that the block size was known by the physicians recruiting subjects for the study. Could this introduce a bias? Why/why not?

7:6 A total of 103 subjects, who were disease-free after treatment for cancers of the head and neck, were included in a randomized trial. The purpose was to study the effect of isotretinoin (a synthetic retinoid) on the risk of second primary tumors. However, the previous treatment was expected to influence the risk of second primary tumors. To avoid imbalance between the isotretinoin and placebo group with regard to previous treatment, subjects were stratified according to their previous treatment (surgery, irradiation, or both) and randomization was performed in blocks within each of the three previous-treatment strata (random permutated blocks within strata).

   A. What is the purpose of using stratified randomization to avoid imbalance between the intervention groups?

   B. Can the purpose of stratified randomization be achieved by a stratified data analysis?

7:7 Mass screening with mammography for early detection and treatment of breast cancer in women may reduce the risk of advanced (stage II +) breast cancer and death from breast cancer. To investigate this, a randomized trial was conducted among all (162,981) women aged 40 years or more and living within two counties in Sweden at the time of randomization. Prior to randomization, "the combined population of the 2 counties was divided into 19 blocks selected to give relative socioeconomic homogeneity within each block."

In one of the two counties, each block was divided into two units of roughly equal size. One of these units was selected at random to receive, and the other not to receive, the screening program.

A. The geographical unit (community), rather than the individual study subject, was the unit of randomization. What are the advantages and disadvantages, respectively, of this approach?

In the other county, each block was divided into three units of roughly equal size. Two of these units were selected at random to receive, and the third not to receive, the screening program. Thus, in this county there were about twice as many women in the intervention group as in the nonintervention group.

B. What are the advantages and disadvantages, respectively, of such unequal randomization?

7:3   A randomized double-blind prevention trial was conducted to determine to what extent folic acid (one of the vitamins in the B group) or a mixture of seven other vitamins, taken around the time of conception, can reduce the risk of neural tube defects in the offspring (cf. Exercise 7:3). A total of 1,817 women were randomly assigned to receive capsules (one capsule a day until 12 weeks of pregnancy) containing either 1) folic acid, 2) other vitamins, 3) folic acid + other vitamins, or 4) placebo. The effect of folic acid was evaluated by comparison of the outcome in groups 1 and 3 (exposed) with that in groups 2 and 4 (unexposed). The effect of other vitamins was evaluated by comparison of the outcome in groups 2 and 3 (exposed) with that in groups 1 and 4 (unexposed). This so-called factorial design is an alternative to random assignment to receive either folic acid, other vitamins, or placebo (3 groups).

A. What are the principal advantages of using a factorial design when studying the effects of two (or more) exposures?
B. What are the principal disadvantages of using a factorial design when studying the effects of two (or more) exposures?

7:9 The effect of beta carotene on the risk of skin cancer was investigated (cf. Exercise 7:2). Subjects were randomly assigned to receive capsules containing either beta carotene or placebo. Plasma levels of beta carotene were determined prior to randomization and annually during follow-up (results not available to the staff or study subjects).

A. Some people may have a high dietary intake of beta carotene and thus relatively high plasma levels of beta carotene both prior to randomization and during follow-up. If such people were included in the trial and assigned to receive placebo, should they be considered as exposed or unexposed to beta carotene when calculating the relative risk?

B. Study subjects should, as far as possible, have a low dietary intake of beta carotene and thus low levels of beta carotene prior to randomization. If such people were assigned to receive beta carotene supplements, but did not take the capsules, they may still have low plasma levels of beta carotene during follow-up. Should they be considered as exposed or unexposed to beta carotene when calculating the relative risk?

7:10 Noncompliance with the intervention is a major limitation of many experimental studies. But the magnitude of the problem is often not recognized because noncompliance is difficult to measure. Counting the number of tablets left in the bottle (pill count) may give an estimate of the total number of tablets taken over a certain period of time, although tablets may be removed but not taken (if, for instance, a pill count is expected). Laboratory analyses of samples of blood or urine to determine the presence of a drug or its metabolites, or a marker substance added to the medication, may reflect compliance at a certain point in time, although compliance tends to increase considerably prior to clinic visits. In several studies as many as 25–50 percent of patients have been found to be noncompliant, but this proportion may be reduced by the subject selection and surveillance in some randomized trials. Questionnaires have usually identified less than half of the subjects found to be noncompliant by other methods. (The answers may be biased by "social desirability;" cf. Exercise 4:12).

The effect of a synthetic retinoid (isotretinoin) on the risk of second primary cancers of the head and neck was investigated in a randomized trial (cf. Exercise 7:6). Compliance was assessed by means of pill counts, and 33 percent of those assigned to receive isotretinoin did not complete the 12-month course of treatment.

A. Considering the consequences of this noncompliance, in what direction would it bias the relative risk calculated on the basis of the random assignments (intention-to-treat analysis)?

Another randomized prevention trial was conducted to study the effect of low-dose aspirin (325 mg. every other day) on the risk of myocardial infarction. The study subjects were sent brief questionnaires asking about their medication compliance. However, several studies comparing questionnaire data with objective data (e.g., pill counts, blood analyses, medication monitors) indicate that less than 50 percent of noncompliant subjects are identified by questionnaire.

B. Considering the consequences of such underestimation of noncompliance, in what direction would it bias the relative risk calculated on the basis of the subjects found to be compliant by questionnaire (on-treatment analysis)?

7:11   The effect of water-sanitation behaviors on the risk of childhood diarrhea in urban Bangladesh was investigated in two different epidemiologic studies.

In a nonexperimental study, families with children under 6 years of age were selected. Examinations were done with regard to water-sanitation behaviors in these families, and the occurrence of diarrhea in the children.

In an experimental study, 51 communities, each comprising 38 families, were randomly assigned to receive or not to receive an educational intervention to alter water-sanitation bahaviors. Children under 6 years of age were then examined for the occurrence of diarrhea.

A. When selecting a suitable study population (Chapter 3), what are the principal differences (if any) between a nonexperimental and an experimental study?
B. When obtaining information on exposures including potential confounders and modifiers (Chapter 4), what are the principal differences (if any) between a nonexperimental and an experimental study?
c. In the follow-up of disease occurrence (Chapter 5), what are the principal differences (if any) between a nonexperimental and an experimental study?

7:12   The effect of dietary cholesterol intake on mortality from ischemic heart disease was investigated in a nonexperimental epidemiologic study (cf. Exercise 3:26). Suppose that an experimental study was planned to investigate this effect.

A. What is the major advantage of conducting an experimental study rather than a nonexperimental study?

B. What is the major disadvantage of conducting an experimental study rather than a nonexperimental study?

7:13 Laboratory findings suggest that fish oil could prevent atherosclerosis. A randomized double-blind trial was done to investigate the possibility of using fish oil to prevent restenosis after surgical treatment for coronary stenosis. Study subjects were randomly assigned to receive capsules containing either fish oil or placebo. The study was double-blind, that is, both the study subjects and the staff (involved in the treatment or follow-up) were kept unaware of which subjects received fish oil and placebo capsules, respectively. During follow-up, restenosis was identified by symptoms and exercise testing and confirmed by X-ray (angiography). What is the purpose of placebo and blinding?

7:14 The possibility that common cold may be prevented by using an intranasal alpha$_2$-interferon spray was investigated in a randomized double-blind trial (cf. Exercise 5:23). Study subjects were assigned to receive nasal sprays with either interferon or placebo. During follow-up, the study subjects used a diary to record any upper respiratory symptoms. When symptoms occurred, a study nurse was called for further examination and diagnosis. The study was double-blind—that is, both the study subjects and the staff (including the study nurse) were kept unaware of whether an individual had received interferon or placebo. The purpose of using placebo and blinding is to improve validity in three respects (cf. Exercise 7:13):

1. To avoid confounding, that may otherwise be introduced by the intervention (or by awareness of the intervention). How would the possibilities of avoiding such bias be influenced:

A. if the staff (including the study nurse) knew the exposure status of individual subjects?

B. if individual study subjects knew their own exposure status?

2. To avoid differences in disease misclassification, that may otherwise be introduced by the intervention (or by awareness of the intervention). How would the possibilities of avoiding such bias be influenced:

c. if the staff (including the study nurse) knew the exposure status of individual subjects?

d. if individual study subjects knew their own exposure status?

3. To avoid differences in selective loss to follow-up, that may otherwise be introduced by the intervention (or by awareness of the intervention). How would the possibilities of avoiding such bias be influenced:

e. if the staff (including the study nurse) knew the exposure status of individual subjects?

f. if individual study subjects knew their own exposure status?

g. How can the purposes of placebo and blinding (1–3) be achieved in nonexperimental research?

7:15   The proposition that vitamin C supplements might reduce the risk of common cold was investigated. Volunteers for a double-blind trial were recruited among National Institutes of Health (NIH) employees who fulfilled certain criteria. A total of 323 study subjects were randomly assigned either capsules containing 500 mg of ascorbic acid or placebo capsules of similar appearance. The maintenance (prophylactic) dose was two capsules three times a day with meals. The drug was dispensed by the pharmacy in bottles of 200, and study subjects were asked to return at monthly intervals with their bottles for refills. At these visits they were interviewed for symptoms of side effects, and the capsules left in the bottle were counted as a check of medication compliance. After 9 months of follow-up the study was stopped because the number of subjects under study had dropped below 200, and because the dropout rate was significantly higher in the placebo group than in the ascorbic acid group.

Why would the dropout rate be significantly higher in the placebo group, and why should this be a reason to stop the trial?

7:16   Considerable attention has been paid to the possibility of preventing the occurrence of acquired immunodeficiency syndrome (AIDS) in subjects infected with human immunodeficiency virus (HIV). In a double-blind trial, 866 subjects with HIV infection were randomly assigned to receive a potentially preventive drug (inosine pranobex) or placebo of similar taste and appearance.

a. During follow-up, 112 of the 429 subjects receiving inosine pranobex reported adverse effects including headache, dizziness, and gastrointestinal symptoms. How could this interfere with the possibility of achieving the purposes of blinding?

B. Routine examinations of study subjects during follow-up included analyses of serum samples for uric acid, which is a metabolite of inosine pranobex. Results were available to the clinical staff. How could this interfere with the possibility of achieving the purposes of blinding?

7:17 The risk of coronary heart disease is considerably increased in subjects with dyslipidemia (high serum levels of low-density lipoprotein and low serum levels of high-density lipoprotein). In a primary-prevention trial of a drug (gemfibrozil) used to normalize serum lipoproteins, 4,081 middle-aged men with dyslipidemia were randomly assigned to receive capsules (twice daily) with either gemfibrozil or placebo. Treatments continued during a 5-year follow-up with regard to coronary heart disease. Dropout rates were recorded, 3-month capsule counts were used to measure compliance, and in addition: "Gemfibrozil was measured in urine to check compliance, and the results were kept blinded for later analysis. A microdose of digoxin (2.2 μg per capsule) was used as a marker in both active and placebo capsules. Urinary digoxin levels were measured in all participants during the last quarter of the third and fifth study years."

Adding the "marker" in both active and placebo capsules (together with the capsule counts) made it possible to study compliance in the placebo group. What interest could there be to study compliance in taking placebo capsules?

7:18 The effect of dietary protein intake on the risk of renal failure in subjects with chronic renal insufficiency was investigated in a trial (cf. Exercise 7:5). The study subjects, who were patients at a renal outpatient clinic, were randomly assigned to receive a protein-restricted or a regular diet. Blinding of study subjects was not feasible. Additional factors that may affect the risk of renal failure include blood pressure and dietary factors other than protein. Each study subject was examined with regard to these factors prior to randomization. Should each subject also be examined with regard to these factors during follow-up? Why/why not?

7:19 In order to prevent the recurrence of duodenal ulcer, attempts have been made to change people's diet and lifestyle. Preventive drug treatment has also been tried. A randomized double-blind trial was conducted to evaluate a drug (ranitidine) in the prevention of duodenal ulcer in people who had recovered from a previous ulcer. Study subjects were randomly assigned to receive long-term treatment with tablets, to be taken nightly, containing either ranitidin or placebo. Efforts were made to keep the study subjects, as well as staff members, unaware of the subjects' exposure status. However, such efforts are not always successful in achieving the purposes of blinding (cf. Exercise 7:14). What signs could indicate a failure to achieve the purposes of blinding?

7:20   The effect of dietary fat intake and smoking on the risk of coronary heart disease (CHD) was studied in a randomized trial. After a screening of 16,202 men aged 40–49 years for coronary risk factors, the trial was entered by 1,232 healthy men with normal blood pressure who were at high risk of CHD. These men were randomly assigned to receive or not to receive an intervention (dietary and antismoking advice). During a 5-year follow-up period, 19 cases of CHD were identified in the intervention group and 36 cases in the nonintervention group (RR = 0.5).

In the absence of placebo and blinding of study subjects, what measures could be taken to deal with:

A. confounding introduced by the intervention?
B. differential disease misclassification?
C. selection bias due to withdrawal from the study?

7:21   A program for reducing perinatal mortality (stillbirths and deaths within 7 days after birth) was evaluated in a trial in Helsinki, Finland. A total of 9,310 women were randomly assigned to participate or not to participate in the program during pregnancy. Blinding was not considered feasible. A total of 69 cases were identified, and the relative risk was RR = 0.5. Only four women were lost to follow-up: one in the intervention group, three in the nonintervention group.

A. In principle, what sources of bias may be introduced by the lack of blinding?
B. In the present study, to what extent is the lack of blinding likely to introduce such bias?

7:22   Epidemiologic findings indicate that calcium intake may be inversely related to the risk of hypertensive disorders of pregnancy. A randomized double-blind trial included women who sought prenatal care before the twentieth week of gestation at three hospitals, fulfilled the eligibility criteria (nulliparous; singleton pregnancy; blood pressure below 140/90; no disease or medications; normal oral glucose-tolerance test), and gave their informed written consent to participate in the trial. A total of 1,194 women entered the trial and were examined with regard to potential confounders and modifiers at baseline. The women were randomly assigned to receive tablets containing either calcium supplementation (500 mg/tablet) or placebo, and each woman was instructed to take four tablets per day. Efforts were made to keep the women, and the clinical staff involved in the care and follow-up, unaware of the assignments. The women were asked to return their medication bottle, in exchange for a new bottle, at each prenatal visit (and the tablets remaining in the old bottle were counted). Follow-up was from the twentieth week of gestation and the women were examined at prenatal visits scheduled during week 23, 25, 27, 31, 35, and then weekly until delivery. The outcome of interest was gestational hypertension ($\geq$ 140 mm Hg systolic and $\geq$ 90 mm Hg diastolic blood pressure on two occasions at least 6 hours apart) or preeclampsia (= gestational hypertension + proteinuria defined as > 0.3 g of protein per liter of urine on two occasions at least 6 hours apart). In addition, information was obtained on possible side effects of treatment and on withdrawals during follow-up. The percentage of women who developed gestational hypertension or preeclampsia was 9.8 percent in the calcium group and 14.8 percent in the placebo group, RR = 0.63 (95% confidence interval: 0.44–0.90). The relative risk was similar for each of the two conditions.

A. Randomization is used to avoid confounding. Is this purpose likely to be achieved in the present study? Why/why not?

B. Could confounding have been introduced by the intervention in the present study? Why/why not?

C. Considering calcium intake as the exposure of interest, what are the potential sources of exposure misclassification in the present study? In what direction is the relative risk likely to be biased by exposure misclassification? What can be done to avoid exposure misclassification?

D. What are the potential sources of disease (hypertension or preeclampsia) misclassification in the present study? In what direction is the relative risk likely to be biased by disease misclassification?

E. Could there be selection bias in the present study? Why/why not?

7:23 Epidemiologic findings suggest that vitamin A deficiency may increase childhood mortality in developing countries, although the results of intervention trials have been somewhat inconsistent. Against this background, the effect of vitamin A supplementation on preschool child mortality was studied in a randomized, double-blind trial in Nepal. The study population was children who lived within 261 wards in the district of Sarlahi, where vitamin A deficiency is endemic. The ward served as the unit of random allocation: all children within a ward were assigned to receive either vitamin A or placebo in identical capsules. All households in a ward were visited by staff every 4 months during the study period (1 year). Children aged 0–60 months were enrolled at the first visit, and children born during the study period were enrolled at subsequent visits. At the time of enrollment, information was obtained on potential confounders including health indicators and maternal history of child mortality. A total of 28,630 children contributed 25,970 child-years at risk and 362 deaths.

A. The mortality was lower in children assigned vitamin A than in children assigned placebo (estimated RR = 0.70). What sources of bias (if any) could explain this finding, if vitamin A deficiency does not increase childhood mortality?

B. Suppose that the mortality was found to be similar in children assigned vitamin A and placebo, respectively (estimated RR = 1). What sources of bias (if any) could explain this finding, if vitamin A deficiency does increase childhood mortality?

7:24 In the largest epidemiological trial ever, the effect of the Salk vaccine on the risk of poliomyelitis was studied in 1.8 million children in the United States. In 1954, all school children in grades 1–3 in the study areas were invited to participate. In some areas, the study was conducted as a double-blind trial, where children were randomly assigned to receive either vaccine or placebo injections. In other areas, it was decided that second grade children should be vaccinated and compared with unvaccinated first and third graders. Of all second graders in the nonrandomized part of the trial, 69.2 percent (245,895) were willing to participate and 62.4 percent received complete vaccinations. Two different possibilities were discussed: 1) to consider only the vaccinated second grade children as exposed; 2) to consider all second graders as exposed, regardless of whether or not they were willing to participate or actually received the vaccine. In both alternatives, the unexposed were all first and third graders regardless of their willingness to participate (according to a parental consent form).

A. What is the principal disadvantage of the first approach (1)?

B. What is the principal disadvantage of the second approach (2)?

C. Could you suggest a third approach, to avoid these disadvantages?

Socioeconomic status was related to the risk of polio. Is socioeconomic status likely to introduce confounding:

D. in the randomized part of the trial?

E. in the nonrandomized part of the trial?

It may be difficult to separate poliomyelitis from other diseases that could give rise to similar symptoms. In the present study, potential cases underwent clinical as well as laboratory examinations. The randomized double-blind part of the trial showed that the vaccine prevented 49 percent of all cases (identified by clinical examination), and 80 percent of the cases from which polio virus was recovered.

F. What is the likely explanation for this apparent difference in effect?

Analyses of blood samples drawn before the vaccination showed that some children had already aquired specific immunity (through polio virus infections with little or no symptoms). In addition, analyses of blood samples drawn after the vaccination showed that some children did not aquire specific immunity as a result of the vaccination.

G. In what direction is this likely to bias the result of the randomized part of the trial?

7:25 The effect of low-dose aspirin on the risk of myocardial infarction was investigated in a randomized double-blind trial (cf. Exercise 7:10B). The study subjects were 22,071 physicians examined with regard to several cardiovascular risk factors and then randomly assigned to receive either low-dose aspirin or placebo. During follow-up, 378 cases of myocardial infarction were identified. As could be expected with the large number of subjects involved in the randomization, the relative risk (RR = 0.56) was not confounded by serum cholesterol or other cardiovascular risk factors at baseline. But interestingly serum cholesterol was found to modify the relative effect of low-dose aspirin: the relative risk was lowest (RR = 0.23) at the lowest level of serum cholesterol ($\leq$ 159 mg per 100 ml), and then increased with increasing levels of serum cholesterol.

Other blood lipids, in addition to cholesterol, could also modify the effect of low-dose aspirin (and might also introduce confounding). However, the laboratory analyses of several lipids in serum samples from 22,071 subjects may be prohibitively expensive. How could effect modification (and potential confounding) by other blood lipids be investigated at a reasonable cost?

7:26 Findings in laboratory research and nonexperimental epidemiology suggest that certain nutritional deficiencies could increase the risk of precursor lesions of cancer of the esophagus. Against this background, a randomized double-blind trial was conducted in a high risk population in the People's Republic of China. A total of 610 subjects were examined with regard to potential confounders and modifiers, and then randomly assigned to receive capsules containing either supplementation (retinol + riboflavin + zinc) or placebo. The capsules were to be taken once a week and "barefoot doctors" delivered the capsules and checked that they were swallowed, in order to avoid noncompliance. At the end of a 13.5-month treatment period, each subject was examined with endoscopy including biopsies to identify precursor lesions of cancer of the esophagus. (Only one endoscopy per subject was considered acceptable.) The prevalence of precursor lesions was found to be similar in the two groups. One possible interpretation of this finding is that, with the doses given and within the limited time period, the supplementation does not prevent precursor lesions of cancer of the esophagus.

A. Should this conclusion be modified, considering the fact that prevalent (rather than incident) cases were identified?

At the time of randomization, the blood levels of retinol were low (deficient) and similar in both groups. During the treatment period, the levels increased among those who received supplementation. But during the same period there was also a substantial increase in the blood levels of retinol among those who received placebo. (This may have been due to seasonal variations in the supply of fresh vegetables and fruit.)

B. How does this influence the interpretation of the result?

7:27 A large randomized trial was conducted to study the effects of interventions against high blood pressure, elevated serum cholesterol, and smoking in middle-aged men. Attention was paid to the risk of coronary heart disease (CHD), stroke, and death. About

30,000 men aged 47–55 years were included in the trial, and randomly allocated to three groups of equal size: one intervention group and two nonintervention groups. All men in the intervention group were invited to a screening for exposures of interest, and 75% (7,495/10,004) participated in this examination. Of these participants, 37% (2,760/7,495) had one or more of the following exposures: hypertension (systolic blood pressure ≥ 175 mm Hg or diastolic blood pressure ≥ 115 mm Hg), high serum cholesterol (≥ 300 mg per 100 ml), or smoking ≥ 15 cigarettes per day. These men were referred to a program for individual intervention against the exposure(s) of interest. (Of the participants, 13% had hypertension and were referred to the program; 33% had serum cholesterol ≥ 260 mg per ml and were referred to the program (serum cholesterol ≥ 300 mg per ml) or to group meetings (serum cholesterol 260–299 mg per ml); 16% smoked ≥ 15 cigarettes per day and were referred to the program, and 34% smoked less than 15 cigarettes per day and received written information on smoking). During more than 10 years' follow-up, the occurrence of CHD, stroke, and death was similar in the intervention group and the nonintervention groups (information available for all subjects).

A. About (100–75) = 25% of the men in the intervention group did not participate in the baseline examinations—and possible subsequent interventions. How can this be expected to influence the observed effect on morbidity and mortality? How could this problem have been handled?

B. About (100–37) = 63% of the participants in the intervention group did not have any of the exposures dealt with in the intervention program. How can this be expected to influence the observed effect on morbidity and mortality? How could this problem have been handled?

7:28   Accidental injuries, common in certain occupations, may partly be due to lack of physical fitness. A randomized trial was conducted to evaluate the effect of physical exercise (flexibility training according to a specified program) on the risk of joint injuries among firefighters. In a city, 469 municipal firefighters working within four fire districts participated in the study. Two of the four fire districts were randomly assigned to receive the training program, and firefighters in the remaining two districts did not receive the program.

A. The purpose of randomization is to avoid confounding. To what extent is this purpose likely to be achieved in the present study?

B. Suppose there had only been two fire districts. To what extent could confounding be avoided by randomization, if one district was randomly assigned to receive (and the other not to receive) the training program?

7:29 In postmenopausal women, osteoporosis is a common cause of fractures. Epidemiologic findings suggest that osteoporosis could perhaps be prevented by physical exercise, calcium supplementation, and estrogen replacement. Postmenopausal women were recruited for a study, and examined with regard to bone density. Of those found to have a bone density above a certain level, a random sample was selected for follow-up without any prior intervention. Women found to have a bone density below that level were randomly assigned to receive one of three interventions prior to follow-up: exercise alone, exercise and calcium tablets, and exercise and estrogen tablets. In these three groups, placebo was used for the tablets not assigned. All four groups were followed for 24 months with regard to bone loss, that is, development of osteoporosis.

One possibility would be to compare each of the three intervention groups with the nonintervention group. Another possibility would be to make comparisons between the three intervention groups. What are the principal differences between these two approaches with regard to possible bias?

7:30 In a WHO cooperative trial, about 10,000 men with high serum cholesterol were randomly assigned to receive a cholesterol-lowering drug (clofibrate) or placebo. During 5 years of treatment and follow-up, information was obtained on the occurrence of myocardial infarction (MI). Prior to follow-up, the subjects were examined with regard to other risk factors for MI—including blood pressure (not influenced by clofibrate). In principle, the study may be used to evaluate the effect of clofibrate, serum cholesterol, and blood pressure on the risk of MI.

In what way, and to what extent, can the randomization be expected to improve the accuracy of the results for:

A. the effect of clofibrate on the risk of MI?

B. the effect of serum cholesterol on the risk of MI?

C. the effect of blood pressure on the risk of MI?

In what ways, and to what extent, can the use of placebo (together with blinding) be expected to improve the accuracy of the results for:

D. the effect of clofibrate on the risk of MI?

E. the effect of serum cholesterol on the risk of MI?

F. the effect of blood pressure on the risk of MI?

G. In what ways (if any) could the accuracy in estimating the effect of serum cholesterol (B and E) differ from that of clofibrate (A and D)?

■ GENERAL QUESTIONS

7:31 What is the major advantage and disadvantage, respectively, of experimental (compared with nonexperimental) study designs in learning about disease causation?

7:32 What are the differences (if any) between an experimental and a nonexperimental study in:

A. selecting a study population?

B. obtaining information on exposures (including potential confounders and modifiers)?

c. follow-up of disease occurrence?

7:33 In a randomized trial, what is the purpose of randomization and on what conditions can this purpose be achieved?

7:34 What is meant by, and what is the purpose of:

A. blocked randomization?

B. stratified randomization?

c. factorial design?

7:35 What is meant by, and what is the purpose of:

A. placebo?

B. single-blinding?

c. double-blinding?

7:36 **A.** What signs may indicate that the blinding is broken?

B. In a randomized double-blind trial, bias may be introduced by differences in side effects between the "active" and placebo treatment. How? Exemplify!

7:37   Even if a trial is not blind, it is essential that staff members are kept unaware of (and cannot predict) the next assignment on the randomization list until the subject has formally entered the trial. Why?

7:38   In a randomized trial, is a bias introduced (and if so, in what direction):

  A. if some of the randomized subjects already have the exposure status induced by the intervention?

  B. if the intervention fails to bring about the intended change in exposure status in all subjects?

7:39   In a randomized trial, does noncompliance with the intervention introduce a bias (and if so, in what direction):

  A. if the result is based on all randomized subjects according to their assignment ("intention-to-treat" analysis)?

  B. if the result is based only on those who comply with the intervention ("on-treatment" analysis)?

7:40   Consider your own recent favorite study. What are the implications for that study of the general problems and possibilities exemplified in the different exercises in this chapter?

8 | *General Exercises*

■■■ **EXERCISE 8:1**

In many countries, a substantial proportion of all women use estrogens to alleviate menopausal symptoms. A study of postmenopausal women in Framingham showed excess risks of cardiovascular diesease (CVD) following estrogen use. But other, previous studies showed no such effect.

The Framingham Study, beginning in 1948, enrolled a probability sample of residents of Framingham, Massachusetts. All study subjects were examined with regard to cardiovascular disease and potential risk indicators for such disease, and were invited to return for routine reexamination every 2 years. The study of estrogen use and CVD, included postmenopausal women over 50 years of age and free of CVD at the twelfth examination (in 1970–1972). The criterion for menopause was cessation of menses more than 1 year earlier. Information on postmenopausal estrogen use, and potential confounders and modifiers, was obtained at the twelfth examination (and to some extent at previous examinations). Of 1,234 study subjects, 302 reported that they had, and 932 that they had not, used postmenopausal estrogens. Follow-up with regard to CVD was from examination 12 through examination 16 (8 years), and was based on findings at the biennial routine examinations, physician reviews of clinic notes, hospital and physician records, and death certificates. A total of 194 cases of CVD were identified, including 45 cases of cerebrovascular disease (RR = 2.27), 51 cases of myocardial infarction (RR = 1.87), and 69 cases of angina pectoris (RR = 2.00).

The general question concerned the effect (if any) of postmenopausal estrogen use on the risk of CVD, and may include several more specific questions.

A:1   Such questions should be specified with regard to the exposure (postmenopausal estrogen use). What aspects of the exposure could be taken into account?

A:2   The questions should also be specified with regard to modifiers. Why?

A:3   In what other respects should the questions be specified?

The study population was a probability sample of women who lived in Framingham. Only postmenopausal women over 50 years of age and free of CVD were included.

B:1   Why were women with previous CVD not included in the study?

B:2   The lower age limit was 50 years. What are the possible advantages and disadvantages, respectively, of using an upper age limit as well?

B:3   Is the validity of the results of the present study likely to be improved by selecting the study population as a probability sample? Why/why not?

B:4   Is the precision of the results (with the present study size) likely to be improved by selecting the study population as a probability sample? Why/why not?

B:5   Is the generalizability of the results of the present study likely to be improved by selecting the study population as a probability sample? Why/why not?

Each woman was classified as either exposed or unexposed to postmenopausal estrogen. A woman was considered as exposed if she ever reported use during examinations 8 through 12. Inquiries at examination 8 included previous use of postmenopausal estrogen.

C:1   The duration of estrogen use, dose of estrogen, or type of estrogen was not taken into account in the present study. In what direction (if any) is this likely to bias the relative risk?

C:2 The use of estrogen during follow-up was not considered. In what direction (if any) is this likely to bias the relative risk?

C:3 The induction time was not taken into account in the data analysis. In what direction (if any) is this likely to bias the relative risk?

C:4 There could be exposure misclassification due to errors in the reporting of estrogen use, for example, because some women did not recall their estrogen use or did not know what type of hormone (drug) they had been taking. In what direction (if any) is this likely to bias the relative risk?

The following potential confounders were considered in the data analysis: age, systolic blood pressure, body-mass index, plasma cholesterol (ratio of total cholesterol to HDL cholesterol), alcohol intake, and cigarette smoking.

D:1 Postmenopausal estrogens are used with the purpose of alleviating certain symptoms, including some cardiovascular symptoms, occurring at menopause. Could such indications for estrogen introduce additional confounding, and if so, in what direction would this bias the relative risk?

D:2 Women at high risk of thrombosis should not use postmenopausal estrogens. Could such contraindications for estrogen introduce additional confounding, and if so, in what direction would this bias the relative risk?

D:3 Women who use postmenopausal estrogens may discontinue their use because they are identified as being at high risk of CVD (thrombosis). Could this introduce additional confounding, and if so, in what direction would this bias the relative risk?

D:4 When cigarette smoking was taken into account as a confounder, all women were classified according to whether or not they had smoked cigarettes regularly during the last year before follow-up (two categories). Could the smoking-adjusted relative risks still be confounded by smoking? Why/why not?

D:5 Estrogen use was found to have a considerable effect on the risk of CVD among smokers (RR = 3.16), but little or no effect among nonsmokers. The confounders that were taken into account were the same as above. Could the observed effect in smokers be confounded by smoking? Why/why not?

In the Framingham Study, efforts were made to identify all incident cases of CVD regardless of whether or not they had been routinely recognized or hospitalized. For example, 35 percent of the identified cases of myocardial infarction would not be recognized in ordinary medical care. Thus, the sensitivity in the disease classification may be higher in the Framingham Study than in previous studies.

E:1   Could this explain the lack of effect in previous studies, if the misclassification (low sensitivity) in these studies was: a) nondifferential, that is, independent of estrogen use; b) differential, with a lower sensitivity in women who had used estrogen; c) differential, with a lower sensitivity in women who had not used estrogen?

E:2   During follow-up, women who use estrogen may be examined by a doctor more often than other women. This could introduce a differential disease misclassification (detection bias). In what direction would this bias the relative risk? How is this potential source of error influenced by the biennial routine examinations in the present study?

E:3   Prior to follow-up, women who use estrogen may be examined by a doctor more often than other women. This could introduce a bias, if women using estrogen were more likely than others to have a CVD diagnosed prior to follow-up and thus not to be included in the study. In what direction would this bias the relative risk? How is this potential source of error influenced by the biennial routine examinations in the present study?

■■■ **EXERCISE 8:2**

The possibility that alcohol intake could increase the risk of breast cancer was investigated, using information collected for the first National Health and Nutrition Examination Survey (NHANES I). This survey was conducted from 1971 to 1975 in a sample of the civilian noninstitutionalized population of the United States, and included a medical examination, a medical and sociodemographic history, and a dietary questionnaire with information on alcohol use. From 1981 to 1984, subjects were traced and interviewed again for the NHANES I Epidemiologic Follow-up Study

(NHEFS). In the present study, hospital records and death certificates were used to identify cases of breast cancer between the initial examination (NHANES I) and the follow-up examination about 10 years later (NHEFS). A total of 121 cases were identified in 7,188 women who participated in both examinations, and were aged 25–74 years at the initial examination.

There is likely to be an interest in several specific questions concerning the effect (if any) of alcohol intake on the risk of breast cancer. But the possibility of answering these questions is influenced by the size (and composition) of the study population as well as by the available information on alcohol intake. The present study was based on information collected for NHANES I, which introduced certain limitations in these respects.

A:1 In what ways could limitations in the size (and composition) of the study population influence the possibility of answering specific questions?

A:2 In what ways could limitations in the available exposure information influence the possibility of answering specific questions?

The subjects selected for NHANES I were a sample of the civilian noninstitutionalized population of the United States in 1971–1975. Subjects were traced and interviewed again for the NHEFS in 1981–1984. Individual follow-up periods were between these two examinations. The study included women aged 25–74 years at the time of NHANES I.

B:1 What are the advantages and disadvantages, respectively, of using information from NHANES I for a study of alcohol intake and breast cancer?

B:2 Women with a history of breast cancer were not included in the present study. Why?

B:3 Women who did not provide information on their alcohol consumption at the initial examination were lost to the present study. In what ways (if any) could this have influenced the validity?

B:4 Women who did not participate in the follow-up examination were lost to the present study. Could this influence the validity in some other way than the loss of women at the initial examination (B:3, above)? Why/why not?

B:5   A total of 1,158 women (about 14%) were lost because they did not participate in the follow-up examination. Suppose that, with these women included, there was no effect (true RR = a*D/b*C = 1). What would the observed relative risk be, if there was a selection bias with loss of: a) 30 percent of the exposed cases, but only 14 percent of the unexposed cases and of all exposed and unexposed women (person-years); b) 30 percent of the unexposed cases, but only 14 percent of the exposed cases and of all exposed and unexposed women (person-years)?

At the initial examination, each woman was asked whether she had had at least one drink of beer, wine, or liquor during the previous year. Women who said they had not, were classified as unexposed. Women who said they had, were asked about the type, quantity, and frequency of alcohol intake. This information was used to estimate the average alcohol intake, and exposed women were classified in three categories: < 1.3; 1.3–4.9; and ≥ 5 g/day.

C:1   Could there be a differential exposure misclassification resulting in an overestimation (or underestimation) of the relative risk? Why/why not?

C:2   What are the principal sources of nondifferential exposure misclassification in the present study?

C:3   There may be exposure misclassification due to a general tendency for people to underreport their alcohol intake. In what direction is this likely to bias the relative risk?

At the initial examination, information was obtained on the following potential confounders: age, smoking, education, body mass index, total dietary fat, parity, age at menarche, and menopausal status. In addition, information on age at first parturition, and family history of breast cancer, was obtained at the follow-up examination. Information on age was available for all women, but information on the other potential confounders was missing for some women (including 33 of the 121 cases).

D:1   What is required for a factor to introduce confounding?

D:2   The risk of breast cancer increases with age, but alcohol consumption was more common in younger than in older women. In what direction did confounding by age bias the relative risk?

D:3   Smoking was found to increase with alcohol consumption. Suppose that smoking increases the risk of breast cancer. In what direction would confounding by smoking bias the relative risk?

D:4   The risk of breast cancer is increased by ionizing radiation, postmenopausal estrogen use, and a history of benign breast disease. No information on these factors was available in the present study. What is required for each of these factors to introduce confounding that would result in a) an overestimation of the relative risk; b) an underestimation of the relative risk?

D:5   Total fat intake, as estimated from a 24-hour recall interview at the initial examination, was taken into account as a confounder. Could there still be confounding by fat intake? Why/ why not?

Follow-up was from the initial examination (NHANES I) in 1971–1975 to the follow-up examination (NHEFS) in 1981–1984. Cases of breast cancer were identified through hospital records or death certificates.

E:1   Most cases were identified through hospital records. They were considered to occur on the date of the first admission for which breast cancer was mentioned as the discharge diagnosis. Could the identification of these cases have introduced a differential disease misclassification? Why/why not?

E:2   Suppose that some of the cases identified through hospital records were cases of early, asymptomatic breast cancer detected at screening examinations and referred to the hospital for treatment. Could the identification of these cases have introduced a differential disease misclassification? Why/why not?

E:3   Some of the cases were identified only through death certificates. They were considered to occur on the date of death. Could the identification of these cases have introduced a differential disease misclassification? Why/why not?

E:4   There is some evidence of differences in etiology between premenopausal and postmenopausal breast cancer. In what ways, if any, should this influence the planning of a study of alcohol intake and breast cancer?

Using your answers to the previous questions, and adding any other sources of bias: What are the sources of error that could introduce a bias towards RR = ∞ in the present study? Try to judge the importance of each of these sources of error, in terms of the extent to which they are likely to introduce such bias.

F.   List the sources of error that could introduce a bias towards RR = ∞. Put the most important sources of error on the top of your list, and the least important at the bottom.

Using your answers to the previous questions, and adding any other sources of bias: What are the sources of error that could introduce a bias towards RR = 0 in the present study? Try to judge the importance of each of these sources of error, in terms of the extent to which they are likely to introduce such bias.

G.   List the sources of error that could introduce a bias towards RR = 0. Put the most important sources of error on the top of your list, and the least important at the bottom.

Using your answers to the previous questions, and adding any other sources of bias: What are the sources of error that could introduce a bias towards RR = 1 in the present study? Try to judge the importance of each of these sources of error, in terms of the extent to which they are likely to introduce such bias.

H.   List the sources of error that could introduce a bias towards RR = 1. Put the most important sources of error on the top of your list, and the least important at the bottom.

▄▄▄ EXERCISE 8:3

It has been suggested that a low dietary intake of selenium may increase the risk of certain cancers. The effect of selenium on the risk of thyroid cancer was investigated in a case-referent study. During the period 1972–1986 more than 100,000 subjects, living in four counties in Norway, had their sera stored in the JANUS serum bank. At the same time, a self-administered questionnaire on diet was answered by about 90 percent of the subjects in three of the four counties. Since 1952, all cancers diagnosed in Norway are to be reported to a national cancer registry. Unique personal identification numbers made it possible to link this source of information to a data file on all subjects who had their sera stored in JANUS, in order to identify all cancers diagnosed in these subjects between their entry in the serum bank and the end of 1985. For each case of thyroid cancer, three referents were selected from the JANUS file. The referents were selected among subjects free from cancer, and were individually matched to the cases by sex, age, calendar year for blood sampling, and county of residence. The sera of cases and referents were identified and analyzed with regard to selenium. Similarly, the questionnaires of cases and referents were identified and examined with regard to dietary sources of selenium.

The study was designed to answer questions concerning the effect of selenium on the risk of thyroid cancer. Information was obtained on serum levels of selenium as well as on dietary intake of selenium.

A:1   Is there a primary interest in the effect of serum selenium—or should the serum levels of selenium be thought of only as a measure of dietary intake?

A:2   What difference would this make with regard to the questions addressed in the present study?

The study population used to study the effect of serum selenium may be defined as all subjects who had their sera stored in the JANUS serum bank between 1972 and the end of 1985. When studying the effect of dietary intake of selenium, only subjects living in three of the four counties were included, and about 90 percent of these subjects answered the diet questionnaire at entry.

B:1   Define the study population used to study the effect of dietary intake of selenium.

B:2   Define a) the study period, and b) the individual follow-up periods.

B:3   Define the study base used to study the effect of a) serum selenium, and b) dietary intake of selenium.

B:4   Suppose that, in a study base of one million person-years at risk, 20 percent had high levels of serum selenium (unexposed), and the incidence rate of thyroid cancer was 5 cases per 100,000 person-years at risk. How many unexposed cases should be expected, if there was no effect (RR = 1)?

Referents were selected as a sample of the study base. Three referents were matched to each case. Exposure information was obtained only for the cases and referents, by analyzing their sera and questionnaires (collected from all subjects prior to follow-up).

C:1   What is the purpose of selecting referents?

C:2   Costs are reduced by using information from the cases and referents, rather than from all subjects in the study population. Suppose that 50 cases occurred, and 150 referents were selected, in a study population of 100,000 subjects. By how much are the costs reduced, if the cost was a) 50 USD for analyzing each serum sample, and b) 5 USD for analyzing each questionnaire?

C:3   Precision is also reduced by using information from the cases and referents, rather than from all subjects in the study population. By how much is the precision reduced, if three times as many referents as cases were selected?

C:4   In what ways, if any, could the validity be influenced by using information from the cases and referents, rather than from all subjects in the study population?

Serum samples were collected from all subjects in the study population as they entered the study, and were kept frozen at $-25°C$. When the cases had been identified, and the referents had been selected, their serum samples were thawed and analyzed with regard to selenium concentration. Similarly, the self-administered questionnaires on diet (answered by study subjects at entry) were identified for the cases, and referents and examined with regard to major sources of selenium intake (bread, fish, meat).

D:1   A differential exposure misclassification could be introduced by differences between laboratories or examiners, differences by time of examination, or by the examiner's awareness that a questionnaire (or serum sample) represents a case or a referent. How can this be avoided?

D:2   Serum selenium was measured in a single serum sample, collected at the beginning of follow-up. The questionnaire provided information on three sources of dietary selenium intake: the current number of meat dinners per week, fish dinners per week, and slices of bread per day. What are the principal sources of non-differential exposure misclassification?

D:3 Some thyroid cancers grow very slowly. Suppose that such tumors may reduce the dietary intake and serum levels of selenium, even before they are diagnosed. In what direction would this bias the relative risk (considering subjects with a low intake, or low serum level, as exposed)? How should this problem be handled?

D:4 Suppose that some of the questionnaires and serum samples collected prior to follow-up were lost at a later stage. Could this introduce selection bias?

The incidence of thyroid cancer varies by age and sex. In addition, there were differences in incidence between the four counties where the study subjects lived. Age, sex, and county of residence were taken into account as potential confounders in the present study.

E:1 Radiation has been found to increase the risk of thyroid cancer. What else is required for radiation to introduce confounding in the present study?

E:2 Other diseases of the thyroid gland, including goiter, have been suggested as risk factors for thyroid cancer. How should this possible source of confounding be handled?

E:3 Dietary intake of iodine has also been suggested as a risk factor for thyroid cancer. How should this possible source of confounding be handled?

Follow-up was achieved by a record linkage, using information from the JANUS file and the national cancer registry. Efforts were made to identify all cases of thyroid cancer diagnosed in the study population during follow-up.

F:1 The utilization of register data for follow-up has advantages with regard to cost and convenience. What are the most important disadvantages, if any?

F:2 Suppose that some cases of thyroid cancer were not identified and reported to the cancer registry, but that the underreporting was independent of selenium intake and serum levels. In what direction, if any, would this bias the relative risk?

F:3   Thyroid cancers may be classified as papillary, follicular, medullary, or anaplastic, according to their appearance. Suppose that selenium would only affect the risk of one of these types of thyroid cancer. How would this influence a relative risk based on all cases of thyroid cancer?

F:4   In the present study, the identified thyroid cancers were reviewed by microscopic examination and classified in accord with the principles of the World Health Organization. Benign tumors and medullary tumors were excluded. Could a differential disease misclassification be introduced at these examinations, and if so, how should this be avoided?

When studying the effect of serum selenium, a total of 45 cases of thyroid cancer were identified (after exclusion of one benign tumor, and one medullary tumor). For two of these cases, no information on serum selenium could be obtained because the amount of serum was insufficient. In a matched analysis, based on the remaining 43 cases and 129 matched referents, the estimated relative risk (with 95% confidence interval) was 7.7 (1.3–44.7) at low levels, and 6.1 (1.3–28.0) at moderate levels of serum selenium (compared with high levels of serum selenium). When the time since the serum sample was collected (possible induction time) was taken into account, there was an effect during the first 6 years but not thereafter. Considering possible sources of error (including B-F, above):

G.   What conclusion can be drawn concerning the effect of serum selenium on the risk of thyroid cancer?

When studying the effect of dietary intake, there were 29 cases and 87 referents. The findings did not suggest any association between thyroid cancer and the three major sources of selenium intake. Considering possible sources of error (including B-F, above):

H.   What conclusions can be drawn from this?

■ EXERCISE 8:4

A study was initiated against the background of clinical observations, suggesting that elderly people developing a bleeding peptic ulcer had often been using certain drugs: non-aspirin non-steroidal anti-inflammatory drugs (NANSAID). Over a 2-year period at two hospitals in Nottingham, England, a total of 903 patients were admitted for suspected hematemesis (bloody vomiting) or melena (bloody stools), or both. A bleeding peptic (gastric or duodenal) ulcer was diagnosed in 406 of these patients, of which 290 were 60 years of age or older (cases). For every case, two age- and sex-matched referents were selected, one from among other patients in the same acute medical intake (hospital referent) and one from the practice register of the general practice to which the case belonged (community referent). All interviews were carried out by a single trained interviewer using the same questionnaire. Habits such as drug use "were regarded as those prevailing on the day of interview" for the community referents (interviewed in their homes) and "on the day of the event causing admission" for the cases and hospital referents (interviewed in the hospital). The nonresponse for the interviews was 21 percent (cases), 0 percent (hospital referents), and 10 percent (community referents), respectively.

The study was initiated against the background of observations, suggesting that elderly people who developed a bleeding peptic ulcer often had been using certain drugs (NANSAID).

A:1   What was the general question?

A:2   This general question includes several more specific questions. In what respects should these questions be specified? Exemplify!

In a case-referent study, the referents should provide information on the occurrence of the exposure in the study base (or study population). The possibility of a referent selection bias can only be judged by considering the referents in relation to the study base (or study population).

B:1   Define the study population and the study base of the present study.

B:2   What sources of bias could be avoided by restrictions when selecting the study population? Exemplify!

B:3   If the study could have been performed elsewhere, would there be any reasons to look for some other source population for the study than people living in the Nottingham area? What reasons?

For every case, two age and sex-matched referents were selected, one from among other patients in the same acute medical intake (hospital referent) and one from the practice register of the general practice to which the case belonged (community referent).

C:1   Could a referent selection bias have been introduced by the community referents? Why/why not?

C:2   Could a referent selection bias have been introduced by the hospital referents? Why/why not?

C:3   What is the purpose of matching referents to the cases on a confounder, such as age or sex? In what circumstances can this purpose be achieved?

C:4   What are the possible disadvantages of matching referents to the cases on a confounder, such as age or sex?

Subjects were classified as exposed or unexposed on the basis of their reported drug (NANSAID) use on the day of the interview (community referents, interviewed in their homes), or on the day of the event causing admission to the hospital (cases and hospital referents, interviewed in the hospital). All interviews were carried out by a single trained interviewer using the same questionnaire.

D:1   Exposure information was collected as the cases were identified, rather than prior to follow-up. In what ways could this influence exposure misclassification?

D:2   Considering the possibility of differential exposure misclassification, what are the principal differences between the hospital referents and the community referents?

D:3   Exposure information was not obtained for 21 percent of the cases (and 10% of the community referents). What additional information would be useful, in judging whether this is likely to introduce a bias?

The questionnaire provided information on potential confounders, including age, sex, social class, alcohol, tobacco, previous diseases, and other drugs.

E:1   What other drugs deserve special attention as potential confounders?

E:2   Suppose that the medical conditions for which NANSAID was taken, or the general health status of subjects who use NANSAID, would affect the risk of bleeding peptic ulcer. If so, there would be confounding by these conditions (or by general health status). How could such confounding be avoided in a study of NANSAID use and bleeding peptic ulcer?

E:3   A previous peptic ulcer may increase the risk of bleeding peptic ulcer. If so, what else is required for confounding by previous peptic ulcer resulting in: a) overestimation of the relative risk (bias towards $RR = \infty$), or b) underestimation of the relative risk (bias towards $RR = 0$)?

E:4   Age could be a confounder, or a modifier, or both. What is the difference between confounding and effect modification by age?

During a 2-year period, cases of bleeding peptic ulcer were identified at two hospitals in Nottingham among patients aged ≥ 60 years, admitted for suspected hematemesis or melena, or both.

F:1   Could a bias have been introduced by the way in which the cases were identified, if the study base is defined as the person-time at risk contributed by subjects aged ≥ 60 years and recorded in the practice registers?

F:2   Would this bias be avoided by defining the study base secondary to the cases (i.e., as the person-time at risk contributed by subjects aged ≥ 60 years who, if they had developed a bleeding peptic ulcer, would have been identified at the two hospitals)?

F:3   NANSAID users are more likely than nonusers to see a physician regularly. Could this be a source of differential disease misclassification? Why/why not?

Suppose that, when using the hospital referents, the results suggested that NANSAID use increases the risk of bleeding peptic ulcer—but that no such effect was seen when using the community referents.

G:1   What sources of bias could result in an overestimation of the relative risk when using the hospital referents, but not when using the community referents?

G:2   What sources of bias could result in an underestimation of the relative risk when using the community referents, but not when using the hospital referents?

Suppose that, when using the community referents, the results suggested that NANSAID use increases the risk of bleeding peptic ulcer—but that no such effect was seen when using the hospital referents.

H:1   What sources of bias could result in an overestimation of the relative risk when using the community referents, but not when using the hospital referents?

H:2   What sources of bias could result in an underestimation of the relative risk when using the hospital referents, but not when using the community referents?

The relative risks (with 95 percent confidence intervals) were 2.7 (1.7–4.4) and 3.8 (2.2–6.4) when using information from the community and hospital referents, respectively. An excess risk was found for both gastric and duodenal ulcer, in men as well as in women. The number of subjects was considered too small to calculate relative risks associated with the specific drugs involved.

I:1   What sources of bias could result in an overestimation of the relative risk both when using the community referents and the hospital referents?

I:2   What conclusions can be drawn from the findings of the present study?

■■■ **EXERCISE 8:5**

Intervention to reduce smoking, hypertension, and elevated serum cholesterol in "high risk" men aged 35–57 years was evaluated in the Multiple Risk Factor Intervention Trial (MRFIT). A purpose was to investigate to what extent (if any) this reduces the risk of death from coronary heart disease (CHD). A total of 361,662 men were initially recruited at 22 clinical centers, for example, by offering voluntary screening to industry and government employee groups. Only men who fulfilled certain eligibility criteria, including a high risk score, were invited to participate in the trial. The risk score was based on smoking, blood pressure, and serum cholesterol. Thus, for instance, some of the high risk men were smokers and others were nonsmokers (but had a high risk score due to their blood pressure or serum cholesterol, or both). Eligibility was determined at three successive screening visits. The 12,866 men who were eligible and willing to participate were examined with regard to potential confounders and randomly allocated to two groups of about equal size. One group received a special intervention, urging men who smoked cigarettes to quit, men with hypertension to follow a stepped-care protocol including treatment with antihypertensive drugs, and men with elevated serum cholesterol to follow dietary advice, including reduced intake of cholesterol and saturated fat. The other group did not receive this special intervention but was referred for usual care. During 6 years of follow-up with regard to deaths from CHD, men in both groups were asked to return for annual examinations, including smoking habits, blood pressure, and serum cholesterol.

Several general questions are addressed in this study. There are questions concerning the effect of the intervention program (or components thereof) on smoking habits, blood pressure, and serum cholesterol. These questions may, however, be answered in a much smaller and less expensive trial. More important, there are questions concerning effects on the risk of death from CHD, including: 1) the overall effect of the intervention program; 2) the separate effects of the intervention against a) smoking, b) hypertension, and c) elevated serum cholesterol; and 3) the effects of a) smoking, b) hypertension, and c) elevated serum cholesterol. (At the time, there was some experimental evidence concerning the effect of hypertension, but little such evidence concerning the effects of smoking and serum cholesterol on CHD mortality).

A:1   Obviously, the overall intervention effect (1) depends upon the separate intervention effects (2a-c). What else determines the overall intervention effect (1)?

A:2   Obviously, the separate intervention effects (2) depend upon the effect of the corresponding exposure (3). What else determines the separate intervention effects (2a-c)?

A:3   The effects of smoking, hypertension, and elevated serum cholesterol (3a-c) were investigated in high risk men. Are these effects likely to depend upon the extent to which these factors are associated (e.g., smokers have hypertension, elevated serum cholesterol, or both) in any particular population of high risk men? Why/why not?

The study population was 12,866 men, aged 35–57 years, who fulfilled certain eligibility criteria, including a high risk score based on smoking, blood pressure, and serum cholesterol. Men with serum cholesterol $\geq$ 350 mg/dl, or diastolic blood pressure $\geq$ 115 mm Hg, were not included because of their "therapeutic requirements." During 6 years of follow-up with regard to CHD mortality, men in the intervention group participated in the intervention program, and men in both groups were examined annualy with regard to smoking, blood pressure, and serum cholesterol.

B:1　The study was restricted to men aged 35–57 years at the initial examination. CHD mortality increases with age. Would it be more efficient to restrict the study to men over 57 years of age: a) if the absolute effect was not modified by age; or b) if the relative effect was not modified by age?

B:2　Subjects were not eligible if they had a history of (or symptoms and signs of, treatments for) diabetes, angina pectoris, or myocardial infarction, or if they had a body weight $\geq$ 150 percent of "desirable weight." Why?

B:3　Subjects were not eligible if they had illnesses or disabilities likely to impair full participation in the trial, diets incompatible with the MRFIT food pattern (dietary advice), or expected geographic mobility. Why?

B:4　Subjects who were already under treatment with antihypertensive medications were included as having hypertension (regardless of their blood pressure level). Those randomized to the intervention group were usually transferred (with the permission of their private physicians) to the MRFIT intervention against hypertension. Those randomized to the nonintervention group usually continued their previous antihypertensive treatment. In what direction, if any, does this bias the relative risk? How could this source of bias be avoided?

B:5　The effect, if any, on CHD mortality of a change in exposure status (smoking cessation, or lowering of elevated blood pressure or serum cholesterol) may occur only after a certain induction time. Suppose that (for one of these factors) the induction time would be a) 0; b) 2 years; c) 5 years; d) 10 years. How would this influence the results of the present study?

After a baseline examination with regard to exposures (including some potential confounders and modifiers), the study subjects were randomly allocated to the intervention and nonintervention group. The randomization was performed in blocks of four to six subjects, after stratification by clinic. The assignment was obtained by the local clinic coordinator by telephone from the coordinating center only after a subject had been found to be eligible and willing to participate and had formally entered the trial.

C:1   What is the principal advantage and disadvantage, respectively, of conducting a randomized experiment (rather than a nonexperimental study)?

C:2   Why was the randomization performed in blocks of four to six subjects? What would be the disadvantages (if any) of using a) a smaller block size; b) a larger block size?

C:3   The randomization list was kept at the coordinating center, and the clinic was informed about the assignment only after the subject had formally entered the trial. Why?

C:4   The results could be based on all subjects included in the randomization according to their assignment (intention-to-treat analysis), or on those who complied with the intervention and changed their exposure status. What is the difference with regard to accuracy and sources of error?

C:5   In the present trial it was not possible to use a sham intervention (placebo) for subjects in the nonintervention group. What difference could this make in terms of accuracy and sources of error?

At baseline, current cigarette smoking was reported by 59 percent of the men in each group. At the annual examinations during follow-up, this proportion was 32–36 percent in the intervention group and 46–56 percent in the nonintervention group. Similarly, there were reductions in blood pressure and serum cholesterol levels in the intervention group—and to some extent also in the nonintervention group.

D:1   Although the proportion of smokers was reduced in the intervention group, there were still 32–36 percent current cigarette smokers in this group during follow-up. In what direction, if any, does this bias the relative risk of death from CHD?

D:2   There was also some reduction in the proportion of smokers in the nonintervention group. This was not anticipated by the investigators. a) What reasons could there be for this reduction, and for similar reductions in blood pressure and serum cholesterol in the nonintervention group? b) In what direction, if any, does this bias the relative risk of death from CHD?

D:3 All study subjects participated in the baseline examination. But all subjects did not participate in the annual examinations during follow-up. Could this have resulted in an overestimation of the changes in smoking, blood pressure, and serum cholesterol due to the MRFIT intervention?

D:4 Among those who participated in the annual examinations during follow-up, there may be misclassification with regard to smoking, blood pressure, and serum cholesterol. Could this have resulted in an overestimation of the changes in smoking, blood pressure, and serum cholesterol due to the MRFIT intervention?

Potential confounders are to be found among factors that increase or reduce the risk of death from CHD—for example, dietary habits, alcohol intake, body mass, and physical exercise. Subjects may be examined with regard to risk factors at baseline and during follow-up.

E:1 Could there be confounding by such factors at baseline: a) in an intention-to-treat analysis; b) in an analysis based on those who changed their exposure status? Why/why not?

E:2 Could there be confounding by such factors during follow-up: a) in an intention-to-treat analysis; b) in an analysis based on those who changed their exposure status? Why/why not?

E:3 Men with both hypertension and elevated serum cholesterol were assigned intervention against both (intervention group) or neither (nonintervention group). Does this introduce confounding by blood pressure when evaluating the effect of serum cholesterol?

Efforts were made to identify all deaths that occurred in the study population during the study period. A total of 525 deaths were identified. By the end of the period, there were 30 subjects (15 in each group) whose survival status remained unknown. For each death, the cause of death was determined by a panel of cardiologists who reviewed the available information—for example, death certificates, clinic and hospital records. Of all deaths, 239 were identified as deaths from CHD.

F:1 What are the possible sources of differential disease misclassification? What could be done to avoid differential disease misclassification?

F:2 Suppose that there would be an effect on the risk of death from myocardial infarction (MI), but not on the risk of death from other CHD. How would this influence the relative risk of death from CHD?

F:3 Is there likely to be a selection bias due to selective loss to follow-up? Why/why not?

There were 115 deaths from CHD in the intervention group, and 124 in the nonintervention group (RR = 0.93; 0.75–1.15, 90% confidence interval). The relative risk (and the number of deaths from CHD in the intervention and nonintervention group, respectively) by exposure status at baseline was: smoking RR = 0.96 (86 and 89 deaths), nonsmoking RR = 0.84 (29 and 35 deaths); hypertensive RR = 1.01 (80 and 79 deaths), nonhypertensive RR = 0.79 (35 and 45 deaths); serum cholesterol ≥ 250 mg/dl RR = 0.90 (66 and 73 deaths), serum cholesterol < 250 mg/dl RR = 0.97 (49 and 51 deaths). Considering possible sources of error in the present study (including B-F, above):

G:1 What conclusions can be drawn from these results, with regard to each of the three effects discussed previously (A): 1) the overall intervention effect, 2) the separate intervention effects, and 3) the effects of smoking, hypertension, and elevated serum cholesterol on the risk of death from CHD?

G:2 What additional information on the methods and findings of the present study would be useful in answering the above question? In what ways could this information be expected to influence the interpretation of the results?

Suppose that you were asked to design a trial to evaluate the effect on CHD mortality of smoking cessation, and lowering of elevated blood pressure and serum cholesterol, respectively.

H. In what ways, if any, would this trial be different from the present study?

9 | *Answers to Exercises*

CHAPTER 2

2:1   *Aspects:* Quantity and frequency—for example, average number of cigarettes smoked per day. Type of cigarettes—for example, by size, filter, and content of active components. Type of smoking behavior—for example, depth of inhalation, and size of the cigarette end left. Patterns, timing, and duration of smoking could also be of interest depending upon the suggested mechanism of action.

Categories: Exposed categories are usually defined on the basis of the average number of cigarettes smoked per day (e.g., 1–4, 5–14, 15–24, 25–34, 35–44, 45+). It could be useful to make a categorization for different time periods, but this is often made only for current smoking while considering "past smokers" as a single category. Other aspects, for example, type of cigarettes and smoking behavior, may be considered separately. The unexposed category should only include those who have never smoked.

Coldiz GA, Bonita R, Stampfer MJ, et al. Cigarette smoking and risk of stroke in middle-aged women. *N. Engl. J. Med.* 318(1988):937–941.

2:2   *Exposure:* breast feeding. *Unexposed category:* no breast feeding. However, the alternative to breast feeding is not simply "no breast feeding," but rather some other way of feeding the baby. These alternatives may include, for instance, cow's milk and powdered milk drunk from a bottle or spoon that may or may not be kept clean. For the scientific purpose of learning about the causation of infant death from diarrhea, as well as for the practical purpose of preventing such deaths, it may be useful to separate the different alternatives to breast feeding. In addition, there may be different aspects of breast feeding worth considering.

Victoria CG, Smith PG, Vaughan JP, et al. Infant feeding and deaths due to diarrhea: a case-control study. *Am. J. Epidemiol.* 129(1989):1032–1041.

2:3 The investigated exposure was "occupational exercise," and the highly exposed were subjects with little or no physical exercise during working hours. However, there is no reason to believe that the effect of physical exercise during working hours would be any different from that of other physical exercise. Thus, the exposure of interest is "physical exercise" rather than physical exercise during working hours. The highly exposed should be subjects with little physical exercise (a sedentary life) rather than those with little physical exercise during working hours (a sedentary job).

Vena JE, Graham S, Zielezny M, et al. Lifetime occupational exercise and colon cancer. *Am. J. Epidemiol.* 122(1985):357–365.

2:4A *Exposure:* use of fenoterol by MDI. *Unexposed category:* no use of fenoterol by MDI. However, in the treatment of asthma, the alternative to use of fenoterol by MDI is not likely to be simply no such use, but rather the use of some other drug or alternative treatment. This should be taken into account when defining the unexposed category, since the effect will depend upon the alternative. (Of course, it may also be useful to consider different aspects of fenoterol use by MDI, e.g. quantity, frequency, and duration of use.)

2:4B *Exposure:* dietary intake of protein. The effect of a high intake will, of course, depend upon the alternative, that is, the unexposed category. This is likely to be a specified "low" intake of protein. However, a lower protein intake also means a lower intake of calories—or a higher intake of some other source of calories. (In addition, other aspects of protein intake may have to be considered. For instance, foods rich in protein, such as meat, are cooked in different ways, and when grilled or fried at high temperatures they produce substances that may be carcinogenic.)

Crane J, Pearce N, Flatt A, et al. Prescribed fenoterol and death from asthma in New Zealand, 1981–83: case-control study. *Lancet* 1(1989):917–922.

Gerhardsson de Verdier M, Hagman U, Steineck G, et al. Diet, body mass and colorectal cancer: a case-referent study in Stockholm. *Int. J. Cancer* 46(1990):832–838.

2:5A The "exposure" of interest could be "family history of leukemia" if the purpose of the study was simply to identify people at high risk of leukemia. But if there is an interest in the causation of leukemia, a family history of leukemia may be regarded as an indicator of genetic and environmental factors shared by members of the same family.

2:5B "Maternal smoking" could refer to maternal smoking during pregnancy (i.e., exposure of the fetus in utero) or after giving birth (i.e., exposure of the newborn baby to passive smoking), or both.

Linet MS, Van Natta ML, Brookmeyer R, et al. Familial cancer history and chronic lymphocytic leukemia: a case-control study. *Am. J. Epidemiol.* 130(1989):655–664;

Malloy MH, Kleinman JC, Land GH, Schramm WF. The association of maternal smoking with age and cause of infant death. *Am. J. Epidemiol.* 128(1988):46–55.

2:6A Information was obtained on the husband's smoking habits. But the exposure of interest is likely to be passive smoking, that is, the inhalation of smoke from other people's smoking. Passive smoking may or may not be reflected by the husband's smoking habits.

2:6B To the extent that the inhalation of tobacco smoke (active and passive smoking) is considered as one exposure, the result suggests that smoking (active or passive) should be compared to no inhalation of tobacco smoke, that is, no active *or* passive smoking.

2:6C Hair color was used as an indicator of pigmentation. But pigmentation of the skin is more likely to be the exposure of interest, depending upon the mechanism for the effect of pigmentation.

Hirayama T. Non-smoking wives of heavy smokers have a higher risk of lung cancer: a study from Japan. *Br. Med. J.* 282(1981): 183–185;

Beitner H, Norell SE, Ringborg U, et al. Malignant melanoma: aetiological importance of individual pigmentation and sun exposure. *Br. J. Dermatol.* 122(1990):43–51.

2:7 From a practical (clinical or public health) point of view, there is primarily an interest in the effect of vitamin E intake. But for the scientific purpose of learning about the etiology of cancer there may, in addition, be an interest in the effect of serum levels of vitamin E. (To the extent that serum levels reflect the dietary intake of vitamin E, the effects would be similar.)

> Knekt P, Aromaa A, Maatela J, et al. Serum vitamin E and risk of cancer among Finnish men during a 10-year follow-up. *Am. J. Epidemiol.* 127(1988):28–41.

2:8 For the purpose of learning about the causation of death from ischemic heart disease, the exposure of interest is the actual dietary intake of, for example, fatty fish. (Dietary advice may fail to alter long-term dietary habits, but this should be considered as a source of exposure misclassification.)

> Burr ML, Fehily AM, Gilbert JF, et al. Effects of changes in fat, fish, and fibre intakes on death and myocardial reinfarction: diet and reinfarction trial (DART). *Lancet* 2(1989):757–761.

2:9 Any potential vehicle for L. monocytogenes infection. (The study identified a special brand of Mexican style soft cheese as a main source of infection, RR = 8.5 (2.4–26.2, 95% confidence interval), and a laboratory study showed that such cheese was contaminated by one phage type of L. monocytogenes.)

> Linnan MJ, Mascola M, Lou XD, et al. Epidemic listeriosis associated with Mexican-style cheese. *N. Engl. J. Med.* 319(1988):823–828.

2:10 Type of benzodiazepines, for example those of long versus short elimination half-life (duration of sedative effect). Amount, frequency, and patterns of drug intake, for example, low dose every day versus high dose once or twice a week. Timing in relation to physical activity, for example daytime use versus at bedtime only. Duration of treatment (benzodiazepine use) could also be relevant.

> Ray WA, Griffin MR, Downey W. Benzodiazepines of long and short elimination half-life and the risk of hip fracture. JAMA 262(1989): 3303–3307.

2:11 There may be differences between America and Europe in one or more aspects of "pipe smoking"—for example, type and amount of pipe tobacco smoked, or patterns and duration of smoking. For instance, it has been estimated that only about 4 percent of pipe smokers in the United States are deep inhalers, whereas the corresponding figures in Europe are much higher (up to 85%). Differences in the effect of pipe smoking, that is, effect modification, is a less likely explanation.

Hartge P, Hoover R, Kantor A. Bladder cancer risk and pipes, cigars and smokeless tobacco. *Cancer* 55(1985):901–906.

Steineck G, Norell SE, Feychting M. Diet, tobacco and urothelial cancer. A 14-year follow-up of 16,477 subjects. *Acta Oncol.* 77(1988):323–327.

2:12   There may be differences between the two countries as regards certain aspects of the exposure under study, for example, type of oral contraceptives or patterns of use. Another possibility is that oral contraceptive use would have different effects in the two countries, that is, effect modification, although this seems unlikely if the two countries were similar.

Lund E, Meirik O, Adami H-O, et al. Oral contraceptive use and premenopausal breast cancer in Sweden and Norway: possible effects of different pattern of use. *Int. J. Epidemiol.* 18(1989):527–532.

2:13A   Any effect of vitamin supplements depends upon the dietary intake of vitamins. In addition, an effect of vitamins could be modified by other characteristics of the population.

2:13B   The investigated exposure was "multivitamins or folate-containing supplements." But for the purpose of learning about the causation of neural-tube defects, there is an interest in the total intake (diet + supplements) of specific vitamins.

Mills JL, Rhoads GG, Simpson JL, et al. The absence of a relation between the periconceptional use of vitamins and neural-tube defects. *N. Engl. J. Med.* 321(1989):430–435.

2:14   Exposed categories:

1. exposed to both alcohol and aflatoxin

2. exposed to alcohol but not to aflatoxin

3. exposed to aflatoxin but not to alcohol

Unexposed category:
• Neither exposed to alcohol nor to aflatoxin

General questions:

• Does alcohol and aflatoxin (1)/ alcohol (2)/ aflatoxin (3) increase the risk of primary liver cancer—and if so, by how much?

Bulatao-Jayme J, Almero EM, Castro Ma CA, et al. A case-control study of primary liver cancer risk from aflatoxin exposure. *Int. J. Epidemiol.* 11(1982):112–119.

2:15 There were 15 exposed categories (1–15) and one unexposed category:

	tobacco	*alcohol*
1.	high	high
2.	high	medium
3.	high	low
4.	high	none
5.	medium	high
6.	medium	medium
7.	medium	low
8.	medium	none
9.	low	high
10.	low	medium
11.	low	low
12.	low	none
13.	none	high
14.	none	medium
15.	none	low
Unexposed category:	none	none

General questions:

• Does 1/2/3/4/5/6/7/8/9/10/11/12/13/14/15 increase the risk of laryngeal cancer—and if so, by how much? (With a large number of categories, precision may be low due to a small number of cases in each category.)

Flanders WD, Rothman KJ. Interaction of alcohol and tobacco in laryngeal cancer. *Am. J. Epidemiol.* 115(1982):371–379.

2:16 To the extent that these characteristics are effect modifiers. For instance, age and sex could very well modify the effect of smoking on mortality. But if there is little or no effect modification by occupation (or nationality), the results would also apply to men from other occupations (or nationalities), and there would be no point in restricting the general question in this respect.

Doll R, Peto R. Mortality in relation to smoking: 20 years' observations on male British doctors. *Br. Med. J.* 2(1976):1525–1536.

2:17 If the effect is modified by race, questions should be asked separately about the effects in different races. But to be able to answer these questions with adequate precision, there should be a sufficient number of exposed and unexposed cases of gallbladder cancer in each race. Otherwise the study, and the questions, should be restricted to races where the number of cases is expected to be sufficient. If the effect is not modified by race, it would make no difference that the study was interracial (although race could still introduce confounding).

Lowenfels AB, Walker AM, Althaus DP, et al. Gallstone growth, size, and risk of gallbladder cancer: an interracial study. *Int. J. Epidemiol.* 18(1989):50–54.

2:18 If an effect is modified by sex, questions should be asked separately about the effect in men and women. But to be able to answer these questions with adequate precision, there should be a sufficient number of exposed and unexposed cases in each sex. If an effect is not modified by sex, the effect would be no different if both sexes were included (but sex could still introduce confounding).

Most people with an occupational exposure to wood dust are likely to be men. The number of exposed cases among women may not be sufficient to estimate the effect in women separately. If so, it may be preferable to study this effect in men only. Similarly, most people with an occupational exposure to textile fibers are likely to be women, and it may be preferable to study this effect in women only.

Brinton LA, Blot WJ, Becker JA, et al. A case-control study of cancers of the nasal cavity and paranasal sinuses. *Am. J. Epidemiol.* 119(1984): 896–906.

2:19 Questions should be asked separately for men and women of different age groups, because age and sex modify the absolute or relative effect, or both. Since the incidence of CHD among non-smokers varies with age and sex, either the absolute or relative effect (or both) is modified by age and sex. (Cf. Chapter 1: Generalizability and Effect Modification.)

Willett WC, Green A, Stampfer MJ, et al. Relative and absolute excess risks of coronary heart disease among women who smoke cigarettes. *N. Engl. J. Med.* 317(1987):1303–1309.

2:20 Yes, in respect of the outcome, that is, death. Weight gain is likely to have different effects on the mortality from different diseases. (In the study, weight gain was found to increase mortality from cancer but not from other diseases.)

Hamm P, Shekelle RB, and Stamler J. Large fluctuations in body weight during young adulthood and twenty-five-year risk of coronary death in men. *Am. J. Epidemiol.* 129(1989):312–318.

2:21 The general question may be specified with regard to exposure (type of partial gastrectomy), disease, and potential modifiers (e.g., age, sex). When there is uncertainty about the induction time, questions may be asked concerning the effect in different "time windows" following surgery. (In Amsterdam, follow-up was continued 5–14 years after surgery: RR = 4.1, 15–24 years after surgery: RR = 9.4, and 25–46 years after surgery: RR = 55.6).

Tersmette AC, Goodman SN, Offerhaus GJA, et al. Multivariate analysis of the risk of stomach cancer after ulcer surgery in an Amsterdam cohort of postgastrectomy patients. *Am. J. Epidemiol.* 134(1991): 14–21.

2:22 The general question may be specified with regard to exposure (e.g., number of pregnancies), disease (type of gallstone disease), potential modifiers (e.g., age), and induction time. (When attention was paid to the effect in different "time windows" following pregnancy, the risk of gallstone disease was found to be increased 0–5 years after pregnancy: RR = 2.4.)

Thijs C, Knipschild P, and Leffers P. Pregnancy and gallstone disease: an empiric demonstration of the importance of specification of risk periods. *Am. J. Epidemiol.* 134(1991):186–195.

2:23 Questions should be asked separately concerning the effect in different "time windows" following a *change* in exposure status—that is, from unexposed to exposed or vice versa. (In a study, this was approximated by "interval since first use" and "interval since last use" of oral contraceptives.)

> The Cancer and Steroid Hormone Study of the Centers for Disease Control and the National Institute of Child Health and Human Development. The reduction in risk of ovarian cancer associated with oral-contraceptive use. *N. Engl. J. Med.* 316(1987):650–655.

2:24   Information on the absolute effects—or the occurrence of deep-vein thrombosis and excessive bleeding, respectively. (The incidence proportion of deep-vein thrombosis was reduced by 13 per 100 patients, while the incidence proportion of excessive bleeding increased by only 2 per 100 patients. In addition, information on the severity of these conditions as well as on other effects, side effects, and costs would be of interest.)

> Collins R, Scrimgeour A, Yusuf S, and Peto R. Reduction in fatal pulmonary embolism and venous thrombosis by perioperative administration of subcutaneous heparin: overview of results of randomized trials in general, orthopedic, and urologic surgery. *N. Engl. J. Med.* 318(1988):1162–1173.

2:25A   It would make a difference if the effect of alcohol intake is modified by age or sex. If there is effect modification by sex, questions should be asked separately for men and women, respectively (and the answers to these questions would be different). Similarly, if there is effect modification by age, questions should be asked separately for different age groups.

2:25B   If alcohol (ethanol) alone is the exposure of interest: quantity and frequency of consumption, for example, average alcohol intake in grams per day; patterns, timing, and duration of alcohol intake may also be of interest depending upon the suggested mechanism of action. If there is an interest in the effect of different kinds of alcoholic beverages (e.g., beer, wine, liquor), questions should be asked separately for each kind of alcoholic beverage.

Exposed categories may be defined on the basis of average daily alcohol intake (e.g., < 1.5; 1.5–4.9; 5.0–14.9; 15.0–24.9; 25+ g/day, depending upon the level where an effect could be expected to occur). Other aspects of alcohol intake may be considered separately. The unexposed are subjects with no alcohol intake.

2:25C If there could be differences in the effect of alcohol intake between different kinds of stroke—for example, between stroke due to thrombosis and stroke due to hemorrhage—questions should be asked separately for each type of stroke. (Strokes may be classified, for instance, as in the U.S. National Survey of Stroke.)

Walker AE, Robins M, and Weinfeld FD. The National Survey of Stroke: clinical findings. Stroke 12, Suppl 1(1981):13–44.

Stampfer MJ, Colditz GA, Willett WC, et al. A prospective study of moderate alcohol consumption and the risk of coronary disease and stroke in women. *N. Engl. J. Med.* 319(1988):267–273.

2:26A It would make a difference if there is effect modification by age or health status. Otherwise the results would apply equally to other age groups and to people who are not healthy.

2:26B The exposure was vaccination with inactivated influenza virus vaccine. The type and quantity of vaccine, as well as the vaccination procedure, should be specified. The number of vaccinations (doses) given should also be specified.

2:26C The illness ("influenza") may be specified by anatomic location (e.g., upper respiratory illness; lower respiratory illness) and by the type, severity, and duration of symptoms. The disease may also be specified on the basis of the virus isolated from the cases, and the rise in specific antibody titer levels in the cases.

Keitel WA, Cate TR, and Couch RB. Efficacy of sequential annual vaccination with inactivated influenza virus vaccine. *Am. J. Epidemiol.* 127(1988):353–364.

2:27 The question should be specified with regard to:
- effect measure(s)—for example, relative risk, risk difference;
- exposure: type—for example, caffeine-containing versus decaffeinated coffee; quantity and frequency—for example, average number of cups per day; patterns, timing, and duration of coffee intake may also be of interest;
- induction time—for example, current and past coffee drinking;
- disease—for example, first myocardial infarction;
- modifiers: the incidence of myocardial infarction varies considerably—for example, with age and sex. Thus, either the absolute or relative effect (or both) is modified by age and sex.

Rosenberg L, Werler MM, Kaufman DW, and Shapiro S. Coffee drinking and myocardial infarction in young women: an update. *Am. J. Epidemiol.* 126(1987):147–149.

2:28   No. The purpose is to evaluate the effect of HDL cholesterol levels during an etiologically relevant period of time, although information was only available on HDL cholesterol at one point in time. The difference may be an important source of exposure misclassification (cf. Chapter 1: Misclassification).

Jacobs DR Jr, Mebane IL, Bangdiwala SI, et al. High density lipoprotein cholesterol as a predictor of cardiovascular disease mortality in men and women: the follow-up study of the Lipid Research Clinics Prevalence Study. *Am. J. Epidemiol.* 131(1990):32–47.

2:29A   The average duration of the disease, until (recovery or) death. (In addition, the prevalence is influenced by any migration of cases (or noncases) into and out of the population. Cf. Chapter 1: Measures of Disease Occurrence.)

2:29B   The risk of developing chronic bronchitis is reflected by the incidence (incidence proportion). Smoking and grain farming may increase the incidence of the disease. But smoking and grain farming may reduce the duration of the disease (by increasing the death rate in people with chronic bronchitis). The prevalence of chronic bronchitis reflects both its incidence and duration.

Chen Y, Horne SL, McDuffie HH, and Dosman JA. Combined effect of grain farming and smoking on lung function and the prevalence of chronic bronchitis. *Int. J. Epidemiol.* 20(1991):416–423.

2:30   It could, in principle at least, be explained as a consequence of the induction time, or of effect modification from menopausal status, or by considering pre- and postmenopausal breast cancer as different diseases.

Hildreth NG, Shore RE, and Dvoretsky PM. The risk of breast cancer after irradiation of the thymus in infancy. *N. Engl. J. Med.* 321(1989): 1281–1284.

■ CHAPTER 3

3:1   The disease, as well as the exposure, may affect the probability of being included in the study population. If the exposure under study would increase the risk of fetal death among those who were to be born with cardiac malformations, the relative risk would be biased towards RR = 0 (and vice versa).

Zierler S, and Rothman KJ. Congenital heart disease in relation to maternal use of Bendectin and other drugs in early pregnancy. *N. Engl. J. Med.* 313(1985):347–352.

3:2A Prevalent cases. At screening, each woman is examined at one point in time to see whether or not she has a breast cancer at that time. (When each woman is examined repeatedly, this may under certain conditions provide information on the incidence of screening-detectable breast cancer between examinations.)

3:2B The presence of (symptoms of) breast cancer, as well as the exposure under study, may influence the probability of attending the screening and thus of being included in the study population. This would introduce selection bias. (In the present study, "symptomatic" women who came for their first screening were about five times as likely to have breast cancer as other women.)

3:2C *Advantage:* The availability of a large number of women examined for the presence of breast cancer.
Disadvantages: The possibility of selection bias (see B, above). In addition, prevalence reflects the duration as well as the incidence of the disease. Thus, a bias is introduced if the exposure is related to the duration of (screening-detectable) breast cancer.

Koenig KL, Pasternack BS, Shore RE, and Strax P. Hair dye use and breast cancer: a case-control study among screening participants. *Am. J. Epidemiol.* 133(1991):985–995.

3:3 Subjects suspecting that they have been infected with HIV could be less (or more) inclined to return for follow-up visits. Thus, occurrence of the disease (outcome) under study could terminate follow-up before the case is identified. This would introduce selection bias. A selective termination of follow-up could, in addition, be different in the exposed (e.g., syringe sharing) and unexposed. (In general, follow-up periods should be defined in such a way that the termination of follow-up is independent of the occurrence of the disease under study.)

Nicolosi A, Musicco M, Saracco A, et al. Incidence and risk factors of HIV infection: a prospective study of seronegative drug users from Milan and northern Italy, 1987–1989. *Epidemiology* 1(1990):453–459.

3:4A *Advantage:* avoids the efforts and costs necessary to trace and interview those who moved out.

   Disadvantage: selection bias is introduced if the tendency to move out of the area is influenced (increased or reduced) by respiratory disease.

3:4B *Advantage:* if those who moved in were similar to those who moved out, both in number and with regard to passive smoking and respiratory disease, they could neutralize any selection bias introduced by those who moved out.

   Disadvantage: if, on the other hand, those who moved in were different from those who moved out, their inclusion could have introduced additional selection bias.

Chen Y, Li W, Yu S, and Quian W. Chang-Ning epidemiological study of children's health: I Passive smoking and children's respiratory diseases. *Int. J. Epidemiol.* 17(1988):348–355.

3:5 When the study population was selected, the cases had already appeared. Thus the selection of subjects for the study could be influenced by the disease, introducing selection bias. This may be avoided if the study population is selected from a list of festival participants prepared before the cases appeared (e.g., as a random sample). In addition, if some kinds of participants are more likely than others to provide information on exposure and disease, restrictions could be used to avoid selection bias due to selective lack of information. (The investigators selected one-third of all festival participants who lived in the United States, from a complete mailing list.)

Lee LA, Ostroff SM, McGee HB, et al. An outbreak of Shigellosis at an outdoor music festival. *Am. J. Epidemiol.* 133(1991):608–615.

3:6A Restriction was used to avoid confounding by these conditions. Cardiac disease is likely to introduce confounding, because it is likely to influence (reduce) physical exercise and increase the risk of myocardial infarction during follow-up.

3:6B   It should be a risk factor (or risk indicator) for myocardial infarction among the unexposed, and be associated with physical exercise in the study base (cf. Chapter 1: Confounding).

3:6C   To the extent that body mass is influenced by exercise, it is not a confounder but a mediator of the effect of physical exercise. (On the other hand, body mass may also be associated with exercise in some other way and thus introduce confounding. It could be useful to estimate the effect of physical exercise both with and without taking body mass into account as a confounder.)

> Donahue RP, Abbott RD, Reed DM, and Yano K. Physical activity and coronary heart disease in middle-aged and elderly men: the Honolulu Heart Program. *Am. J. Pub. Health* 78(1988):683–685. Copyright: American Public Health Association.

3:7   No. To the extent that smoking during pregnancy increases the risk of low birth weight and preterm delivery, and these factors increase the risk of death during the first year of life, they are mediators of the effect of smoking during pregnancy on infant mortality. If so, birth weight and gestation should not be taken into account as confounders. If they were, the results would reflect the effect (if any) of smoking during pregnancy on infant mortality except for the effect mediated by low birthweight and preterm delivery.

> Kleinman JC, Pierre MB Jr, Madans JH, et al. The effects of maternal smoking on fetal and infant mortality. *Am. J. Epidemiol.* 127(1988): 274–282.

3:8A   The relative risks would be overestimated (biased towards RR = ∞). The magnitude of this bias would increase with the amount of alcohol consumed, if smoking increases with alcohol intake. (In the study, confounding by smoking masked the protective effect of moderate alcohol intake. The presented relative risks are adjusted for smoking.)

3:8B   Mortality in the unexposed would be overestimated, and relative risks at different levels of alcohol intake would be underestimated. This might explain the reduced risks found in the present study.
   To deal with this problem, only men who were healthy (not classified as sick) at enrollment were included in a separate analy-

sis. However, there were no substantial changes in relative risks. In addition, the first 6 years of follow-up were omitted in a separate analysis. But again, there were no major changes in the relative risks for total and CHD mortality.

Boffetta P, and Garfinkel L. Alcohol drinking and mortality among men enrolled in an American Cancer Society prospective study. *Epidemiology* 1(1990):342–348.

3:9A There is likely to be a considerable association between the number of sex partners of a woman and that of her current mate. Thus, each of these factors is likely to be an important confounder when estimating the effect of the other. (For women with ≥10 sex partners, the relative risk was reduced from 8.99 to 4.86 when the number of sex partners of her current mate was taken into account. For women having a current mate with ≥10 sex partners, the relative risk was reduced from 8.62 to 3.96 when the number of sex partners of the woman was taken into account.)

3:9B Women with a history of hysterectomy were not included because (in principle at least) a woman is no longer at risk of cervical cancer after surgical removal of the uterus.

3:9C To avoid confounding by race. If there is effect modification by race, precision is not likely to be sufficient to estimate effects is nonwhites (less than 5 percent of the population).

Slattery ML, Overall JC Jr, Abbott TM, et al. Sexual activity, contraception, genital infections, and cervical cancer: support for a sexually transmitted diesase hypothesis. *Am. J. Epidemiol.* 130(1989):248–258.

3:10A Higher (RR = 9.1 after adjustment for parity). This is because women aged 18–19 had given birth to fewer children and thus appeared to have a lower risk of SIDS.

3:10B Lower (RR = 1.0 after adjustment for income and education). The risk of SIDS appeared to be higher in infants of black mothers because they more frequently had a low income and education.

3:10C Single mothers more often had a low income.

3:10D Higher (RR = 3.6 after adjustment for maternal age). Mothers who had given birth to three or more children were older and thus appeared to have a lower risk of SIDS.

> Kraus JF, Greenland S, and Bulterys M. Risk factors for sudden infant death syndrome in the U.S. Collaborative Perinatal Project. *Int. J. Epidemiol.* 18(1989):113–120.

3:11A If these factors increase the risk of CHD, confounding results in overestimation of the relative risk. (All these factors, except alcohol, increase the risk of CHD.)

3:11B Expected total number of MI cases: $100,000 * 5 * 0.0015 = 750$. Expected number of MI cases in the highly exposed: $750 * 0.04 = 30$.

> Klatsky AL, Friedman GD, and Armstrong MA. Coffee use prior to myocardial infarction restudied: heavier intake may increase the risk. *Am. J. Epidemiol.* 132(1990):479–488.

3:12A The occurrence of the exposure—that is, the proportion that was exposed among men and women, respectively.

3:12B One possibility is that men with "any alcohol consumption" (exposed men) tend to have a higher alcohol intake (be more highly exposed) than women with "any alcohol consumption" (exposed women). Another possibility is, of course, effect modification by sex.

3:12C For women, the precision would be insufficient at some levels of alcohol intake. For instance, the number of cases (total = 48) with a high intake of alcohol (1.2 percent of all women) is likely to be too small to estimate the effect at this level separately.

For men, the distribution is more likely to provide a sufficient number of subjects (and cases) at each level of alcohol intake. But, at least for some levels, precision will be low. (The relative risk (with 95 percent confidence interval) at high, medium, and low alcohol intake was 5.42 (2.24—13.99), 3.83 (1.55—12.10), and 2.03 (0.54—7.32), respectively).

> Hirayama T. Association between alcohol consumption and cancer of the sigmoid colon: observations from a Japanese cohort study. *Lancet* 2(1989):725–727.

3:13   If the relative effect is similar in the two age groups, the precision would be higher among men aged 50–59 years. But if the absolute effect is similar in the two age groups, precision would be higher among men aged 35–49 years.

In addition, there could be differences in the distribution of serum triglycerides between the two age groups. A distribution with a high proportion of subjects at each extreme (i.e., with high and low levels) would give the highest precision.

> Tverdal A, Foss OP, Leren P, et al. Serum triglycerides as an independent risk factor for death from coronary heart disease in middle-aged Norwegian men. *Am. J. Epidemiol.* 129(1989):458–465.

3:14A   If "a large range of dietary habits" means that a large proportion of the study population is highly exposed and a large proportion is unexposed with regard to the dietary factor of interest, this will improve precision (with any particular study size). But confounding by other dietary factors may increase if there is a large variability with regard to other dietary habits. Confounding by smoking is reduced if there are few smokers. (In general, precision increases with a high variability of the exposure, but validity increases with a low variability of confounders.)

3:14B   When studying the effect of a medication, a large variability with regard to dietary factors will increase any confounding by these factors. But confounding by smoking is reduced if there are few smokers. (Precision is influenced by the proportion using the medication.)

3:14C   The maximum number of person-years at risk (if all subjects could be followed for the entire 6-year period) was 6*34,198. With an incidence rate of $7*10^{-5}$ per year, the total number of cases of kidney cancer would be about $6*34,198*7*10^{-5} = 14$ cases. Thus, precision will be low unless there is a strong effect and a favorable distribution of the exposure under study.

3:14D   *Adventists:* It would be possible to identify a sufficiently large unexposed group with a low frequency of intake (<1 day/week), but the possibility of studying the effect at high frequencies of intake is likely to be limited due to low precision (e.g., only 5.8% exposed at 7 days/week).

Non-Adventists: It would be difficult to identify a sufficiently large unexposed group with a low frequency of intake (only 2.2% at <1 day/week). Thus, in order to improve precision, exposed subjects —for example, at 1–3 days/week (9.0%)—may have to be included among the "unexposed." On the other hand, it would be possible to identify a sufficiently large group that is highly exposed.

Fraser GE, Phillips RL, and Beeson WL. Hypertension, antihypertensive medication and risk of renal carcinoma in California Seventh-day Adventists. *Int. J. Epidemiol.* 19(1990):832–838.

Snowdon DA, Phillips RL, and Choi W. Diet, obesity, and risk of fatal prostate cancer. *Am. J. Epidemiol.* 120(1984):244–250.

3:15A No, the study population should not be selected to reflect the distribution of the exposure (malnutrition) in the general population. If it were, the number of cases is likely to be insufficient to estimate the effect of moderate and severe malnutrition with adequate precision. In order to improve precision (with a certain study size), each exposure level should be represented by a similar number of children. (In the present study, no children with severe malnutrition were included since the number of such children was insufficient.)

3:15B There is likely to be confounding by previous diarrhea. Children who had diarrhea previously are more likely to have new episodes of diarrhea during follow-up. Since previous diarrhea also increases the risk of malnutrition, it is likely to introduce confounding.

3:15C A high variability of the exposure (high proportion of children with malnutrition) would reduce the size and cost of the initial screening necessary to enroll a sufficient number of children with malnutrition. But high variability of potential confounders is not desirable, since this would increase the amount of confounding in the study.

Sepulveda J, Willett W, and Muñoz A. Malnutrition and diarrhea. A longitudinal study among urban Mexican children. *Am. J. Epidemiol.* 127(1988):365–376.

3:16A To the extent that the (absolute or relative) effect is modified by age, sex, or occupation, the generalizability of the results are limited in these respects. However, these limitations are not introduced by restrictions when selecting the study population, but reflect true differences in the effect of the exposure between different subgroups of the population. The generalizability and usefulness of the results are improved by restrictions with regard to modifiers (cf. Chapter 1: Generalizability and Effect Modification).

3:16B Prevent any confounding by sex and occupation, and reduce confounding by age. In addition the comparability, accuracy, and completeness of information may very well have been improved by these restrictions.

3:16C Body mass is related to coronary heart disease and cancer. In addition, the closer surveillance of people with such diseases could increase the probability of having a diabetes diagnosed (i.e., introduce differential disease misclassification).

Coldiz GA, Willett WC, Stampfer MJ, et al. Weight as a risk factor for clinical diabetes in women. *Am. J. Epidemiol.* 132(1990):501–513.

3:17A The selection of subjects for the study may be influenced by the disease, introducing selection bias. Selection may be differential— that is, different in the exposed and unexposed. For instance, obese women could be more (or less) likely to be members of the TOPS club if, in addition, they had diabetes. This would result in an overestimation (underestimation) of the occurrence of diabetes in obese women, and of the relative risk.

3:17B Nonresponse to the 1969 questionnaire may be influenced by the disease (diabetes) as well as by the exposure (obesity, family history), introducing selection bias. (In addition, the exposure information may be influenced by the disease, introducing differential exposure misclassification.)

3:17C Prevalence depends on incidence and duration (Chapter 1). In a study based on prevalence, cases with a long duration are more likely to be included than cases with a short duration. This will bias the results if the exposure under study (obesity, family history) is related to the duration of the disease (diabetes). For instance, the duration of diabetes could be shorter in very obese people, due to a higher mortality.

3:17D *Advantage:* the availability of information on exposure and disease from the 1969 survey.

Disadvantages: see above (A-C). In addition, members of a weight loss club are likely to make special efforts to reduce their weight. Thus, there could be considerable variations in weight over time among members of the TOPS club.

Morris RD, Rimm DL, Hartz AJ, et al. Obesity and heredity in the etiology of non-insulin-dependent diabetes mellitus in 32,662 adult white women. *Am. J. Epidemiol.* 130(1989):112–121.

3:18A The study population should be representative of the total population of the five metropolitan areas: The incidence (and prevalence) of major depression among the study subjects should reflect that of all residents aged 18–44. In addition, there may be an interest in the occurrence of major depression in other age groups.

3:18B The study population should be selected to reflect the occurrence of major depression in different population subgroups, rather than in the general population. Each subgroup of interest should be represented by a sufficiently large number of subjects and cases to provide adequate precision in estimating the occurrence of major depression, and other subgroups should not be included. (In the present study, the number of incident cases identified by race/ethnicity was: 121 white, 47 black, 19 hispanic, and 6 other minority. Further subdivision, e.g., by sex, may be of interest.)

3:18C The accuracy and generalizability of the results can usually be improved by restrictions when selecting the study population (see Chapter 1, and Chapter 3: Introduction). This means that the study population should usually not be representative of the general population.

Anthony JC, and Petronis KR. Suspected risk factors for depression among adults 18–44 years old. *Epidemiology* 2(1991):123–132.

3:19A When a subject's decision to participate in the screening is influenced by symptoms or signs of the disease, their inclusion in the study may introduce selection bias. This is avoided if the study is restricted to screening participants who have not experienced any symptoms or signs that could be related to the disease under study. (However, awareness of the screening results may influence the decision not to include subjects on the basis of their symptoms. In order to avoid this source of selection bias, restrictions should be made "blind"—that is, without knowledge of the screening result.)

3:19B When a subject's tendency to recall and report past exposure is influenced by the experience of symptoms or signs of the disease under study, differential exposure misclassification may be introduced. This is avoided if the study is restricted to screening participants who have not experienced any symptoms or signs that could be related to the disease under study. (However, awareness of the screening result may influence the study subject or the interviewer, or both. In order to avoid these sources of differential exposure misclassification, study subjects and interviewers should be kept unaware of the screening result until the interview is completed.)

Dawson DA, Hendershot GE, and Bloom B. Trends in routine screening examinations. *Am. J. Pub. Health* 77(1987):1004–1005. Copyright: American Public Health Association.

3:20 *Advantages:* Precision will be higher, since the number of unexposed employees was relatively small. In addition, the information is available at a low cost.

Disadvantages: Possible confounding by, for instance, general health status ("healthy worker effect"), area of residence (could perhaps be reduced by using rates for London, rather than national rates), and socioeconomic status (could also be reduced, if rates for specific socioeconomic groups were available). Information on other potential confounders, such as smoking habits, may not be available. In addition, the "unexposed" (all men in the country) will include all exposed men, but this will introduce little or no bias if only a small proportion of all men in the country were exposed to amosite asbestos. Finally, there may be differences in the accuracy of information on death from (specific types of) cancer between the exposed workers and all men in the country, introducing differential misclassification.

Acheson ED, Gardner MJ, Winter PD, and Bennett C. Cancer in a factory using amosite asbestos. *Int. J. Epidemiol.* 13(1984):3–10.

3:21A Unexposed children were matched to the exposed with regard to, for example, age and sex, to avoid confounding by these factors. (Matching of unexposed to exposed subjects should not be confused with matching of referents to the cases, discussed in Chapter 6.)

3:21B *Age and sex:* In order to avoid confounding by age and sex, specific rates were used in (3), and matching of unexposed to the exposed in (1) and (2). But for siblings (2) the limited number of children in each family reduces the possibility of close age and sex matching.

Place of origin and time of immigration: The unexposed group that was most similar to the exposed in these respects is likely to be (2), followed by (1), while (3) was matched for "ethnic origin" with no mentioning of country or year of immigration.

Residential area and socioeconomic characteristics: Children who received their X-ray treatment at the four treatment centers could be different in these respects from Israeli children of the same age, sex, and ethnic origin. Of the three unexposed groups, (2) was similar to the exposed with regard to these and other family characteristics.

3:21C   When the exposure under study is a medical treatment, the possibility of confounding by other treatments (and examinations) for the same condition, by the condition itself, or by indications (or contraindications) for the treatment, should always be considered. In addition, there may be confounding by general health status if subjects with the disease or treatment at issue tend to have a poor general health ("unhealthy patient effect"). But this may not have been an issue in the present study.

3:21D   The third unexposed group (3) includes all exposed children, and this would bias the relative risk towards RR = 1 if a substantial fraction of (3) had been exposed.

3:21E   Of the three unexposed groups, the highest precision was offered by (3), with information available for 10,834 exposed and a large number of unexposed subjects; followed by (1), with 10,834 exposed and a similar number of unexposed; and finally (2), with only about half as many exposed and unexposed subjects.

Ron E, Modan B, and Boice JD Jr. Mortality after radiotherapy for ringworm of the scalp. *Am. J. Epidemiol.* 127(1988):713–725.

3:22   Bias towards RR = ∞, which could explain the observed excess risk. Subjects with an early, asymptomatic cancer at the time of the initial examination would tend to have a low serum cholesterol at that time and to develop a more advanced, symptomatic cancer during follow-up. If so, the association between serum cholesterol and cancer is likely to be strongest during the first years of follow-up, especially for fast-developing cancers (as found in the present study). If the induction time is unknown, the problem may be dealt with by considering the effect in different "time windows" following the initial examination.

Knekt P, Reunanen A, Aromaa A, et al. Serum cholesterol and risk of cancer in a cohort of 39,000 men and women. *J. Clin. Epidemiol.* 41(1988):519–530.

3:23 Nationality, sex, and occupation could be:

- confounders. If so, restriction to male British doctors prevents confounding by nationality, sex, and occupation.
- factors that influence the accuracy of information on exposure (smoking habits) or disease (cause of death). If so, restriction to male British doctors may increase the comparability (and perhaps also the accuracy) of information.
- effect modifiers. If so, the effect should be investigated in each subgroup (cf. Exercise 2:16), and restriction to one subgroup (male British doctors) increases precision at any particular study size. (In addition, precision is influenced by the occurrence of smoking, and by the mortality and strength of the effect, in male British doctors compared to any alternative population subgroup).

Doll R, Peto R. Mortality in relation to smoking: 20 years' observation on male British doctors. *Br. Med. J.* 2:(1976):1525–1536.

3:24A 1. The occurrence of the exposure: The highest precision would be obtained with a U-shaped distribution, where a high proportion of the subjects have very low and very high levels, respectively, of vitamin D (provided that the effect increases with the level of exposure).

2. The occurrence of the disease and the strength of the effect: For instance, the incidence of MI increases with age. If age does not modify the absolute effect, precision would be higher in middle-aged than in elderly people. But if age does not modify the relative effect, precision would be higher in the elderly.

3:24B The accuracy and completeness of information (on exposure, disease, and potential confounders) that can be obtained is likely to be better before the age of 65 than in elderly people. Precision may or may not be higher in middle-aged than in elderly people (cf. A, above).

Scragg R, Jackson R, Holdaway IM, et al. Myocardial infarction is inversely associated with plasma 25-hydroxyvitamin D3 levels: a community-based study. *Int. J. Epidemiol.* 19(1990):559–563.

3:25A   At least two assumptions: 1) that the particular oral contraceptive that was dispensed (or one with the same estrogen and progestin potency) was used by the woman during the subsequent 56-day period, and 2) that the induction time is equal to zero.

3:25B   *Advantages* include the availability (at a relatively low cost) of computerized information for a large study population on exposure (COC:s dispensed, recorded before the cases appeared), disease (hospitalizations with diagnosis, prescriptions for anticoagulants), and some potential confounders. In addition, to the extent that Medicaid enrollees are similar with regard to certain potential confounders, such as socioeconomic status, confounding by these factors is avoided or reduced by restricting the study to Medicaid enrollees.

Disadvantages include possible incompleteness and inaccuracy of the available information for the purpose of the present study. In addition, complete information on potential confounders was not available from the register, and the possibilities of obtaining supplementary information from study subjects was limited.

3:25C   Advantages: 1) confounding due to restrictions in the prescription of oral contraceptives is avoided (unless women at high risk of thrombosis are more likely to receive low-estrogen-potency than high-estrogen-potency oral contraceptives); 2) the identification of cases will not be influenced by exposure status (unless the probability of having a thrombosis diagnosed is related to the estrogen-potency of an oral contraceptive, which seems unlikely).

Disadvantages: By using a low level of exposure as the "unexposed" category, no information is obtained on the effect of low versus no exposure, and the effect of intermediate or high versus no exposure is likely to be underestimated.

Gerstman BB, Piper JM, Freiman JP, et al. Oral contraceptive estrogen and progestin potencies and the incidence of deep venous thromboembolism. *Int. J. Epidemiol.* 19(1990):931–936.

3:26A   These restrictions will prevent any confounding by sex, and reduce confounding by age, employment, and area of residence. If there was effect modification by these factors, a study of the same size may not have been sufficient to estimate the effect in different subgroups—for example, among men and women in different age groups or among people with different employments and living in different regions.

3:26B For the purpose of the present study, further restrictions to improve validity, or to improve precision (with the same study size), may have been preferable to selecting a random sample. However, participants were originally selected for several purposes of the Western Electric Study.

3:26C To the extent that serum cholesterol is a mediator of the effect of dietary cholesterol intake, serum cholesterol should not be taken into account as a confounder. (However, the results of the present study suggest that a high cholesterol intake may increase the risk of death from ischemic heart diease at any particular level of serum cholesterol.)

Shekelle RB, and Stamler J. Dietary cholesterol and ischemic heart disease. *Lancet* 1(1989):1177–1179.

3:27A To save cost and time. Serum samples had been collected for the Hypertension Detection and Follow-up Program and were available for analysis of serum vitamins.

3:27B To the extent that blood pressure or antihypertensive treatment could be associated with serum vitamins and the risk of cancer, there may be confounding by these factors (taken into account in the data analysis in the present study). The variability of other potential confounders, and modifiers, may also have been higher than when selecting a study population in some other way. The variability of the exposure (serum vitamins) may have been lower than when selecting a study population in some other way.

3:27C If the occurrence of cancer during follow-up could have influenced the order of storage (the freezer used for storage), the breakdown of a freezer could introduce selection bias. Otherwise the most important consequence may have been a reduction in study size and thus in precision.

Willett WC, Polk BF, Underwood BA, et al. Relation of serum vitamins A and E and carotenoids to the risk of cancer. *N. Engl. J. Med.* 310(1984):430–434.

3:28A Because information on serum lipids including HDL cholesterol and some potential confounders was already available from the Lipid Research Clinics Prevalence Study. This reduces the cost for obtaining exposure information in the present study.

3:28B The wide age range and considerable geographic, socioeconomic, and occupational heterogeneity are likely to increase confounding and perhaps also differential misclassification. For the purpose of the present study, restrictions would have been preferable considering the accuracy as well as the generalizability of the results (cf. Chapter 1). However, subjects were initially selected for the purpose of the Lipid Research Clinics Prevalence Study.

The distribution of HDL cholesterol in these subjects is not likely to be optimal for the purpose of the study of HDL cholesterol and CHD mortality. The highest precision would be obtained with a U-shaped distribution (a high proportion of subjects with unusually high and unusually low HDL cholesterol levels) or, to be able to study the effect at different levels, with the addition of a sufficient number of subjects at an intermediate level.

3:28C To the extent that these subjects had more extreme levels of HDL cholesterol, this will increase the variability of the exposure and thus improve precision in the present study. On the other hand these subjects had more extreme levels of other serum lipids, likely to be confounders in the present study.

3:28D Restriction may be used to avoid confounding by race and by coronary heart disease, without substantially reducing the size of the study. Thus, nonwhites and subjects who had coronary heart disease at the beginning of follow-up were not included in the study of HDL cholesterol and CHD mortality.

> Jacobs DR Jr, Mebane IL, Bangdiwala SI, et al. High density lipoprotein cholesterol as a predictor of cardiovascular disease mortality in men and women: the follow-up study of the Lipid Research Clinics Prevalence Study. *Am. J. Epidemiol.* 131(1990):32–47.

3:29A *Advantage:* Individual matching (unexposed/exposed twin) is used to avoid confounding by genetic, and to some extent also environmental, factors. (It has been suggested that genetic factors may influence both smoking habits and mortality.)

Disadvantage: A considerable reduction in study size and thus in precision. (Information is contributed only by smoking-discordant twin pairs where at least one subject died.) The lack of precision is even more evident when studying the effect at different exposure levels, or the effect on mortality from specific diseases such as myocardial infarction or lung cancer.

3:29B Study size, and thus precision, would be reduced. (In addition, the occurrence of potential confounders and the possibilities of obtaining complete and accurate information could be different).

3:29C Study subjects are enrolled only after the cases (deaths) have occurred. Thus, not only the exposure (smoking) but also the outcome (death) could influence the probability of being included. This would introduce selection bias. (In addition to B, above).

Floderus B, Cederlöf R, and Friberg L. Smoking and mortality: a 21-year follow-up based on the Swedish Twin Registry. *Int. J. Epidemiol.* 17(1988):332–340.

3:30A The study population was children who were born alive and survived until October 1, 1950 or until the time of the supplementary survey in 1960. But the exposure may have caused deaths in utero, stillbirths, or deaths before October 1, 1950 or the time of the 1960 survey. Those who were less susceptible and survived may also have been less susceptible to the carcinogenic effect of radiation. This would tend to reduce the relative risks.

3:30B It may have introduced selection bias, since the occurrence of cancer before 1960 may have influenced the probability of being identified in the 1960 survey and thus of being selected for the study.

Yoshimoto Y, Kato H, and Schull WJ. Risk of cancer among children exposed in utero to A-bomb radiations, 1950–84. *Lancet* 2(1988): 665–669.

▄▄▄ CHAPTER 4

4:1A Centrally deposited fat, peripherally deposited fat, and overall obesity—during an etiologically relevant period of time. (More detailed theoretical definitions may be desirable, and should be based on a proposed mechanism of action.)

4:1B Subscapular skinfold, triceps skinfold, and body mass index (= weight/height^2)—at one point in time.

4:1C   There are two principal sources of exposure misclassification:

1. Any discrepancy between (A) and (B). Such discrepancies could be expected for each of the three aspects of obesity that were investigated. (For example, it could be argued that body mass does not only reflect obesity, and that subscapular skinfold does not reflect intra-abdominal fat, which is a large and metabolically important central fat depot.)

2. Errors in the measurement of (B). Such errors could be expected for each of the three aspects of obesity, but to a different extent. (While the measurement of weight and height is likely to be fairly accurate, there may be errors in the measurement of skinfold thickness.)

Selby JV, Friedman GD, and Quesenberry Jr CP. Precursors of essential hypertension: the role of body fat distribution pattern. *Am. J. Epidemiol.* 129(1989):43–53.

4:2   When exposure information is collected only after the cases appear, there is always the possibility that the disease could influence the accuracy of the exposure information. For example, some subjects may not report their intake of gravy, but the experience of illness after the banquet could increase their tendency to recall and mention gravy when answering the questionnaire. This would result in an overestimation of the relative risk, and the results might show an excess risk even if gravy did not increase the risk of illness. (Although the possibility of such recall bias is sometimes exaggerated, it is usually not possible to demonstrate its absence (or presence) or to take it into account in the data analysis.)

If exposure information had been collected before the cases appeared, the illness could not have influenced the accuracy of exposure information. Thus, the principal difference is that this source of differential exposure misclassification would be eliminated.

Petersen LR, Mshar R, Cooper Jr GH, et al. A large Clostridium perfringens foodborne outbreak with an unusual attack rate pattern. *Am. J. Epidemiol.* 127(1988):605–611.

4:3A   Sensitivity = 0.90 means that 90 percent of the exposed were classified as exposed. Thus, 10 percent of the exposed were classified as unexposed ("false negatives"), both among the cases and among the noncases (nondifferential misclassifcation):

	Classified as:	
	Exposed	*Unexposed*
Cases	269.10	136.90
Noncases	4,052.70	2,762.30
All men	4,321.80	2,899.20
Incidence proportion (*1000)	62.27	47.22

The incidence proportion in the exposed is the same as in the original table, where there was no misclassification. This is because the same proportion (10%) has been removed from cases and noncases. However, the incidence proportion in the unexposed is biased towards that in the exposed, since some (10%) of the exposed have been added to the unexposed.

$$RR = 62.27/47.22 = 1.32$$

The relative risk is biased towards RR = 1 (from 1.41 to 1.32) by this nondifferential misclassification.

4:3B Specificity = 0.70 means that 70% of the unexposed were classified as unexposed. Thus, 30% of the unexposed were classified as exposed ("false positives"), both among the cases and among the noncases (nondifferential misclassifcation):

	Classified as:	
	Exposed	*Unexposed*
Cases	331.10	74.90
Noncases	5,196.60	1,618.40
All men	5,527.70	1,693.30
Incidence proportion (*1000)	59.90	44.23

The incidence proportion in the unexposed is the same as in the original table, since the same proportion (30%) has been removed from cases and noncases. However, the incidence proportion in the exposed is biased towards that in the unexposed, since some (30%) of the unexposed have been added to the exposed.

$$RR = 59.90/44.23 = 1.35$$

The relative risk is biased towards RR = 1 (from 1.41 to 1.35) by this nondifferential misclassification.

4:3C Now there is a misclassification in both directions, with 10% false negatives (10% of the 299 exposed cases, and 10% of the 4,503 exposed noncases, are classified as unexposed) and 30% false positives (30% of the 107 unexposed cases, and 30% of the 2,312 unexposed noncases, are classified as exposed). The numbers of misclassified subjects are the sum of those in A and B, above:

	Classified as:	
	Exposed	*Unexposed*
Cases	301.20	104.80
Noncases	4,746.30	2,068.70
All men	5,047.50	2,173.50
Incidence proportion (*1000)	59.67	48.22

$$RR = 59.67/48.22 = 1.24$$

The relative risk is biased towards RR = 1 (from 1.41 to 1.24) by this nondifferential misclassification.

4:3D Among noncases, sensitivity = 0.90 (as in A, above). However, among cases there was no misclassification:

	Classified as:	
	Exposed	*Unexposed*
Cases	299	107
Noncases	4,052.70	2,762.30
All men	4,351.70	2,869.30
Incidence proportion (*1000)	68.71	37.29

$$RR = 68.71/37.29 = 1.84$$

The relative risk is overestimated (biased towards RR = ∞) by this differential misclassification.

4:3E Among noncases, specificity = 0.70 (as in B, above). However, among cases there was no misclassification:

	Classified as:	
	Exposed	*Unexposed*
Cases	299	107
Noncases	5,196.60	1,618.40
All men	5,495.60	1,725.40
Incidence proportion (*1000)	54.41	62.01

$$RR = 54.41/62.01 = 0.88$$

The relative risk is underestimated (biased towards RR = 0) by this differential misclassification. Although misclassification is reduced compared with B (no misclassification among men with CHD), the bias due to misclassification is increased.

4:3F Now there is misclassification in both directions, with 10% false negatives and 30% false positives (as in C, above), but only among noncases:

	Classified as:	
	Exposed	*Unexposed*
Cases	299	107
Noncases	4,746.30	2,068.70
All men	5,045.30	2,175.70
Incidence proportion (*1000)	59.26	49.18

$$RR = 59.26/49.18 = 1.20$$

Donahue RP, Abbott RD, Reed DM, and Yano K. Physical activity and coronary heart disease in middle-aged and elderly men: the Honolulu Heart Program. *Am. J. Pub. Health* 78(1988):683–685. Copyright: American Public Health Association.

4:4A Among noncases, 5% of the exposed were classified as unexposed. But among cases there was no misclassification:

	Classified as:		
	Exposed	*Unexposed*	*Total*
Cases	41	253	294
Noncases	50.35	326.65	377
All subjects	91.35	579.65	671

$$RR = 41*579.65/253*91.35 = 1.03$$

4:4B Among noncases, 5% of the exposed were classified as unexposed. But among cases there was no misclassification. This would give the following table (which is similar to the findings of the present study):

Classified as:

	Exposed	Unexposed	Total
Cases	290	4	294
Noncases	353.40	23.60	377
All subjects	643.40	27.60	671

$$RR = 290*27.60/4*643.40 = 3.11$$

In general, a reduction in sensitivity has little effect when a small proportion is exposed (A), but a strong effect when a large proportion is exposed (B). Conversely, a reduction in specificity has little effect when a small proportion is unexposed, but a strong effect when a large proportion is unexposed.

Petersen LR, Mshar R, Cooper Jr GH, et al. A large Clostridium perfringens foodborne outbreak with an unusual attack rate pattern. *Am. J. Epidemiol.* 127(1988):605–611.

4:5A The first approach. Marriage to a smoker is not the only source of passive smoking. Even a detailed questionnaire is unlikely to cover all sources and aspects of passive smoking. But the gap between the exposure of interest (theoretical definition, e.g., inhaled smoke from other peoples' smoking) and what is being measured (the empirical definition) is likely to be much wider when marriage to a smoker is used as an indicator of passive smoking.

4:5B The second approach. The accuracy of information on marriage to a smoker is likely to be relatively high. The accuracy of information on various sources and aspects of passive smoking may be much lower. Thus, the measurement error is likely to be smaller for the indicator (marriage to a smoker).

4:5C The second approach. The disease is likely to influence the accuracy of measurement rather than the gap between definitions. Using the indicator may reduce the amount of differential exposure misclassification (recall bias). When using a detailed questionnaire, a separate analysis may sometimes be based only on "hard" items (where recall bias is less likely).

4:5D Yes, sources of passive smoking other than marriage to a smoker may be more important among women in the United States. This is likely to introduce nondifferential exposure misclassification (bias towards RR = 1).

Hirayama T. Non-smoking wives of heavy smokers have a higher risk of lung cancer: a study from Japan. *Br. Med. J.* 282(1981):183–185.

Garfinkel L. Time trends in lung cancer mortality among nonsmokers and a note on passive smoking. *JNCI* 66(1981):1061–1066.

Repace JL. Consistency of research data on passive smoking and lung cancer. *Lancet* 1(1984):506.

4:6A Even in the absence of measurement errors, considerable exposure misclassification may be introduced by a gap between the empirical and theoretical definition of the exposure of interest. Serum cotinine is used as an indicator of passive smoking, and the cotinine level in a single blood specimen may not reflect the inhalation of environmental tobacco smoke during a relevant period of time. (For instance, with a serum half-life of 17 hours, considerable differences in serum cotinine could be expected between blood specimens drawn in the morning and in the afternoon, or before and after a weekend or holiday. In addition, serum cotinine levels may be influenced by differences in nicotine metabolism between subjects.)

4:6B No. Serum cotinine in a blood specimen collected after the child has developed symptoms of respiratory disease could very well be influenced by the disease. For instance, children with symptoms of respiratory disease may be protected from environmental tobacco smoke. If so, differential exposure misclassification would bias the relative risk towards RR = 0.

Chen Y, Li W, Yu S, and Quian W. Chang-Ning epidemiological study of children's health: I Passive smoking and children's respiratory diseases. *Int. J. Epidemiol.* 17(1988):348–355.

Wall MA, Johnson J, Jacob P, and Benowitz NL. Cotinine in the serum, saliva, and urine of nonsmokers, passive smokers, and active smokers. *Am. J. Pub. Health* 78(1988):699–701.

Jarvis MJ, McNeill AD, Bryant A, Russell MAH. Factors determining exposure to passive smoking in young adults living at home: quantitative analysis using saliva cotinine concentrations. *Int. J. Epidemiol.* 20(1991):126–131.

4:7 1. Towards RR = 1. (To the extent that any risk indicators for colon cancer that could influence the exposure information were taken into account in the data analysis.)

2. Towards RR = 1. (If the strategies were successful in avoiding any differences between cases and noncases.)

3. Towards RR = 1.

4. Towards RR = 1. (Unless nutrient levels were influenced by an early, undiagnosed cancer. Cf. Exercise 3:22.)

5. Towards RR = 1.

Schober SE, Comstock GW, Helsing KJ, et al. Serologic precursors of cancer. I. Prediagnostic serum nutrients and colon cancer risk. *Am. J. Epidemiol.* 126(1987):1033–1041.

4:8 The use of a single measurement is likely to introduce a large amount of nondifferential exposure misclassification, and bias relative risks towards RR = 1. This bias may be avoided by measuring the levels at different times and different locations to assess individual exposures.

Brunekreef B, Noy D, and Clausing P. Variability of exposure measurements in environmental epidemiology. *Am. J. Epidemiol.* 125(1987): 892–898.

4:9 It is likely to introduce a bias towards RR = 0. The accuracy of exposure information is improved among the cases. However, the comparability of exposure information is reduced (unless similar information was available for the noncases). Differential exposure misclassification will bias the relative risk towards RR = 0 when "false positives" are re-classified as unexposed among the cases but still classified as exposed among the noncases.

Ray WA, Griffin MR, and Downey W. Benzodiazepines of long and short elimination half-life and the risk of hip fracture. *JAMA* 262(1989): 3303–3307.

4:10 Less than 10%. Of women with mild dysplasia, 27 percent (23/86) developed carcinoma in situ within 4 years. Thus, to obtain 30 cases (= all exposed cases in the present study) during a 4-year period, there should be 30/0.27 = 111 women with mild dysplasia. This is about 10% of the 1,107 women identified as exposed to HPV in the present study. Taking into account that the period of follow-up was 6 rather than 4 years (and that RR = 1 with about 30/15 = 2 exposed cases), less than 10% would be required.

> Mitchell H, Drake M, and Medley G. Prospective evaluation of risk of cervical cancer after cytological evidence of human papillomavirus infection. *Lancet* 1(1986):573–575.

4:11A If smoking was reduced by symptoms of the disease, the cases would tend to underestimate (retrospectively) their smoking at the time when they fell ill. This would result in a bias towards RR = 0. (Conversely, if symptoms of the disease tends to increase smoking, the relative risk would be overestimated).

4:11B If exposure information was collected at the time when the first symptoms of disease appeared, this source of bias would be avoided. For ulcerative colitis and Crohn's disease, this may be difficult to achieve, since considerable time may elapse from the initial symptoms to diagnosis. But for many other diseases, it may be possible to collect exposure information shortly after the first symptoms of disease. (For other reasons, however, it is sometimes unsuitable to collect the information during the first days or even weeks of a serious illness.)

> Persson P-G, and Norell SE. Retrospective versus original information on cigarette smoking: implications for epidemiologic studies. *Am. J. Epidemiol.* 130(1989):705–712.
>
> Persson P-G, Ahlbom A, and Hellers G. Inflammatory bowel disease and tobacco smoke—a case-control study. *Gut* 31(1990):1377–1381.

4:12A The mortality in nondrinkers would be overestimated and could even appear to be higher than at one drink/day. If so, the J-shaped distribution could be explained as a distortion (due to exposure misclassification) of a gradual increase in mortality with increasing alcohol intake. (In the present study, however, mortality from liver cirrhosis, and other diseases known to be associated with alcohol intake, was found to be lowest among those classified as nondrinkers.)

4:12B Yes, the gap between true and reported exposure that is introduced by social desirability could be reduced by the presence of disease. Suppose that, due to social desirability, women would tend to underestimate their number of sex partners and genital infections. But having a cervical cancer diagnosed might increase a woman's motivation to provide accurate information on her number of sex partners and history of genital infections. This would result in a differential exposure misclassification with overestimation of relative risks.

Boffetta P, and Garfinkel L. Alcohol drinking and mortality among men enrolled in an American Cancer Society prospective study. Epidemiology 1(1990):342–348.

Slattery ML, Overall Jr JC, Abbott TM, et al. Sexual activity, contraception, genital infections, and cervical cancer: support for a sexually transmitted disease hypothesis. *Am. J. Epidemiol.* 130(1989):248–258.

4:13 Yes, an obvious possibility is that vasectomy was underreported by Catholic men, but that Catholic men who had a testicular cancer were less likely to underreport vasectomy. This would result in a differential exposure misclassification that would bias the relative risk towards RR = ∞ among Catholic men. (An alternative, but less likely, explanation is a difference between Catholic and Protestant men in the effect of vasectomy.)

Strader CH, Weiss NS, and Daling JR. Vasectomy and the incidence of testicular cancer. *Am. J. Epidemiol.* 128(1988):56–63.

4:14 Yes, as pointed out in the subsequent discussion, exposure information from the questionnaires completed for the National Asthma Mortality Survey was only available for those who died, that is, for the cases. Differences in the accuracy of exposure information obtained from different sources could have introduced a differential exposure misclassification and resulted in overestimation of the relative risk. (In response to this criticism, another study was conducted using the same source of exposure information for all subjects. However, the second study showed a similar result with RR = 5.8 (1.6–21.0, 95% confidence interval) among patients on oral corticosteroids).

Crane J, Pearce N, Flatt A, et al. Prescribed fenoterol and death from asthma in New Zealand, 1981–83: case-control study. *Lancet* 1(1989): 917–922.

Pearce N, Grainger J, Atkinson M, et al. Case-control study of prescribed fenoterol and death from asthma in New Zealand, 1977–81. *Thorax* 45(1990):170–175.

4:15A Yes, information from the medical records is likely to increase the accuracy of information on antihypertensive medications, and thus reduce the amount of exposure misclassification among the cases.

4:15B No, since this source of information was available only for the cases, it is likely to introduce a difference in exposure misclassification between cases and noncases (i.e., a differential exposure misclassification). If the information from medical records would increase sensitivity, relative risks would be overestimated (and if the information would increase specificity, relative risks would be underestimated. Cf. Exercise 4:3).

4:15C Since medical records were available only for the cases, they should be used only as a source of information on the disease (as in the present study), and not as a source of information on exposure.

> Fraser GE, Phillips RL, and Beeson WL. Hypertension, antihypertensive medication and risk of renal carcinoma in California Seventh-day Adventists. *Int. J. Epidemiol.* 19(1990):832–838.

4:16A The information in the obstetric records had been collected before the cases were identified. Thus, the disease could not have influenced the exposure information in the obstetric records.

However, information was abstracted from the records only after the cases had been identified. Thus, knowledge of the infant's disease status could influence the abstraction of information from the records and the exposure classification. This source of differential exposure misclassification can be avoided if all handling of the records, processing of exposure information and classification in respect of exposure is done blind, that is, without knowledge of disease status.

4:16B More detailed and complete information on exposure and potential confounders may be obtained by interview, since information in the obstetric records is likely to be incomplete. (In the study, a separate classification in respect of exposure to Bendectin was done using information from interviews and obstetric records, respectively. This permitted a comparison of results influenced by the potential errors linked to each of the two sources of exposure information.)

> Zierler S, and Rothman KJ. Congenital heart disease in relation to maternal use of Bendectin and other drugs in early pregnancy. *N. Engl. J. Med.* 313(1985):347–352.

4:17A   If the proportion that is identified as exposed by interview is the same among infants identified as exposed in the records as among truly exposed infants (including those with missing information in the obstetric records).

4:17B   The relative risk would be overestimated.

4:17C   An increased tendency to accurate reporting of exposure that is not documented in the medical record. (Many infants may be classified as unexposed simply because there was no information on exposure in the medical record.)

4:17D   The type of exposure, the questions asked, the time and method of questioning, and characteristics of the study population (or respondents). In addition, the impression (among the cases) of an exposure's hazards could be important. (For example, in the study on malformations, the only large difference in recall "sensitivity" was for "use of birth control after conception" and, as suggested by the investigators, this could be "because of publicity of the putative hazards of spermicides, oral contraceptives, and intrauterine devices").

Werler MM, Pober BR, Nelson K, and Holmes LB. Reporting accuracy among mothers of malformed and nonmalformed infants. *Am. J. Epidemiol.* 129(1989):415–421.

Drews CD, Kraus JF, and Greenland S. Recall bias in a case-control study of Sudden Infant Death Syndrome. *Int. J. Epidemiol.* 19(1990): 405–411.

4:18A   Yes. Since surrogate respondents have to be used for the cases, similar surrogate respondents should also be used for the noncases in order to improve the comparability of exposure information (avoid differential exposure misclassification).

4:18B   The study population may be restricted to subjects with available surrogate respondents, using the same criteria for cases and noncases. (But the possibility of selection bias may have to be considered if the availability of surrogate respondents is influenced by the disease.)

4:18C   The study population may be restricted to subjects with available surrogate respondents of a certain kind. (The present study was restricted to subjects who had been married for at least 10 years, using the spouse as surrogate respondent.)

4:18D The presence of the disease could increase the tendency to report a suspected cause: spouses of cases could be more likely than spouses of noncases to report head trauma. If so, the relative risk would be overestimated due to differential exposure misclassification (recall bias).

4:18E Yes. Recall bias is more likely for mild head injury, while an effect on the risk of Alzheimer's disease is likely to be more pronounced for severe head injury. (The relative risk was found to be 2.9 for severe, and 5.5 for less severe, head injury.)

> Graves AB, White E, Koepsell TD, et al. The association between head trauma and Alzheimer's disease. *Am. J. Epidemiol.* 131(1990): 491–501.

4:19 The basic condition is that any recall bias would be similar for the exposure and the distractor items. In addition, there should be no (positive or negative) association between the distractor items and the disease under study. (Proposals for assessment and control of recall bias have been made, using "fake exposures" unrelated to the disease but with a perceived risk similar to that of the exposure under study.)

> Walter SD, Marrett LD, From L, et al. The association of cutaneous malignant melanoma with the use of sunbeds and sunlamps. *Am. J. Epidemiol.* 131(1990):232–243.
>
> Raphael K. Recall bias: a proposal for assessment and control. *Int. J. Epidemiol.* 16(1987):167–170.

4:20A If the virus infection had given rise to symptoms, or had been diagnosed previously.

4:20B Measurement of current exposure was used to reflect past exposure (serum cholesterol). But if the exposure had been influenced by the disease, current exposure would no longer reflect past exposure. Benign colorectal polyps may not influence serum cholesterol or the accuracy by which it is measured (but in a similar study of asymptomatic colon cancer, serum cholesterol could have been influenced by the disease. Cf. Exercise 3:22).

4:20C Among cases with symptomatic or previously diagnosed gallstone disease, the disease could influence the exposure information. If the subjects—or the interviewer (examiner)—knew the result of the ultrasonography at the time of the interview (examination), this could also influence the exposure information.

4:20D The exposure information is unlikely to be influenced by previously unrecognized hypertension. But for the 89 subjects with previously known hypertension, this could have influenced their recall (knowledge) of hypertension among relatives. In addition, it could have influenced the "exposure" (family history) itself, since hypertension may be more likely to be diagnosed among family members of a case with known hypertension.

Kjaer SK, Engholm G, Teisen C, et al. Risk factors for cervical human papillomavirus and herpes simplex virus infections in Greenland and Denmark: a population-based study. *Am. J. Epidemiol.* 131 (1990):669–682.

Demers RY, Neale AV, Demers P, et al. Serum cholesterol and colorectal polyps. *J. Clin. Epidemiol.* 41(1988):9–13.

Maurer KR, Everhart JE, Knowler WC, et al. Risk factors for gallstone disease in the Hispanic populations of the United States. *Am. J. Epidemiol.* 131(1990):836–844.

Mao Y, Morrison H, MacWilliam L, et al. Risk factors for hypertension: results from a cross-sectional survey. *J. Clin. Epidemiol.* 41(1988): 411–415.

4:21 Yes. Noncases may select a day for the interview when they are not bothered by pain and illness, and thus less likely to take analgesics. If so, relative risks would be overestimated.

Somerville K, Faulkner G, and Langman M. Non-steroidal anti-inflammatory drugs and bleeding peptic ulcer. *Lancet* 1(1986): 462–464.

4:22A Awareness of disease status could (unintentionally) influence the processing (encoding, etc.) of exposure information in the questionnaire. This may introduce differential exposure misclassification.

In studies where this could be a source of bias, investigators processing the returned questionnaires should be kept unaware of the disease status of study subjects when handling exposure information. (Similarly, they should be kept unaware of the subjects' exposure status when handling information on the disease under study.) Such "blinding" can only be achieved if all questionnaires look alike. In addition, information on exposure and disease (outcome) may be confined to separate parts of the questionnaire labeled with a code number for each subject (selected to make it impossible to identify a subject's disease or exposure status from the code number). Thus, the two parts of the questionnaire can be separated before handling the information on exposure and disease, respectively. The procedures should be described in the final report.

4:22B It may be necessary to make appointments at the subjects' convenience in order to maintain a high participation in the interviews. However, it should be kept in mind that certain exposures (perhaps not those in the present study) may vary considerably over time, and that the exposure information may be related to "convenience" (cf. Exercise 4:21).

> Rolnick SJ, Gross CR, Garrard J, and Gibson RW. A comparison of response rate, data quality, and cost in the collection of data on sexual history and personal behaviours: mail survey approaches and in-person interview. *Am. J. Epidemiol.* 129(1989):1052–1061.

4:23A Blinding in respect of disease status is the primary concern to avoid differential exposure misclassification. (However, it may be more difficult to keep the interviewer unaware of a subject's disease status than of the expected findings of the study.)

4:23B In studies of early, asymptomatic disease—usually prevalent cases identified at screening (cf. Exercise 4:20).

4:23C When processing (encoding, etc.) exposure information after the cases have been identified (cf. Exercise 4:22A).

> Kelly JP, Rosenberg L, Kaufman DW, and Shapiro S. Reliability of personal interview data in a hospital-based case-control study. *Am. J. Epidemiol.* 131(1990):79–90.
>
> Zierler S, and Rothman KJ. Congenital heart disease in relation to maternal use of Bendectin and other drugs in early pregnancy. *N. Engl. J. Med.* 313(1985):347–352.
>
> Koenig KL, Pasternack BS, Shore RE, and Strax P. Hair dye use and breast cancer: a case-control study among screening participants. *Am. J. Epidemiol.* 133(1991):985–995.
>
> Mills JL, Rhoads GG, Simpson JL, et al. The absence of a relation between the periconceptional use of vitamins and neural-tube defects. *N. Engl. J. Med.* 321(1989):430–435.

4:24 Yes, the amount of exposure misclassification is likely to depend upon the number of study subjects that are close to the cut-off points. Suppose that more subjects smoke about 10, or about 20 cigarettes (= one pack) per day than any other particular numbers. If so, a reporting error of ± 1 or 2 cigarettes per day would result in more people being misclassified with alternative 2 than with alternative 1. (Cut-off points should also be selected with regard to precision at each level of exposure and, of course, the levels at which the exposure can be expected to have an effect. In a questionnaire, it may be useful to collect information on the exact (average) number of cigarettes smoked per day.)

Willett WC, Green A, Stampfer MJ, et al. Relative and absolute excess risks of coronary heart disease among women who smoke cigarettes. *N. Engl. J. Med.* 317(1987):1303–1309.

4:25 For scientific as well as for practical purposes, there is an interest in being as specific as possible. Any reduction in the intake of saturated fat may or may not be accompanied by a corresponding increase in caloric intake from other sources of energy. Associations between different components of the diet makes it important to consider confounding by other dietary factors. Similarly, total energy intake (including that contributed by saturated fat) should be taken into account as a potential confounder. Sometimes the effect of, for instance, saturated fat is estimated both with and without adjustment for total energy intake.

Maclure M, and Willett W. A case-control study of diet and risk of renal adenocarcinoma. *Epidemiology* 1(1990):430–440.
Willett WC, and Stampfer MJ. Total energy intake: implications for epidemiologic analyses. *Am. J. Epidemiol.* 124(1986):17–27.

4:26 A method may be selected to avoid differential and nondifferential exposure misclassification and selection bias. There is primarily an interest in the accuracy of the study results (e.g., relative risks), rather than in the accuracy of the exposure information. The comparability of exposure information should be given a high priority in order to avoid differential exposure misclassification that could result in an over- or underestimation of relative risks. For instance, when the subjects are approached only after the cases have been identified, records prepared before the cases appeared may provide exposure information that is not influenced by the disease under study. Similarly, the completeness of information is important in studies where lack of information could be influenced by the disease under study (possible selection bias). Finally, exposure information of low accuracy may result in a considerable underestimation of the strength of the association (bias towards RR = 1) due to nondifferential exposure misclassification.

Siemiatycki J, Dewar R, and Richardson L. Costs and statistical power associated with five methods of collecting occupation exposure information for population-based case-control studies. *Am. J. Epidemiol.* 130(1989):1236–1246.

4:27A Mortality in the total study population will be underestimated, since mortality was higher in nonparticipants. (This may be due to an excess of one or more factors that increase mortality, e.g., smoking, obesity, illness, or poor general health.)

4:27B One or more factors that increase mortality were more common in nonparticipants than in participants.

- If such a factor is associated with the exposure of interest, it may introduce confounding. Thus, there could be differences in confounding between the participants and the selected study population. However, there is not necessarily more confounding among the participants than in the total study population. (There may in fact be less confounding among the participants if they show less variability with regard to general health status and other potential confounders.)
- If such a factor is a modifier of the effect under study, there is a true difference in effect between the participants and the selected study population (no bias). However, there is an interest in specific rather than average effects (Chapter 1: Generalizability and Effect Modification). An average based on the distribution of modifiers in the selected study population is not likely to be more useful than that in the participants.

Benfante R, Reed D, MacLean C, and Kagan A. Response bias in the Honolulu Heart Program. *Am. J. Epidemiol.* 130(1989):1088–1100.

4:28A The amount of confounding may be different due to differences in the occurrence of confounders. (With more variability of confounders there would be more confounding among respondents. But to the extent that these confounders were taken into account in the data analysis, this would not bias the results.)

4:28B There is, in addition, the possibility that the nonresponse is influenced by the disease under study. This may introduce selection bias.

Criqui MH, Austin M, and Barrett-Connor E. The effect of non-response on risk ratios in a cardiovascular disease study. *J. Chron. Dis.* 32(1979):633–638.

4:29A Relative risk = 1.01. Let N be the size of the study population, where 62% (= 0.62*N) were exposed and 38% (0.38*N) unexposed. With 351 exposed and 214 unexposed cases, RR = 351*(0.38*N)/214*(0.62*N) = 1.01 (This is similar to the estimated relative risk in the present study.)

4:29B The relative risk would have been overestimated.

4:29C Relative risk = 0.85 (suggesting a 15% protective effect of multivitamins). Adding 133 exposed and 133 unexposed cases gives RR = (133+351)*(0.38*N)/(133+214)*(0.62*N) = 0.85.

4:29D Relative risk = 0.45 (suggesting a 55% protective effect of multivitamins). Adding 266 unexposed cases gives RR = 351*(0.38*N)/(266+214)*(0.62*N) = 0.45.

Mills JL, Rhoads GG, Simpson JL, et al. The absence of a relation between the periconceptional use of vitamins and neural-tube defects. *N. Engl. J. Med.* 321(1989):430–435.

4:30A Response (% returning questionnaire or participating in interview) among the cases. Missing data: answers to one or more questions may be missing in a returned questionnaire (or completed interview). Accuracy and comparability of information. Cost and time necessary to collect the information.

4:30B "Social desirability" could be more likely to influence the answers given in face-to-face interviews than in questionnaires (cf. Exercise 4:12). If so, there may be less misclassification (with regard to certain exposures) in questionnaires than in face-to-face interviews. If this tendency is similar in cases and noncases, nondifferential misclassification is introduced. However, the gap between true and reported exposure that is introduced by social desirability could be reduced by the presence of disease (depending upon the severity of the disease and other circumstances). This may result in differential exposure misclassification (bias towards RR = ∞).

Rolnick SJ, Gross CR, Garrard J, and Gibson RW. A comparison of response rate, data quality, and cost in the collection of data on sexual history and personal behaviours: mail survey approaches and in-person interview. *Am. J. Epidemiol.* 129(1989):1052–1061.

■ **CHAPTER 5**

5:1A The effect of physical activity is likely to be different for death from different kinds of diseases and accidents. When considering total mortality, an effect on the mortality from a certain disease is mixed with the effect, or "diluted" by the absence of an effect, on the mortality from other diseases. The size (precision) of any particular study limits the possibility of evaluating the effect on more specific (rare) outcomes. But from a scientific point of view, as well as for practical and public health purposes, there is an interest in the effect on mortality from specific diseases. (In addition, there is an interest in total health effects, including morbidity as well as mortality and perhaps also other effects.)

5:1B Yes, the effect of vitamin A intake may be different for different types of primary lung cancer. (For instance, when considering different histologic subtypes of lung cancer, a high vitamin A intake was found to reduce the risk of squamous cell carcinoma, but not the risk of adenocarcinoma of the lung.)

5:1C Yes, the effect of serum cholesterol may be different for different types of stroke. (In the present study, a high serum cholesterol was found to reduce the risk of hemorrhagic stroke, but increase the risk of nonhemorrhagic stroke. At the highest serum cholesterol level, the relative risk was RR = 0.16 for stroke due to subarachnoid hemorrhage, RR = 0.38 for stroke due to intracranial hemorrhage, and RR = 2.57 for nonhemorrhagic stroke.)

5:1D Yes, to the extent that the etiology could be different for different types of gallstones. (For instance, cholesterol stones and pigmented stones differ in chemical composition and perhaps also in etiology. But, unless the stones are removed surgically, it may be difficult or impossible to identify the specific type of gallstones. Thus, a relative risk may reflect a mix of the effects of an exposure on the risk of different types of gallstones.)

Paffenbarger RS, Hyde RT, Wing AL, and Hsieh C-C. Physical activity, all-cause mortality, and longevity of college alumni. *N. Engl. J. Med.* 314(1986):605–613.

Byers T, Vena J, Mettlin C, et al. Dietary vitamin A and lung cancer risk: an analysis by histologic subtypes. *Am. J. Epidemiol.* 120(1984): 769–776.

Iso H, Jacobs DR, Wentworth D, et al. Serum cholesterol levels and six-year mortality from stroke in 350,977 men screened for the Multiple Risk Factor Intervention Trial. *N. Engl. J. Med.* 320(1989): 904–910.

Maclure KM, Hayes KC, Colditz GA, et al. Weight, diet, and the risk of symptomatic gallstones in middle-aged women. *N. Engl. J. Med.* 321(1989):563–569.

5:2A Sensitivity = 0.90 means that 90% of those who developed diabetes were classified as cases. Thus, 10% of those who developed diabetes were classified as noncases ("false negatives"), both among the exposed and among the unexposed (nondifferential misclassification):

Classified as:	Exposed	Unexposed
Cases	140.40	112.50
Noncases	20,286.60	9,757.50
All women	20,427	9,870
Incidence proportion ($*10^4$)	68.73	113.98

Both in the exposed and in the unexposed, the number of cases is 10% lower than in the original table, where there was no misclassification. But the number of women at risk is the same as in the original table. Thus the incidence proportion is underestimated by 10%, both in the exposed and in the unexposed.

$$RR = 68.73/113.98 = 0.60$$

The relative risk (IP ratio) is not biased by a nondifferential disease misclassification, where only the sensitivity is reduced. However, the number of identified cases will be lower, and this tends to reduce precision. (In studies based on incidence rates, the IR ratio is slightly biased towards RR = 1, but this effect is negligible unless the incidence of the disease is very high.)

5:2B Specificity = 0.99 means that 99% of those who did not develop diabetes were classified as noncases. Thus, 1% of those who did not develop diabetes were classified as cases ("false positives"), both among the exposed and among the unexposed (nondifferential misclassification):

Classified as:	Exposed	Unexposed
Cases	358.71	222.45
Noncases	20,068.29	9,647.55
All women	20,427	9,870
Incidence proportion ($*10^4$)	175.61	225.38

$$RR = 175.61/225.38 = 0.78$$

The relative risk is biased towards RR = 1 (from 0.60 to 0.78) by this nondifferential misclassification.

5:2C Now there is a misclassification in both directions, with 10% false negatives (10% of the cases are classified as noncases) and 1% false positives (1% of the noncases are classified as cases), both in the exposed and in the unexposed. The numbers of misclassified subjects are the sum of those in A and B, above:

Classified as:	Exposed	Unexposed
Cases	343.11	209.95
Noncases	20,083.89	9,660.05
All women	20,427	9,870
Incidence proportion ($*10^4$)	167.97	212.72

$$RR = 167.97/212.72 = 0.79$$

The relative risk is biased towards RR = 1 (from 0.60 to 0.79) by this nondifferential misclassification.

5:2D There is a similar misclassification as in A, above, but only among the exposed:

Classified as:	Exposed	Unexposed
Cases	140.40	125
Noncases	20,286.60	9,745
All women	20,427	9,870
Incidence proportion ($*10^4$)	68.73	126.65

$$RR = 68.73/126.65 = 0.54$$

The relative risk is underestimated (biased towards RR = 0) by this differential misclassification. Although misclassification is reduced compared with A (no misclassification among the unexposed), this has actually introduced a bias.

5:2E There is a similar misclassification as in B, above, but only among the exposed:

Classified as:	Exposed	Unexposed
Cases	358.71	125
Noncases	20,068.29	9,745
All women	20,427	9,870
Incidence proportion ($*10^4$)	175.61	126.65

$$RR = 175.61/126.65 = 1.39$$

The relative risk is overestimated (biased towards RR = ∞) by this differential misclassification, even to the extent that alcohol intake now appears to increase the risk of diabetes (reversed direction of effect).

5:2F There is a similar misclassification as in C, above, but only among the exposed:

Classified as:	Exposed	Unexposed
Cases	343.11	125
Noncases	20,083.89	9,745
All women	20,427	9,870
Incidence proportion ($*10^4$)	167.97	126.65

$$RR = 167.97/126.65 = 1.33$$

Stampfer MJ, Colditz GA, Willett WC, et al. A prospective study of moderate alcohol drinking and risk of diabetes in women. *Am. J. Epidemiol.* 128(1988):549–558.

5:3A Among the exposed, 5% of the noncases were classified as cases. But among the unexposed there was no misclassification:

Classified as:	Exposed	Unexposed
Cases	121.60	40
Noncases	30.40	183
All subjects	152	223

$$RR = 4.46 \text{ (true value: } 4.40).$$

5:3B   Among the exposed, 5% of the noncases were classified as cases. But among the unexposed there was no misclassification:

Classified as:	Exposed	Unexposed
Cases	19	4
Noncases	133	219
All subjects	152	223

RR = 6.97 (true value: 4.40).

In general, the amount of bias that is introduced by a certain reduction in specificity is inversely related to the occurrence of the disease. Conversely, the amount of bias (if any) that is introduced by a certain reduction in sensitivity increases with the occurrence of the disease.

Lee LA, Ostroff SM, McGee HB, et al. An outbreak of Shigellosis at an outdoor music festival. *Am. J. Epidemiol.* 133(1991):608–615.

5:4A   BB or RAE:
   sensitivity = $8/(8 + 17)$ = 0.32 (or 32%)
   specificity = $185/(185 + 6)$ = 0.97 (or 97%)
   RespR > 60:
   sensitivity = $15/(15 + 10)$ = 0.60 (or 60%)
   specificity = $139/(139 + 52)$ = 0.73 (or 73%)
   T > 38.5:
   sensitivity = $15/(15 + 10)$ = 0.60 (or 60%)
   specificity = $156/(156 + 35)$ = 0.82 (or 82%)

5:4B   No. Sensitivity and specificity are not characteristics of a certain method, but rather of a method applied in a certain way to a certain kind of population. In the present study, different methods (signs) were used to identify cases of severe LRI (lobar consolidation) among children with symptoms of respiratory infection. In the absence of lobar consolidation, each of the three signs is more common among such children than among healthy children. Thus, the specificity will be lower than in a population where most children are healthy.

5:4C   Sensitivity would be improved if the presence of either one is sufficient to identify a case. This is likely to increase the number of "true positives" and thus the sensitivity (but reduce the number of "true negatives" and thus the specificity).

5:4D The sign, or combination of signs, that would be most useful in an epidemiolologic study depends upon their impact on the accuracy of the results (e.g., relative risk). This could mean, for instance, that a method that is unlikely to be influenced by the exposure under study (and thus introduce differential misclassification), is preferred even if this would increase the amount of misclassification. The choice of sign, or combination of signs, to identify children suitable for a certain treatment is based on other considerations, such as the consequences of not providing the treatment for children with severe LRI (resulting from low sensitivity) and perhaps also of providing the treatment for children without severe LRI (resulting from low specificity).

Campbell H, Byass P, Lamont AC, et al. Assessment of clinical criteria for identification of severe acute lower respiratory tract infections in children. *Lancet* 1(1989):297–299.

Armstrong JRM, Campbell H. Indoor air pollution exposure and lower respiratory infections in young Gambian children. *Int. J. Epidemiol.* 20(1991):424–429.

5:5A The sensitivity would be higher, and the specificity would be lower, than that of palpation of pulses alone (unless there is complete overlapping of misclassification). This is because when only one "positive" sign (questionnaire or palpation of pulses) is required for diagnosis, there is likely to be an increase in the number of "true positives" (and thus in sensitivity), but a decrease in the number of "true negatives" (and thus in specificity).

5:5B The sensitivity would be lower, and the specificity would be higher, than that of the questionnaire alone (unless there is complete overlapping of misclassification). This is because when two "positive" signs (questionnaire and palpation of pulses) are required for diagnosis, there is likely to be a decrease in the number of "true positives" (and thus in sensitivity), but an increase in the number of "true negatives" (and thus in specificity).

Fowkes FGR. The measurement of atherosclerotic peripheral arterial disease in epidemiological surveys. *Int. J. Epidemiol.* 17(1988): 248–254.

5:6A A sensitivity < 1 does not bias the relative risk, provided that the disease misclassification is nondifferential (cf. Exercise 5:2A). However, it may be useful to consider the possibility that the exposure of interest could be related to a subject's tendency to seek medical care (or to be thoroughly examined). This would introduce bias due to differential disease misclassification.

5:6B Cf. A, above. An exposure might increase the risk of dying from an MI. If so, the relative risk would be underestimated if only nonfatal cases of MI were included.

Wong ND, Cupples LA, Ostfeld AM, et al. Risk factors for long-term coronary prognosis after initial myocardial infarction: the Framingham Study. *Am. J. Epidemiol.* 130(1989):469–480.

5:7A Such misclassification is likely to be nondifferential. If so, a sensitivity < 1 would not bias the relative risk, but a specificity < 1 would introduce a bias towards RR = 1.

5:7B If there could be differences between the exposed and the unexposed with regard to hospital, laboratory, physicians, and so on, the possibility of a differential misclassification should be considered. Otherwise: cf. A, above.

5:7C If the autopsy rate, or the availability of ECG and enzyme data, could be related to the exposure under study, the possibility of a differential misclassification should be considered. Otherwise: cf. A, above.

Beaglehole R, Stewart AW, and Butler M. Comparability of old and new World Health Organization criteria for definite myocardial infarction. *Int. J. Epidemiol.* 16(1987):373–376.

Tuomilehto J, and Kuulasmaa K. WHO MONICA Project: assessing CHD mortality and morbidity. *Int. J. Epidemiol.* 18(Suppl.1)(1989): S38-S45.

5:8A Prevalent cases. For each subject there was only information about the presence or absence of meningococci at one point in time. The prevalence is influenced by the incidence as well as by the duration of meningococcal carriage.

5:8B Prevalent cases. Each subject was examined for the presence of oral cleft at one point in time: at birth. The development of malformations during fetal life (incident cases) may or may not result in malformed infants being born alive (prevalent cases).

5:8C Symptom-free cases identified at screening are prevalent cases of asymptomatic disease. Each woman is examined at one point in time, and the examination is not initiated by the occurrence of symptoms of the disease. (But for certain diseases, subjects may attend a screening clinic or other clinic due to increasing symptoms of the disease under study. Such cases are incident cases of symptomatic disease.)

5:8D   Deaths from other causes, but with the disease present at the time of death, are prevalent cases. Deaths from the disease are incident cases of fatal disease.

Stuart JM, Cartwright KAV, Robinson PM, and Noah ND. Effect of smoking on meningococcal carriage. *Lancet* 2(1989):723–725.

Khoury MJ, Weinstein A, Panny S, et al. Maternal cigarette smoking and oral clefts: a population-based study. *Am. J. Pub. Health* 77(1987): 623–625. Copyright: American Public Health Association.

Wassertheil-Smoller S, Romney SL, Wylie-Rosett J, et al. Dietary vitamin C and uterine cervical dysplasia. *Am. J. Epidemiol.* 114(1981): 714–724.

Chan CK, Josephy BR, Wells CK, and Feinstein AR. An analysis of gastric and oesophageal cancers found with epidemiological necropsy during 1953–1982. *Int. J. Epidemiol.* 18(1989):315–319.

5:9   An incident case is the event when a disease episode reaches a certain stage of development (cf. Fig. 1–1). Like many other diseases, cervical cancer has a gradual onset. Incident cases may be defined on the basis of the first (visible) signs of the disease, for example, the transition to carcinoma in situ. But the detection of such cases would require continuous screening of a study population. Alternatively, incident cases may be defined on the basis of some later event in the disease process, for example, the transition to invasive cervical cancer. But even so, many incident cases would remain undetected, at least for some time.

Another approach that has been used (sometimes implicitly) is to define incident cases of a disease on the basis of the development of symptoms. The incidence of "symptomatic disease" usually refers to the appearance of "symptoms severe enough to make the subject see a doctor." The evaluation of symptoms may vary between subjects, but the consequences of this are usually acceptable as long as the tendency to see a doctor is not related to the exposure under study.

Finally, incident cases may be defined as deaths from the disease. In practice there may sometimes be difficulties to make a clear distinction between death from the disease, and death from other causes but with the disease present at the time of death. The latter are not incident cases (but may be prevalent cases, depending upon the definition used).

Occasionally, incident cases of a disease have been defined as "newly diagnosed cases." But this may not be appropriate since, for instance, prevalent cases identified at screening would be considered as "incident." An incident case is the event when the disease reaches a certain stage of development, rather than when it is being diagnosed.

Beral V, Hannaford P, and Kay C. Oral contraceptive use and malignancies of the genital tract. Results from the Royal College of General Practitioners' Oral Contraception Study. *Lancet* 2(1988):1331–1335.

5:10A Towards RR $= \infty$. If, among the exposed, prevalent cases of asymptomatic endometrial cancer are added to incident cases of symptomatic disease, the relative risk would be overestimated.

5:10B 150 cases. Person-years contributed by 10,000 women from 45 to 75 years of age: $10,000 * (75 - 45) = 300,000$ person-years. Incidence rate (women ≥ 45 years): 5 cases per 10,000 person-years. Number of cases: $300,000 * 5 / 10,000 = 150$.

5:10C 30 cases.

5:10D Towards RR $= 0$. Detection of early endometrial cancers in women examined before receiving a prescription of estrogen may result in depletion of cases-to-be in the exposed.

5:10E Towards RR $= 0$. When women are considered as exposed only after using estrogen for several months, but are examined because of vaginal bleedings due to estrogen during the first months of treatment, there may be additional depletion of cases-to-be in the exposed.

Horwitz RI, Feinstein AR, Horwitz SM, and Robboy SJ. Necropsy diagnosis of endometrial cancer and detection-bias in case/control studies. *Lancet* 2(1981):66–68.

5:11A No, if women who had a tubal sterilization or hysterectomy were more likely to have an ovarian cancer diagnosed during follow-up, relative risks would be overestimated. This could not explain the risk reductions found in the present study.

5:11B Yes. Asymptomatic ovarian cancers and premalignant conditions could give rise to symptomatic cancer during follow-up. If only exposed women would have such asymptomatic conditions identified and treated (removed) prior to follow-up, relative risks would be underestimated. (In principle, this source of bias could be assessed by a review of surgical records.)

In general, the identification and treatment of subjects with asymptomatic disease may affect the occurrence of symptomatic disease (and death). This is a potentially important source of bias whenever the identification and treatment of asymptomatic disease is related to the exposure under study.

Irwin KL, Weiss NS, Lee NC, and Peterson HB. Tubal sterilization, hysterectomy, and the subsequent occurrence of epithelial ovarian cancer. *Am. J. Epidemiol.* 134(1991):362–369.

5:12A If the association was explained by detection bias, it is likely to be the result of (1): routine examinations of patients being treated for (chronic or recurrent) heart disease. In principle, it may be possible to identify such asymptomatic prevalent cases in a review of the medical records.

5:12B The main difficulty in identifying incident cases of symptomatic prostate cancer is (2): cases of prostate cancer detected in patients admitted for diseases that give rise to symptoms similar to those seen in prostate cancer. In practice, it may be difficult or impossible to know if the symptoms are due to the prostate cancer or to the coexisting condition—for example, benign enlargement of the prostate gland. (This may introduce detection bias when studying the effect of exposures related to the probability of being examined for conditions with symptoms similar to those of the disease under study.)

Thompson MM, Garland C, Barrett-Connor E, et al. Heart disease risk factors, diabetes, and prostatic cancer in an adult community. *Am. J. Epidemiol.* 129(1989):511–517.

5:13A If the exposed, more often than the unexposed, would be examined for other diseases during follow-up. (Or if the unexposed, more often than the exposed, would be examined for other diseases prior to follow-up; cf. Exercise 5:11.)

5:13B A review of medical records could, in principle at least, identify prevalent cases of asymptomatic disease (cf. Exercise 5:12A). The problem may be avoided by restrictions when selecting the study population, for instance by not including subjects with chronic diseases (cf. Exercise 3:16C).

5:13C It would introduce a bias towards RR = ∞ due to differential disease misclassification. To avoid this source of bias, no weight criterion should be used in the diagnosis of diabetes when studying the effect of obesity on the risk of diabetes.

Colditz GA, Willett WC, Stampfer MJ, et al. Weight as a risk factor for clinical diabetes in women. *Am. J. Epidemiol.* 132(1990):501–513.

National Diabetes Data Group. Classification and diagnosis of diabetes mellitus and other categories of glucose intolerance. *Diabetes* 28(1979):1039–1057.

5:14A The discussion in the media is likely to attract much attention among women who had a spontaneous abortion after working with VDTs. As a consequence, women could be more likely to recall and report spontaneous abortions if they had been working with VDTs. This would introduce a differential misclassification, and result in overestimation of the relative risk.

5:14B Differential misclassification in respect of spontaneous abortion is avoided—unless VDT use was related to the probability that a woman would be admitted to the gynecological hospital units if she had a spontaneous abortion. (The results showed no association between VDT use and the risk of spontaneous abortion.)

Bryant HE, and Love EJ. Video display terminal use and spontaneous abortion risk. *Int. J. Epidemiol.* 18(1989):132–138.

Wilcox AJ, and Horney LF. Accuracy of spontaneous abortion recall. *Am. J. Epidemiol.* 120(1984):727–733.

5:15A When the disease is being diagnosed, the physician usually knows whether or not the patient is a smoker, and that smoking is important in the etiology of chronic bronchitis. Thus, patients with mild or even moderate symptoms could be more likely to be diagnosed with chronic bronchitis if they are smokers. This would introduce a differential disease misclassification, resulting in overestimation of the relative risk.

5:15B Differential disease misclassification is avoided—unless the accuracy of the information on respiratory symptoms in the questionnaire was related to the subjects' smoking habits.

Chen Y, Horne SL, McDuffie HH, and Dosman JA. Combined effect of grain farming and smoking on lung function and the prevalence of chronic bronchitis. *Int. J. Epidemiol.* 20(1991):416–423.

5:16A *Advantage:* follow-up is facilitated, since cases can be identified by scanning hospital records and death certificates.

Disadvantage: many injuries will not lead to care or evaluation at a hospital surveillance site or result in death. To the extent that this is determined by the severity of an injury, it would not cause much concern (although light injuries would be missed). But if the decision to visit a hospital is influenced by factors other than the severity of the injury, this may introduce differential misclassification.

5:16B Only if the misclassification (low sensitivity) was different for the exposed and unexposed (cf. Exercise 5:2).

Grisso JA, Wishner AR, Schwarz DF, et al. A population-based study of injuries in inner-city women. *Am. J. Epidemiol.* 134(1991):59–68.

5:17 The outcome of interest is respiratory diseases, rather than diagnoses or hospitalizations. Most episodes of respiratory disease are, of course, mild and unlikely to be diagnosed by a physician or lead to hospitalization. In the interview, these cases can only be identified by asking the parents about signs of respiratory disease. However, parents may not recall every episode of mild respiratory disease over an 18-month period. Any differences in recall between smoking and nonsmoking families would result in differential misclassification.

Episodes of respiratory disease diagnosed by a physician, or leading to hospitalization, are likely to be more severe cases. In addition, a visit to a doctor or a hospitalization is likely to enhance recall. Thus, differences in recall may be less likely for respiratory diseases diagnosed by a physician or leading to hospitalization. On the other hand, physician diagnosis or hospitalization may not only reflect the type and severity of respiratory disease. Should the probability of physician diagnosis or hospitalization of cases of respiratory disease be related to family smoking habits, differential misclassification would be introduced. (In the present study, information was collected on respiratory diseases diagnosed by a physician or leading to hospitalization.)

Chen Y, Li W, Yu S, and Quian W. Chang-Ning epidemiological study of children's health: I Passive smoking and children's respiratory diseases. *Int. J. Epidemiol.* 17(1988):348–355.

5:18 A nondifferential underreporting (sensitivity < 1) of diarrhea would not bias the relative risks. However, any differences between the exposed and unexposed in respect of the length of the intervals between visits when diarrheal episodes are reported, would introduce a differential disease misclassification and result in an over- or underestimation of relative risks. (Even with identical intervals between visits there could, of course, be differences between mothers of exposed and unexposed children in their ability to recall episodes of diarrhea.)

> Alam N, Henry FJ, and Rahaman MM. Reporting errors in one-week diarrhea recall surveys: experience from a prospective study in rural Bangladesh. *Int. J. Epidemiol.* 18(1989):697–700.

5:19A Information that can be used to identify each subject in the DCR and in the complementary data file. Such identifiers are needed for any individual record linkage, and should be unique, permanent, and universal. (The identifier used by the DCR was based on the subject's name and date of birth, and was replaced in 1968 by a "universally used, unique personal identification number provided to all Danish citizens, containing information on day, month, year and century of birth, and sex.")

5:19B The apparent deficit could be due to underreporting of cases from the clinics to the DCR, or to linkage failure due to incomplete or incorrect identifiers. (It was found that nearly 18 of the 20% deficit was explained by incomplete or incorrect identifiers.)

> Storm HH. Completeness of cancer registration in Denmark 1943–1966 and efficacy of record linkage procedures. *Int. J. Epidemiol.* 17 (1988):44–49.

5:20A Yes, any risk factor for death from cardiovascular disease would also appear to increase the risk of death from diabetes. (This is a potential source of bias in studies of death from any particular disease, when there are two or more causes of a single death.)

5:20B Yes, differential misclassification (with regard to death from diabetes) would be introduced if the exposure under study is associated with cardiovascular disease. (Misclassification occurs when diabetes is mentioned on the death certificate but was not a contributing cause of death, or when diabetes is not mentioned on the death certificate but was a contributing cause of death.)

5:20C No, precision would be reduced considerably since diabetes was seldom mentioned as the underlying cause of death. Furthermore, the bias introduced by A and B (above) may not be avoided since cardiovascular (and other) diseases could still be contributing causes of death (and may appear as "other mentions" on the death certificate).

> Crews DE, Stamler J, and Dyer A. Conditions other than underlying cause of death listed on death certificates provide additional useful information for epidemiologic research. *Epidemiology* 2(1991): 271–275.

5:21A When the exposed and unexposed differ with regard to factors that influence the choice of diagnosis (and these factors are not taken into account in the data analysis). A nondifferential misclassification between different diagnostic categories could, in principle at least, bias the relative risk towards RR = ∞ (or RR = 0) if the exposure increases (or reduces) the risk of other cardiovascular disease but not of chronic heart disease.

5:21B When the exposed and unexposed do not differ with regard to factors that influence the choice of diagnosis (or when these factors are taken into account in the data analysis).

5:21C It may be useful to consider, and perhaps review death certificates with regard to, alternative diagnoses. In addition, when selecting a study population, restrictions can be made with regard to race, sex, area of residence, and other factors that may influence the choice between diagnoses.

> Sorlie PD, and Gold EB. The effect of physician terminology preference on coronary heart disease mortality: an artifact uncovered by the 9th revision ICD. *Am. J. Pub. Health* 77(1987):148–152. Copyright: American Public Health Association.

5:22A Differential misclassification due to between-observer variation may be avoided if each observer is assigned a similar proportion of X-rays from exposed and unexposed subjects. Differential misclassification due to within-observer variation may be avoided if X-rays from exposed and unexposed subjects are examined under similar conditions, for instance as regards their distribution over time. Another aspect of this is that the observer should be kept unaware of the exposure status of the subjects ("blinding" of observers).

5:22B The extent to which a certain criterion, or combination of criteria, predicts pain and disability could be evaluated. (In the present study, where 2% of all hips had a minimal joint space $\leq$ 1.5 mm, hip pain was reported by 56.0% of men with minimal joint space $\leq$ 1.5 mm and by 28.6% of all men who answered the questionnaire.)

5:22C To the extent that different radiologic features could be related to conditions which differ in etiology, it may be useful to study such features separately (and in different combinations) in epidemiologic studies.

> Croft P, Cooper C, Wickham C, and Coggon D. Defining osteoarthritis of the hip for epidemiologic studies. *Am. J. Epidemiol.* 132(1990): 514–522.

5:23A If the study subjects had been aware of their own exposure status, this could influence their reporting of respiratory symptoms in the diary (and their tendency to call the study nurse). "Blinding" of study subjects was used to avoid this source of differential disease misclassification.

5:23B If the staff members had been aware of the exposure status of study subjects, this could influence their handling and coding of the information on respiratory symptoms in the diary. "Blinding" of staff members was used to avoid this source of differential disease misclassification.

> Douglas RM, Moore BW, Miles HB, et al. Prophylactic efficacy of intranasal alpha$_2$-interferon against rhinovirus infections in the family setting. *N. Engl. J. Med.* 314(1986):65–70.

5:24 Misclassification of panic attacks with cardiovascular symptoms (i.e., history of disease) as "cardiac symptoms" (i.e., exposure) at the first interview, and perhaps also misclassification of symptoms of heart disease as "panic attacks with cardiovascular symptoms" at the second interview. (Another possibility is, of course, that there was no misclassification and that cardiac symptoms increased the risk of panic attacks with cardiovascular symptoms).

> Keyl PM, and Eaton WW. Risk factors for the onset of panic disorder and other panic attacks in a prospective, population-based study. *Am. J. Epidemiol.* 131(1990):301–311.

5:25 Selection bias may be introduced by nonparticipation in the second (follow-up), but not in the first (baseline), interview. The disease under study (= first-time depression during the year of follow-up) could influence participation in the second interview. For instance, people may be less willing to participate if they experienced a depression (cases). This tendency may or may not be different in exposed and unexposed subjects.

Anthony JC, and Petronis KR. Suspected risk factors for depression among adults 18–44 years old. *Epidemiology* 2(1991):123–132.

5:26A No bias is introduced.

In the example, 60% of the exposed and 90% of the unexposed participated in the follow-up examinations (regardless of whether or not they developed diabetes):

	Exposed	*Unexposed*
Cases	0.6*a	0.9*b
Person-years	0.6*C	0.9*D

Incidence rate in the exposed: 0.6*a/0.6*C = a/C
Incidence rate in the unexposed: 0.9*b/0.9*D = b/D
Relative effect (IR ratio): (a/C)/(b/D) = a*D/b*C
Absolute effect (IR difference): a/C–b/D

5:26B The relative effect is unbiased. But the absolute effect is biased (IR difference underestimated by 33% in the example).

	Exposed	*Unexposed*
Cases	0.6*a	0.6*b
Person-years	0.9*C	0.9*D

Incidence rate in the exposed: 0.6*a/0.9*C = 0.67*a/C
Incidence rate in the unexposed: 0.6*b/0.9*D = 0.67*b/D
Relative effect (IR ratio): (0.67*a/C)/(0.67*b/D) = a*D/b*C
Absolute effect (IR difference): 0.67 * (a/C–b/D)

5:26C The relative effect is biased (IR ratio underestimated by 33% in the example). The absolute effect is also biased (IR difference underestimated in the example).

	Exposed	*Unexposed*
Cases	0.6*a	0.9*b
Person-years	0.9*C	0.9*D

Incidence rate in the exposed: $0.6*a/0.9*C = 0.67*a/C$
Incidence rate in the unexposed: $0.9*b/0.9*D = b/D$
Relative effect (IR ratio): $(0.67*a/C)/(b/D) = 0.67*a*D/b*C$
Absolute effect (IR difference): $0.67 * a/C-b/D$

Holbrook TL, Barrett-Connor E, and Wingard DL. A prospective population-based study of alcohol use and non-insulin-dependent diabetes mellitus. *Am. J. Epidemiol.* 132(1990):902–909.

5:27A 3,194 women-years (including a small number of women-years lost because the cases occurred). A 6-year follow-up of 1,107 exposed women would give $6*1,107 = 6,642$ woman-years. But there were only 3,448 woman-years of follow-up. Thus, $(6,642 - 3,448) = 3,194$ woman-years were lost to follow-up. (The 261 women who did not return for their first follow-up visit contributed nearly half of this loss: $6*261 = 1,566$ woman-years.)

5:27B The relative risk would be overestimated if exposed women who developed (symptoms of) a cervical cancer during follow-up were more likely to return for follow-up visits. (This may or may not be balanced by a corresponding loss among the unexposed.)

5:27C The relative risk could be overestimated by up to 90 percent. In the exposed, the observed incidence rate (IR) was $30/3,448 = 0.0087$ per year. The true IR would have been approximately $30/6*1,107 = 0.0045$ per year (if all 30 cases were identified). Thus, the observed IR would be up to $0.0087/0.0045 = 1.9$ times the true IR. Since the relative risk (RR) is the IR in the exposed divided by that in the unexposed, RR would also be overestimated by up to 90 percent. (In the present study, the observed RR was 15.6.)

Mitchell H, Drake M, and Medley G. Prospective evaluation of risk of cervical cancer after cytological evidence of human papillomavirus infection. *Lancet* 1(1986):573–575.

5:28A Results, after loss to follow-up:

	Exposed	Unexposed	Total
Hip fractures	6	12	18
Person-years	6,939	15,600	22,539

Incidence rate $= 18/22,539 = 8.0 * 10^{-4}$ per year. This is an accurate estimate of the incidence rate of hip fracture among the women in Framingham.

5:28B Proportion exposed $= 6,939/22,539 = 30.8\%$. This is an accurate estimate of the occurrence of the exposure among the women in Framingham.

5:28C $RR = 6*15,600/12*6,939 = 1.12$. This is a highly biased estimate of the relative risk (true value: $RR = 2.94$).

> Felson DT, Kiel DP, Anderson JJ, and Kannel WB. Alcohol consumption and hip fractures: the Framingham study. *Am. J. Epidemiol.* 128 (1988):1102–1110.

5:29A The proportion of subjects successfully traced, as well as the cost and time needed to trace subjects. (Tracing by the commercial firm was less expensive and time consuming, and supplied address information on 87% of the subjects. However, a large proportion of these were not current addresses.)

5:29B *Advantage:* Follow-up will be less costly and time consuming.
Disadvantage: Selection bias may be introduced if the decision to move outside the area is influenced by the development of (symptoms of) cardiovascular disease. (If this is a possible source of bias, it may be avoided by including all subjects, although this will increase the cost and time necessary to trace the subjects.)

> Hahn LP, Sprafka JM, Burke GL, and Jacobs Jr DR. Comparison of two procedures for tracing participants in an epidemiologic cohort study. *Epidemiology* 1(1990):157–160.

5:30 Several characteristics of the study population (cf. Chapter 3). For instance, health professionals may be both willing and able to answer a questionnaire on health matters. People aged 40–75 years could be more likely to respond than elderly people. In addition, the follow-up only included the 51,672 subjects who had already answered a six-page questionnaire 2 years earlier. Thus, many of those who were unwilling or unable to answer a questionnaire were not included in the follow-up.

> Rimm EB, Stampfer MJ, Colditz GA, et al. Effectiveness of various mailing strategies among nonrespondents in a prospective cohort study. *Am. J. Epidemiol.* 131(1990):1068–1071.

■ CHAPTER 6

6:1A For the prevalent cases, the denominator is the number of women examined for the presence of breast cancer at their first visit.

For the incident cases, the denominator is the number of person-years contributed by women initially free from breast cancer. (Or, if individual follow-up periods were of the same length, the number of women free from breast cancer at their first visit.)

6:1B   Referents should be selected in such a way that they reflect the occurrence of the exposure (cigarette smoking) in the appropriate denominator (see A, above).

6:1C   Referents are selected to improve cost-efficiency by reducing the cost of obtaining exposure information. In the present study, all women had completed a self-administered questionnaire on smoking and potential confounders. However, there are costs involved in transferring this information from the questionnaire to a computer in a form suitable for data analysis. Even if this would only cost a few dollars per subject, the total cost would be substantial, since there were nearly 60,000 women. Most of this cost is avoided by using information from cases and referents only.

6:1D   Precision is reduced. But precision increases with the sample size—that is, the number of referents selected. The maximum precision is obtained when using exposure information from the entire study population. When using referents, the precision is approximately $r/(r + 1)$ of the maximum, where r = number of referents/number of cases. In the present study, where $r = 3$, the precision was about $3/(3 + 1) = 75\%$ of the highest possible with that number of cases. Cost-efficiency was improved if the costs were reduced more than the precision.

6:1E   Two potential sources of bias are introduced, both of which can be avoided in the present study:

1. A sampling bias (referent selection bias) is introduced if the referents are selected in such a way that they do not reflect the occurrence of the exposure in the appropriate denominator. This is avoided by selecting referents as a random sample of the base.

2. A differential exposure misclassification may be introduced if the investigator is aware of a woman's case-referent status when handling (encoding, etc.) the information in the questionnaire. This is avoided by blinding—that is, if those who

handle the questionnaires are kept unaware of the subjects' case-referent status (cf. Chapter 4).

Schechter MT, Miller AB, Howe GR, et al. Cigarette smoking and breast cancer: case-control studies of prevalent and incident cancer in the Canadian National Breast Screening Study. *Am. J. Epidemiol.* 130(1989):213–220.

6:2A None, provided that the referents gave an unbiased estimate of the occurrence of the exposure in the appropriate denominator. No sampling bias (referent selection bias) is introduced if the referents are selected as a random sample of the base. No additional exposure misclassification is introduced by restricting the vitamin E analyses to the cases and referents. (But the timing of the analyses could influence the accuracy of exposure information—for example, if the quality of frozen serum samples would deteriorate over time.)

6:2B Precision is reduced by about $1/3$ and the cost by 701,250 USD. In a study based on serum vitamin E of all 15,093 women, which would give the maximum precision, the total cost for analyzing serum vitamin E would be $15,093 * 50 = 754,650$ USD. In the present study, the precision is about $2/(2 + 1) = 2/3$ of the maximum precision in a study with that number of cases: $r/(r + 1)$ where $r = 2$ since there were twice as many referents as cases. The cost for analyzing serum vitamin E of 356 cases and $2*356$ referents is $(356 + 2*356) * 50 = 53,400$ USD. (In addition, the timing of the analyses may add cost for storage of sera.)

6:2C

	Precision (% of max.)	Cost (USD)
$r = 1$	50	35,600
$r = 2$	67	53,400
$r = 4$	80	89,000
$r = 8$	89	160,200
$r = 16$	94	302,600

As shown by the table, increasing the number of referents from $r = 1$ to $r = 2$ would improve precision considerably at a cost of $(53,400 - 35,600) = 17,800$ USD. By contrast, increasing the number of referents from $r = 8$ to $r = 16$ would result in only a modest gain in precision at a cost of $(302,600 - 160,200) = 142,400$ USD.

Knekt P. Serum vitamin E level and risk of female cancers. *Int. J. Epidemiol.* 17(1988):281–288.

6:3A When studying the disease with low incidence, there would be 80 cases + 80 referents = 160 subjects, and the cost would be:

$125 * 160 = \$20,000$ using method 1;
$600 * 160 = \$96,000$ using method 5.

6:3B When studying the disease with high incidence, there would be 800 cases + 800 referents = 1,600 subjects, and the cost would be:

$125 * 1600 = \$200,000$ using method 1;
$600 * 1600 = \$960,000$ using method 5.

6:3C The cost of obtaining exposure information for all study subjects was $ 220,000 using method 1, and $ 5,200,000 using method 5. The cost is reduced by:

$\$220,000 - 20,000 = \$200,000$ using method 1 in a study with 80 cases (the disease with low incidence);
$\$5,200,000 - 96,000 = \$5,104,000$ using method 5 in a study with 80 cases (the disease with low incidence);
$\$,220,000 - 200,000 = \$20,000$ using method 1 in a study with 800 cases (the disease with high incidence);
$\$5,200,000 - 960,000 = \$4,240,000$ using method 5 in a study with 800 cases (the disease with high incidence).

These reductions in cost should be related to the total study cost (also including costs for planning, follow-up of disease occurrence, data analysis, and presentation of results).

The precision is approximately $r/(r + 1)$ of the maximum precision, and $r = 1$ in the present study. Thus, the precision is reduced by about 50 percent (regardless of method and disease occurrence).

6:3D The gain in cost-efficiency increases when the occurrence of the disease is low (see C, above).

6:3E The gain in cost-efficiency increases when the cost per subject is high (see C, above).

Siemiatycki J, Dewar R, and Richardson L. Costs and statistical power associated with five methods of collecting occupation exposure information for population-based case-control studies. *Am. J. Epidemiol.* 130(1989):1236–1246.

6:4 In principle, information on recent drug intake may be collected continuously during follow-up from all subjects in a large study population. But this is likley to be very costly and impractical. Referents, selected to represent person-time (persons and time) in the study base, can be used to obtain information on recent drug intake for the study base. In general, referents are useful in obtaining information on current exposure in the study base when there are variations in exposure over time.

Ray WA, Griffin MR, and Downey W. Benzodiazepines of long and short elimination half-life and the risk of hip fracture. JAMA 262(1989): 3303–3307.

6:5A The information may be obtained by interviewing referents, selected as a random sample of the study base, concerning their dietary habits in the past. (In the present study, referents were selected every 4 months during the study period as a random sample from a continuously updated register of the population of Stockholm. As the referents were selected, they were interviewed in the same way as the cases.) In general, referents may be useful in obtaining exposure information from large "open" populations.

6:5B The sampling fraction, that is, the relation between the number of referents and the total number of person-years in the study base.

Gerhardsson de Verdier M, Hagman U, Steineck G, et al. Diet, body mass and colorectal cancer: a case-referent study in Stockholm. *Int. J. Cancer* 46(1990):832–838.

6:6 Women who belonged to the study population, but did not have a household telephone, could not be selected as referents by the method used. Thus, if women with and without a telephone differ in respect of exposure, a referent selection bias is introduced. To address this issue, the investigators reanalyzed the data excluding cases who did not have a telephone—i.e., redefining the study population as women with a telephone aged 20–54 who resided in the eight geographic locations.

In addition, the methods used for sampling should not merely provide a random sample of household telephones but a random sample of the (redefined) study base—that is, the person-time experience of women with a telephone aged 20–54 who resided in the eight geographic locations during the study period. The extent to which this is achieved depends upon the sampling methods used as well as on the extent to which information on household members is obtained for the telephone numbers selected.

Wingo PA, Ory HW, Layde PM, et al. The evaluation of the data collection process for a multicenter, population-based, case-control design. *Am. J. Epidemiol.* 128(1988):206–217.

Longnecker MP. Re: "The evaluation of the data collection process for a multicenter, population-based case-control design" (Letter). *Am. J. Epidemiol.* 129(1989):1311.

Wingo PA, Chu SY, and Lee NC. The authors reply (Letter). *Am. J. Epidemiol.* 129(1989):1311–1312.

6:7A   No referent selection bias is introduced provided that the property tax assessment rolls reflect the study base. If part of the study population (as defined) would not be included in the property tax assessment rolls, the study population could be redefined to include only subjects listed in these rolls. If so, only cases listed in the rolls should be accepted (cf. Exercise 6:6).

6:7B   The possibilty of recall bias may have been reduced by using referents who had skin lesions with an appearance similar to melanoma. Like melanoma, such lesions could be perceived as being associated with the use of sunbeds and sunlamps. (A further step towards avoiding possible recall bias may be to conduct the interviews prior to diagnosis—or before the subjects are informed about their diagnosis, by an interviewer who is kept unaware of the diagnosis.)

6:7C   A referent selection bias is introduced if patients with other skin lesions do not reflect the occurrence of the exposure in the study base. This occurs if the use of sunbeds and sunlamps is associated with other skin lesions or with clinic attendance. For instance, a referent selection bias is introduced if exposure to sunbeds and sunlamps increases the risk of other skin lesions. But a referent selection bias may be introduced even if there is no association between the exposure and the occurrence of other skin lesions. For instance, subjects with other skin lesions (many of which are benign and remain undiagnosed) could be more likely to visit the clinic if they are exposed to sunbeds and sunlamps, for example, because they pay more attention to their skin or because they have heard about the association between UV-exposure and melanoma.

Walter SD, Marrett LD, From L, et al. The association of cutaneous malignant melanoma with the use of sunbeds and sunlamps. *Am. J. Epidemiol.* 131(1990):232–243.

6:8A *Nonmalformed referents:* The occurrence of the exposure among nonmalformed infants is likely to reflect that in the study population, since only a small proportion of newborn babies are malformed. If so, no referent selection bias is introduced when referents are selected as a random sample of nonmalformed infants in the study population.

Malformed referents: A referent selection bias is introduced if these malformed infants differ from the entire study population in their exposure to vitamins. If vitamin intake would reduce the risk of other malformations, the occurrence of the exposure (vitamin intake) would be lower among malformed infants than in the study population, and the relative risk of neural-tube defect associated with vitamin intake would be overestimated when using malformed referents.

6:8B *Nonmalformed referents:* Recall bias is introduced if mothers of infants with a neural-tube defect and mothers of nonmalformed infants differ in their recall and reporting of vitamin intake around the time of conception. If mothers of infants with a neural-tube defect are more likely to recall (report) vitamin intake, the relative risk of neural-tube defect associated with vitamin intake is overestimated—and vice versa.

Malformed referents: Mothers of infants with a neural-tube defect and mothers of infants with other major malformations may have a similar tendency to recall their vitamin intake around the time of conception. If so, potential recall bias would be avoided by using malformed referents.

6:8C One possible interpretation is that vitamin intake reduces the risk of both neural-tube defect and other malformations. If so, the use of malformed referents would result in overestimation of the relative risk due to referent selection bias.

Another possibility is that mothers of infants with neural-tube defects (malformed infants) are less likely than mothers of nonmalformed infants to recall and report periconceptional vitamin intake. If so, the relative risk would be underestimated when using nonmalformed referents, and the results would not suggest that vitamin intake reduces the risk of neural-tube defect.

6:8D These results would suggest that mothers of infants with neural-tube defects (malformed infants) are more likely than mothers of nonmalformed infants to recall and report periconceptional vitamin intake. This would result in an overestimation of the relative risk when using nonmalformed referents, and the results would suggest that vitamin intake reduces the risk of neural-tube defect.

The alternative interpretation, that periconceptional vitamin intake increases the risk of other malformations (but not the risk of neural-tube defect), would seem to be a less likely explanation.

Mills JL, Rhoads GG, Simpson JL, et al. The absence of a relation between the periconceptional use of vitamins and neural-tube defects. *N. Engl. J. Med.* 321(1989):430–435.

6:9A Yes. The study population (i.e., the population that generated the cases) was all subjects aged 20–79 years living in a defined area in England. But these subjects could not be selected as referents unless they were recorded on the Patient Master Index due to hospital attendance. A referent selection bias is introduced if subjects with and without hospital attendance differ with regard to exposure.

6:9B If the referents were sampled from a list of hospital attendances, rather than from a list of subjects with any hospital attendance, subjects with several hospital visits would have a higher probability of being selected as referents. This would introduce additional referent selection bias, if the exposure was related to the number of hospital visits. (In the present study, this was avoided by using a computerized record linkage "to link all records for one individual, so that the probability of selecting an individual is independent of the number of attendances . . .".)

Elwood JM, Whitehead SM, Davison J, et al. Malignant melanoma in England: Risks associated with naevi, freckles, social class, hair colour, and sunburn. *Int. J. Epidemiol.* 19(1990):801–810.

6:10A Yes. As pointed out in the subsequent discussion, the cases were deaths that occurred during 12 months following admission for asthma to a major hospital. Thus, the study population consisted of patients admitted to such hospitals with a subsequent follow-up of 12 months. But the referents were not selected as a random sample of the study base or study population, since they were selected only among those who were hospitalized a second time within 12 months. Any difference in exposure between those who were and those who were not hospialized a second time within 12 months would introduce a referent selection bias.

In response to this criticism, a similar study was conducted for the period 1981–1987 using referents that were selected at random from the study population (i.e., without the additional requirement of a second hospitalization within 12 months). The relative risk with 95 percent confidence interval was RR = 3.8, 1.7–8.5 (RR = 5.8, 1.6–21.0 in the previous study) among patients on oral corticosteroids.

6:10B   Yes, the assessment could be influenced by awareness of the subject's case-referent status. But this source of bias can be avoided by "blind" assessment of exposure based on drug prescriptions documented in the hospital record of each subject prior to follow-up (cf. Chapter 4).

> Pearce N, Grainger J, Atkinson M, et al. Case-control study of prescribed fenoterol and death from asthma in New Zealand, 1977–81. *Thorax* 45(1990):170–175.
>
> Grainger J, Woodman K, Pearce N, et al. Prescribed fenoterol and death from asthma in New Zealand, 1981–7: a further case-control study. *Thorax* 46(1991):105–111.

6:11A   All cases (regardless of their survival) are generated by the study base. No referent selection bias is introduced by living referents selected as a random sample of the study base. But if the exposure is associated with death, a referent selection bias is introduced by selecting referents from deaths occurring in the study base. For instance, smoking increases mortality, and referents selected as a random sample of deaths in the study base can be expected to smoke more than referents selected as a random sample of the study base. If so, the relative risk of kidney cancer associated with smoking is underestimated due to referent selection bias when using dead referents.

On the other hand, there could be differences in the accuracy of exposure information obtained from living referents and from surrogate respondents of dead cases. Selecting dead referents for dead cases may reduce any such differences and thus reduce differential exposure misclassification. (But unless the exposure is unrelated to death, a referent selection bias is introduced.)

6:11B In principle, the differences could represent true differences in exposure, or differences in the accuracy of exposure information, or both. True differences in exposure between referents representing deaths and person-years in the study base means that dead referents would introduce a referent selection bias. (In the present study, several findings suggested that there were true differences in exposure between the two series of referents. Exclusion of subjects with known smoking-related causes of death reduced but did not eliminate the excess of cigarette smokers among the dead referents.)

6:11C Only surviving cases of kidney cancer would be included. But an exposure could increase the risk of dying from a kidney cancer. If so, the relative risk would be biased towards $RR = 0$ (cf. Exercise 5:6B).

McLaughlin JK, Blot WJ, Mehl ES, and Mandel JS. Problems in the use of dead controls in case-control studies. I. General results. *Am. J. Epidemiol.* 121(1985):131–139.

McLaughlin JK, Blot WJ, Mehl ES, and Mandel JS. Problems in the use of dead controls in case-control studies. II. Effect of excluding certain causes of death. *Am. J. Epidemiol.* 122(1985):485–494.

Gordis L. Should dead cases be matched to dead controls? *Am. J. Epidemiol.* 115(1982):1–5.

6:12A The data for men and women together is obtained by adding each number in the table for men to the corresponding number in the table for women:

	Exposed	Unexposed
Cases	48	43
Study population	83,893	181,107

$$RR = 2.4$$

Thus, confounding by sex resulted in a considerable underestimation of the relative risk ($RR = 2.4$ rather than $RR = 4.0$ which is the true value).

6:13B

	Exposed	*Unexposed*
Cases	92	50
Referents	181	245

$$RR = 2.5$$

The relative risk is still biased (RR = 2.3 rather than RR = 4.0, which is the true value). However, this bias is introduced by the matching (since matched referents do not reflect the occurrence of the exposure in the total study population) and does not merely represent the original confounding.

6:12C No, the relative risk is still biased (see B, above). Confounding by sex may be controlled in the data analysis, regardless of whether or not the referents are matched to the cases on sex.

6:12D The purpose is to improve efficiency (rather than to control confounding, which may be achieved in the data analysis regardless of matching). Efficiency may be improved if there is a strong association between the matching factor and the disease under study. Otherwise matching may reduce efficiency (so-called overmatching).

Hirayama T. Association between alcohol consumption and cancer of the sigmoid colon: observations from a Japanese cohort study. *Lancet* 2(1989):725–727.

6:13A

	Exposed	*Unexposed*
Cases	92	50
Study population	83,893	181,107

$$RR = 4.0$$

There is no confounding by sex, because sex is unrelated to the occurrence of the disease among the unexposed.

6:13B

	Exposed	*Unexposed*
Cases	92	50
Referents	181	245

$$RR = 2.5$$

The relative risk is biased (RR = 2.5 rather than RR = 4.0, which is the true value).

6:13C A bias is introduced by matching referents to the cases. This is because matched referents represent a distortion of the study population according to the (sex) distribution of the cases. (A proper stratified analysis will remove the bias, although there may be loss of precision.)

> Hirayama T. Association between alcohol consumption and cancer of the sigmoid colon: observations from a Japanese cohort study. *Lancet* 2(1989):725–727.

6:14A Matching may improve efficiency if there is a strong association between the matching factor and the disease under study. This requirement is met in the present study: the incidence is about 30 times higher in the oldest age group than in the youngest age group (RR = 114*140/12*41 = 32). But in many other studies, and for many other sociodemographic variables, there is not a strong association with the disease. In these situations, matching should be avoided since it may reduce efficiency (overmatching). Unless there is a strong association, a moderate increase in the number of unmatched referents may be sufficient to provide at least as many referents as cases in each stratum (age group).

6:14B Unmatched referents may be selected if the cost of including 10 times as many referents is low or moderate. In the age group < 65 years, the number of referents would increase from 140 to about 1,400, with only 41 cases. Although this is a waste of referents, it may be acceptable if the cost per subject is low. But if the cost per subject is high, matching may improve cost-efficiency.

> Felson DT, Kiel DP, Anderson JJ, and Kannel WB. Alcohol consumption and hip fractures: the Framingham Study. *Am. J. Epidemiol.* 128 (1988):1102–1110.

6:15 *Potential problems:* Individual matching may virtually double the number of subjects lost due to nonresponse (since matched pairs should be analyzed together), or introduce bias because pairs are not analyzed together or because referents that have been lost are replaced by others (who may be different with regard to exposure). This may be avoided in studies where exposure information is available for all potential referents (e.g., Exercise 6:2). In other studies, these problems are avoided if referents are not individually matched to the cases.

Limitations: Whenever matching is used, the study cannot be utilized to investigate how the risk of disease is influenced by a factor on which subjects have been matched (e.g., maternal age, race, income). This limitation is avoided if referents are not matched to the cases. In addition, if there are two or more diseases (e.g., SIDS and other infant deaths) in the same study, individual matching means that new referents have to be matched to the cases of each disease. This is avoided if refrents are not individually matched to the cases. (Cf. Introduction, Chapter 6.) (In the present study, ten times as many referents as cases were selected as an unmatched random sample.)

Kraus JF, Greenland S, and Bulterys M. Risk factors for sudden infant death syndrome in the US collaborative perinatal project. *Int. J. Epidemiol.* 18(1989):113–120.

6:16A No, cases that fail to meet the criteria defining the study base should not be included, even if they were diagnosed at one of the 17 hospitals during the study period.

6:16B Yes, cases identified at a private clinic (or elsewhere) should be included if they occurred in the study population during the study period. If such cases cannot be included, a bias may be introduced.

van't Veer P, Kok FJ, Hermus RJJ, and Sturmans F. Alcohol dose, frequency and age at first exposure in relation to the risk of breast cancer. *Int. J. Epidemiol.* 18(1989):511–517.

6:17A The study base may be defined as the person-time experience of the 300,000 population during the study period.

6:17B Yes. A referent selection bias is introduced unless the use of anti-inflammatory drugs (NSAID) in the study base is reflected by that of the patients admitted as surgical emergencies. If, for some reason, NSAID-users would be more likely than nonusers to be admitted as surgical emergencies, referent selection bias would result in underestimation of the relative risk (and vice versa).

Note that, although this study is "hospital based" in the sense that cases and referents are patients admitted to a hospital, the study population is the 300,000 population that generated the cases (cf. Chapter 1, Study Population and Follow-up Period). Case-referent studies are seldom hospital based in the sense that the study population consists of hospital patients.

Collier DStJ, and Pain JA. Non-steroidal anti-inflammatory drugs and peptic ulcer perforation. *Gut* 26(1985):359–363.

6:18A In principle, this source of bias is avoided by defining the study base according to alternative 2. However, it is not possible to select referents as a random sample of a study base defined in this way. When referents are selected among subjects who seek advice for similar symptoms, a referent selection bias is introduced if the exposure is associated with the conditions that caused the symptoms in the referents. (In addition, it may be difficult to judge whether the exposure is related to the tendency to seek medical advice in a similar way among potential cases and potential referents.)

6:18B Depending upon the circumstances, there may be differences with regard to recall bias and nonresponse (when collecting exposure information) between referents selected according to alternative 1 and 2. Cost and convenience may also have to be taken into account.

The Italian-American Cataract Study Group. Risk factors for age-related cortical, nuclear, and posterior subcapsular cataracts. *Am. J. Epidemiol.* 133(1991):541–553.

6:19A The study base may be defined as the person-time experience of women aged 45–74 years who, if they had suffered a hip fracture during the study period, would have been admitted to one of the four hospitals.

6:19B A referent selection bias is introduced unless the occurrence of the exposure among the women admitted for trauma reflects that in the study base (see A, above). Thus, a referent selection bias is introduced if there is an association between estrogen use and the occurrence of trauma, or the probability of being admitted to a hospital for trauma. (In addition, the study was conducted at four hospitals and a referent selection bias may be introduced if some women from the study base were admitted for trauma to other hospitals, or vice versa.)

Krieger N, Kelsey JL, Holford TR, and O'Connor T. An epidemiologic study of hip fracture in postmenopausal women. *Am. J. Epidemiol.* 116(1982):141–148.

6:20A The probability of being hospitalized varies from nearly 0 to 100 percent for different diseases, and smoking could be associated with the probability of being hospitalized rather than with the occurrence of disease. Whenever hospital referents are selected among patients with diseases where hospitalization is elective, the exposure could be related to the probability of hospitalization. If so, a referent selection bias is introduced (unless this is balanced by a similar association with the probability of hospitalization among potential cases, which seems unlikely for lung cancer and "all other diseases." Cf. Exercise 6:18).

6:20B
$$RR = 13.4*12.1/7.0*8.5 = 2.7$$

A relative risk of 2.7 when using the population sample, would be estimated at RR = 1 when using the hospital referents.

6:20C
$$RR = 35*69/57*23 = 1.8$$

A relative risk of 1.8 when using the population sample, would be estimated at RR = 1 when using the hospital referents.

Doll R, and Hill AB. A study of the aetiology of carcinoma of the lung. *Br. Med. J.* 2(1952):1271–1286.
Haenszel W, Shimkin MB, and Mantel N. A retrospective study of lung cancer in women. *JNCI* 21(1958):825–842.

6:21 The exposure (fluoride in drinking water) could be associated with one or more surgical conditions, or with the probability of being hospitalized for such conditions (or both).

In the present study, it was found that patients with fractures tended to have low levels of fluoride in their drinking water. When such patients were excluded from the hospital referents, the relative risk rose from RR = 2 to RR = 3.

Luoma H, Aromaa A, Helminen S, et al. Risk of myocardial infarction in Finnish men in relation to fluoride, magnesium, and calcium concentration in drinking water. *Acta Med. Scand.* 213(1983):171–176.

6:22A The chronic condition referents.

In general, slowly progressing or recurrent diseases that may lead to hospitalization only in their late stages, may alter individual habits and lifestyle exposures at an early stage. In the present study of coffee use, the occurrence of the exposure was reduced among chronic condition referents. But for other exposures, such as medication use or physical inactivity, the occurrence of the exposure may be elevated among chronic condition referents.

6:22B $$RR = 19*42/35*15 = 1.5$$

A relative risk of 1.0 when using the acute condition referents, would be estimated at RR = 1.5 when using the chronic condition referents.

6:22C Chronic condition referents should not be used if long-standing illness tends to reduce coffee consumption. Such referents are likely to underestimate coffee use in the study base, resulting in overestimation of relative risks (referent selection bias).

Similarly, referents should not be selected as a representative sample of all patients admitted to the same hospital as the cases during the study period. Such hospital referents would to a large extent (5,835/6,815 = 86% in the present study) be patients admitted for chronic conditions, and thus introduce a similar referent selection bias as the chronic condition referents.

Acute condition referents would seem to be the best choice among the hospital referents. To the extent that their conditions and probability of hospitalization are independent of coffee use, they will reflect the coffee consumption in the study base. However, patients admitted for acute conditions may have more previous illnesses (chronic conditions, medical care visits) than subjects in the study base (general population). If so, even the acute condition referents may introduce a referent selection bias resulting in overestimation of relative risks. (Some support for this was found in the present study, where the proportion of coffee drinkers was lower in acute condition referents than in a sample of "community women.")

Rosenberg L, Slone D, Shapiro S, et al. Case-control studies on the acute effects of coffee upon the risk of myocardial infarction: problems in the selection of a hospital control series. *Am. J. Epidemiol.* 113(1981):646–652.

6:23A As suggested by the investigators, selecting referents "from patients with different diseases of the same organ may be inappropriate . . . since agents which cause one disease are often implicated in other diseases of the same organ." Such referent selection bias would lead to underestimation of relative risks when using hospital referents with other gynecological disorders. To the extent that the referents selected among residents of the state were equivalent to a random sample of the study base, no referent selection bias was introduced by these referents.

For certain exposures, perhaps including treatment for venereal disease, differences in the accuracy of reporting could also play a part. But this is unlikely for simple demographic characteristics, such as marital status, where the differences in relative risk estimates were even more pronounced. Similarly, true differences in effect (effect modification) is not a tenable explanation for the findings.

6:23B The results based on all cases and referents selected among all residents (for the reasons mentioned above).

West DW, Schuman KL, Lyon JL, et al. Differences in risk estimations from a hospital and a population-based case-control study. *Int. J. Epidemiol.* 13(1984):235–239.

6:24A Referents are used to estimate the occurrence of the exposure (oral contraceptive use) in the study base.

6:24B Because pregnancy and gynecological conditions may be associated with oral contraceptive use. If so, women admitted to obstetric or gynecological wards will not reflect the use of oral contraceptives in the study base.

6:24C Women admitted for conditions that may be associated with oral contraceptive use should not be selected as referents. These include any conditions that may be caused or prevented by oral contraceptives, and long-standing or recurrent conditions that may influence the use of oral contraceptives (including indications and contraindications for oral contraceptives).

6:24D Yes, they should be accepted as referents. Alternatively, the study should be restricted to women with no history of diabetes or cardiovascular disease—a restriction that would apply equally to cases and referents. If women with a history of diabetes or cardiovascular disease were not accepted as referents, but were accepted as cases, this would introduce a referent selection bias. (In practice, it may be difficult to judge whether the decision to admit a woman for a condition that is unrelated to oral contraceptive use, is influenced by a history of other diseases such as diabetes or cardiovascular disease.)

6:24E The probability of admission to the participating hospitals should be independent of oral contraceptive use. A large proportion of all patients are likely to be admitted electively for various conditions. A referent selection bias is introduced if the probability of admission to the participating hospitals is related to oral contraceptive use (even if the referent disease is unrelated to oral contraceptive use).

In the present study, the 2,432 referents were subdivided into broad diagnostic categories. The percentage who ever used oral contraceptives varied between 42 percent among women admitted for circulatory diseases and 25 percent among women admitted for skin disorders (RR = 42*75/25*58 = 2.2).

WHO collaborative study of neoplasia and steroid contraceptives. Epithelial ovarian cancer and combined oral contraceptives. *Int. J. Epidemiol.* 18(1989):538–545.

Lubin JH, and Hartge P. Excluding controls: misapplications in case-control studies. *Am. J. Epidemiol.* 120(1984):791–793.

6:25A The exposure (BCG vaccination) may be unrelated to AD and BP, and perhaps also to other diseases. However, parents of children with chronic or recurrent illness could be more (or less) inclined to have their children vaccinated than parents of other children. If so, a referent selection bias is introduced by referents hospitalized for chronic or recurrent illness.

In addition, hospitalization is elective for many diseases and the probability of hospitalization may be related to the exposure. For instance, parents who are concerned with health problems may tend to have their children vaccinated and they may also be more inclined than other parents to have their children treated in a hospital. If so, a referent selection bias is introduced by referents admitted electively to the hospital.

If referents were selected among all children admitted to the hospital during the study period, most referents would probably have been admitted electively or for a chronic or recurrent illness. There is nothing to suggest that "on average" no referent selection bias would be introduced by such referents (cf. Exercise 6:22). A referent selection bias may be avoided by selecting referents among children admitted for diseases that are unrelated to the exposure (BCG vaccination) and require hospitalization. To the extent that AD and BP fulfilled these requirements, these referents may be preferable to referents selected among all children admitted to the hospital. (In the present study, 29% of the cases, 67% of the AD referents, and 56% of the BP referents were BCG vaccinated.)

6:25B Yes. For areas outside the metropolitan region, incomplete referral of children with AD and BP (and perhaps also of children with MT) suggests that the referents may not adequately represent the study base—that is, the person-time contributed by all residents aged 0–12 years (or those who would have been referred if they had developed MT) during the study period. This may be avoided by restricting the study to regions with complete, or nearly complete, coverage. (An alternative might be to select referents with a disease that has the same referral pattern as MT, but this may not be feasible in the present study.)

> Camargos PAM, Guimaraes MDC, and Antunes CMF. Risk assessment for aquiring meningitis tuberculosis among children not vaccinated with BCG: a case-control study. *Int. J. Epidemiol.* 17(1988):193–197.

6:26A No, lung cancer may be associated with (although not caused by) alcohol intake. Lung cancer is often caused by smoking, and smokers are more likely than nonsmokers to drink alcohol. Thus, patients admitted for lung cancer are more likely to drink alcohol than people in the study base.

6:26B Yes. For instance, alcohol intake may cause accidents but accident victims were selected as referents. Alcohol intake is associated with smoking, which causes myocardial infarction (cf. A, above), but patients admitted for myocardial infarction were selected as referents.

> Bulatao-Jayme J, Almero EM, Castro Ma CA, et al. A case-control dietary study of primary liver cancer risk from aflatoxin exposure. *Int. J. Epidemiol.* 11(1982):112–119.

6:27A Referent selection bias is avoided only to the extent that the referents reflect the occurrence of sunlight exposure in the study base. But people waiting for a friend or relative at the clinics may not be representative of the study base. (In fact, they may not even belong to the study population, defined as people who would have been admitted to the clinics if they had developed a cataract requiring surgery during the study period.) For instance, people with no full-time employment are likely to be overrepresented among those accompanying friends or relatives to the hospital. Such people may differ from others in the time spent outdoors in the sun. If they tend to be more exposed to sunlight, the relative risk is biased towards $RR = 0$ (and vice versa). This referent selection bias may not be less than that introduced by hospital referents selected among patients admitted for other diseases.

6:27B In a population, some people would be selected by many as their best friend. Such people are more likely than others to be selected as "friend referents." But they may not be representative of the study base. Friend referents tend to be gregarious people who differ from others with regard to several exposures related to habits and lifestyle. This may introduce a referent selection bias ("friendly referent bias").

Dolezal JM, Perkins ES, and Wallace RB. Sunlight, skin sensitivity, and senile cataract. *Am. J. Epidemiol.* 129(1989):559–568.
Flanders WD, and Austin H. Possibility of selection bias in matched case-control studies using friend controls. *Am. J. Epidemiol.* 124(1986): 150–153.
Pike MC, and Robins J. Re: "Possibility of selection bias in matched case-control studies using friend controls" (letter). *Am. J. Epidemiol.* 130(1989):209–210.
Austin H, Flanders WD, and Rothman KJ. Bias arising in case-control studies from selection of controls from overlapping groups. *Int. J. Epidemiol.* 18(1989):713–716.
Siemiatycki J. Friendly control bias. *J. Clin. Epidemiol.* 42(1989):687–688.

6:28A The neighbor referents were selected from the study population during the study period, individually matched to the cases by residence. Referent selection bias is avoided provided that the matching was taken into account in the data analysis. However, some potential problems introduced by matching should be kept in mind (cf. Chapter 6, Introduction: Matching, and Exercises 6:12–15). Any deviation from the strict scheme used to identify referents may introduce a referent selection bias.

6:28B Again, referents were individually matched to the cases. But the referents may not belong to the study population—that is, women who would have been admitted to one of the paricipating hospitals if they had a stroke during the study period. A referent selection bias is introduced if there are differences in exposure between neighbors who would, and neighbors who would not, be admitted to one of the paritcipating hospitals. Other conditions are as above (A).

6:28C There may be differences in exposure between women who were selected as referents but not interviewed, and women replacing such referents. If so, a referent selection bias is introduced by the replacements. (Even if no replacements are permitted, some of the selected households may not provide information on household members, and this could introduce unknown replacements of referents. In a study report, it may be useful to mention the number of households not providing information on household members as well as the number of women not providing exposure information.)

Collaborative group for the study of stroke in young women. Oral contraception and increased risk of cerebral ischemia or thrombosis. *N. Engl. J. Med.* 288(1973):871–878.

6:29A The registry included cancers occurring in the entire population of New Zealand. The study base may be defined as the person-time experience, during the study period, of all men in New Zealand aged 20 years or more (who had a current or past occupation).

6:29B A referent selection bias is introduced if the occurrence of the exposure (most recent occupation = electrical worker) in men with all other types of cancer (selected as referents) was different from that in the study base. A possible source of referent selection bias is that the risk of referent cancers could be higher (or lower) in electrical workers than in men with other occupations. Another possibility would be that the probability of having referent cancers registered is related to electrical work (in a way different from the cancer under study). Thus, in order to avoid a referent selection bias, the occurrence of the referent diseases and the probability of registration should be independent of the exposure under study (cf. the corresponding requirements for hospital referents).

6:29C Convenience and low cost are among the main advantages, since information on cases and referents is available from the same registry. In addition, the accuracy of information on occupation is likely to be similar for cases and referents.

Pearce N, Reif J, and Fraser J. Case-control studies of cancer in New Zealand electrical workers. *Int. J. Epidemiol.* 18(1989):55–59.
Linet MS, and Brookmeyer R. Use of cancer controls in case-control cancer studies. *Am. J. Epidemiol.* 125(1987):1–11.
Smith AH, Pearce NE, and Callas PW. Cancer case-control studies with other cancers as controls. *Int. J. Epidemiol.* 17(1988):298–306.

6:30A The study base was the person-time experience of all U.S. white men aged 20 years or older during the study period.

6:30B The exposed were all pulp and paper mill workers in New Hampshire. Comparisons were made with all men in the United States, considered as unexposed in the present study. (Restriction was made to white males aged $\geq$ 20 years.)

6:30C Potential confounders include residence (state), socioeconomic group, and employment (healthy worker effect). In principle, such confounding could have been avoided by restricting the study to blue-collar workers in New Hampshire (cf. Exercise 3:20). But information for the entire U.S. population was available at a low cost. Additional potential confounders include tobacco, alcohol, and diet.

6:30D If all-cause mortality in the exposed is equal to that in the unexposed. All deaths may be thought of as referents, representing the study base. PMR = $a*d/b*c$, and RR = $a*D/b*C$ where C and D are the number of person-years in the exposed and unexposed, respectively. Thus PMR = RR if $d/c = D/C$, that is, $c/C = d/D$, where c/C and d/D is the all-cause mortality in the exposed and unexposed, respectively.

Schwartz E. A proportionate mortality ratio analysis of pulp and paper mill workers in New Hampshire. *Br. J. Ind. Med.* 45(1988):234–238.

■■■ **CHAPTER 7**

7:1A The possibility of achieving the purpose increases with the number of subjects (or other units) involved in the randomization. With a limited number of subjects (units) involved, differences between the exposed and unexposed may occur by chance. But this becomes increasingly unlikely with an increasing number of subjects (units) involved in the randomization.

7:1B The principal advantage is that confounding by unidentified (unknown) factors, as well as by identified factors, may be avoided by random assignment of exposure.

7:1C No, randomization does not prevent confounding by factors that are introduced or influenced by the intervention (or by awareness of the intervention). In the present study, for instance, subjects receiving a special diet could become more conscious about other risk factors and decide to quit smoking. This may introduce confounding by smoking.

7:1D In order to achieve the purpose of randomization, subjects are considered as exposed or unexposed, depending upon whether or not they were assigned to receive the intervention diet. If some of the men assigned not to receive the intervention diet would still have the diet, this would introduce a bias towards RR = 1. In general, such bias may be introduced when subjects who are exposed regardless of the intervention are included in a trial.

7:1E Awareness of the next assignment (e.g., a tough diet, or a regular diet) could influence subject recruitment, eligibility check, informed consent, or the decision on formal entry. If so, assignments would in practice be decided by those involved in the enrollment of study subjects (e.g., by order of enrollment) rather than by the randomization. This would make the randomization invalid.

In order to avoid this source of bias, subject registration and randomization is usually handled by an independent person (e.g., a statistician) who is not involved in the enrollment, treatment, or follow-up of study subjects. Information about the next assignment should be disclosed to staff members only after the subject has formally entered the trial (or after follow-up in double-blind trials).

Burr ML, Fehily AM, Gilbert JF, et al. Effects of changes in fat, fish and fibre intakes on death and myocardial reinfarction: diet and reinfarction trial (DART). *Lancet* 2(1989):757–761.

7:2A In order to control (or demonstrate the absence of) confounding by these factors due to chance associations with the exposure (assignment), cf. Exercise 7:1A.

7:2B This is possible only for factors on which information is available. But confounding by such factors could be controlled in the data analysis regardless of randomization. The principal advantage of randomization is the possibility of avoiding confounding by unidentified factors. There is no way to check whether this purpose has been achieved.

Greenberg ER, Baron JA, Stukel TA, et al. A clinical trial of beta carotene to prevent basal-cell and squamous-cell cancers of the skin. *N. Engl. J. Med.* 323(1990):789–795.

7:3A To improve validity. Actions were taken to prevent people from entering the trial if they could be unwilling or unable to participate. A bias would be introduced if such people were included in the randomization and, for instance, failed to take their supplements.

7:3B To improve efficiency. Like many diseases, the two conditions (neural tube defect in the offspring, and skin cancer) are uncommon among people not previously affected. Thus, a study would have to include a very large number of such people in order to obtain the number of cases required for adequate precision. The cost per subject is usually high in randomized trials, and a very large trial may be prohibitively expensive. (However, the purpose of improving efficiency may or may not be achieved by selecting a study population where the disease is common. Cf. Chapter 1, Random Error: Improving Efficiency.)

MRC Vitamin Study Research Group. Prevention of neural tube defects: results of the medical research council vitamin study. *Lancet* 338 (1991):131–137.

7:4A Subjects no 3,11, and 12.

7:4B Subjects no 1,2,6,10,11, and 12.

7:4C Blocked randomization is used to improve efficiency, by ensuring that a similar number of subjects are allocated to each group in studies where only a limited number of subjects are involved in the randomization. (In studies with several hundreds of subjects, the number of subjects allocated to each group is likely to be similar without blocking.)

In some studies, the unit of randomization is families, wards, or even communities, rather than individual subjects. Since the number of such units is often limited, blocked randomization may be used to avoid imbalance between groups. (In addition, blocking is sometimes used when the recruitment of study subjects extends over a long period of time, and the outcome could be related to the time of recruitment.)

Ettinger B, Tang A, Citron JT, et al. Randomized trial of allopurinol in the prevention of calcium oxalate calculi. *N. Engl. J. Med.* 315(1986): 1386–1389.

7:5 Yes, if the first study subject was randomly assigned to receive a regular diet, the physicians could predict that (with a block size of two) the next subject recruited would be assigned to receive the protein-restricted diet, and vice versa. This could influence their decision to recruit, or not to recruit, a certain patient as the next study subject. If so, the randomization would be invalid (cf. Exercise 7:1E).

In order to avoid this source of bias, those who recruit study subjects should not know that blocking is being used. In addition, one should usually avoid a block size of two: The simple pattern "one out of two" may easily be revealed even without knowledge that a block size of two is being used.

Ihle BU, Becker GJ, Whitworth JA, et al. The effect of protein restriction on the progression of renal insufficiency. *N. Engl. J. Med.* 321(1989): 1773–1777.

7:6A To avoid confounding by previous treatment that could otherwise be introduced if, by chance, previous treatment was associated with the intervention. (This is unlikely to occur in studies where a large number of subjects, or other units, are involved in the randomization.)

7:6B Yes, a useful alternative may be to control confounding (e.g., by previous treatment) in a stratified data analysis. But if, by chance, there is a strong imbalance, a stratified analysis may become inefficient. Stratified randomization may then serve the purpose of improving efficiency.

Stratified randomization is sometimes used in studies with a relatively small number of subjects (or other units of randomization) when there is an obvious potential confounder (such as "previous treatment" in the present study). In addition, stratification is often made for treatment center (hospital) in multicenter studies.

Hong WK, Lippman SM, Itri LM, et al. Prevention of second primary tumors with isotretinoin in squamous-cell carcinoma of the head and neck. *N. Engl. J. Med.* 323(1990):795–801.

7:7A *Advantages:* cost and convenience in carrying out the screening program. In addition, it may reduce the spill-over effect (bias towards RR = 1) that would occur if women in the nonintervention group would learn about the screening from neighbors who belonged to the intervention group and then decide to see their own doctor for a screening examination.

Disadvantage: the number of units involved in the randomization will be much smaller, and this increases the likelihood of confounding due to chance associations between the intervention (screening) and risk factors for advanced breast cancer.

7:7B *Advantage:* from an ethical point of view there may be an incentive to provide as many women as possible with the screening program, if it is expected to be beneficial.

Disadvantages: efficiency is reduced by unequal randomization (unless the screening program had a very strong preventive effect). In addition, if it turned out that advanced breast cancer was not prevented by the screening program, more women would have been subjected to unnecessary screening examinations and breast operations.

> Tabár L, Fagerberg CJG, Gad A, et al. Reduction in mortality from breast cancer after mass screening with mammography. Randomised trial from the Breast Cancer Screening Working Group of the Swedish National Board of Health and Welfare. *Lancet* 1(1985):829–832.

7:8A Precision is improved with any given study size. In the present study, about 50% of the women were exposed (and 50% were unexposed) to folic acid. Similarly, 50% were exposed (and 50% were unexposed) to other vitamins. With a random assignment to three groups, considering those on placebo as unexposed, about 33% of the women would be exposed to folic acid, 33% to other vitamins, and 33% would be unexposed.

When there is evidence that at least one of the exposures under study has a preventive effect, there may be ethical arguments for reducing the number of subjects receiving placebo (25% of the women with the factorial design, 33% of the women in a study with random assignment to three groups).

In principle, a factorial design would also make it possible to study interaction between the two exposures. But this would require a sufficient number of cases in each group, and thus a large number of study subjects to obtain adequate precision.

7:8B About 50% of the women exposed to folic acid are exposed to other vitamins. This will not introduce any bias (confounding), as long as a similar proportion of those unexposed to folic acid are also exposed to other vitamins (no association between the two exposures). However, the possibility of effect modification should be considered. In addition, there is a possible practical inconvenience of having to administer four, rather than three, alternative treatments. Nontheless, factorial designs are often useful in trials where the effects of two (or more) exposures are being studied.

MRC Vitamin Study Research Group. Prevention of neural tube defects: results of the medical research council vitamin study. *Lancet* 338 (1991):131–137.

7:9A   In order to achieve the purpose of randomization, all subjects assigned to receive placebo should be considered as unexposed (intention-to-treat analysis). Thus, if subjects with a high dietary intake of beta carotene were included in the study, some of those considered as unexposed would actually be exposed and the relative risk is biased towards $RR = 1$.

In an effort to avoid this source of bias, subjects might be considered as unexposed only if they had a low total intake (and low plasma levels) of beta carotene. But then the result would not be based on the random assignments, and the purpose of avoiding confounding by randomization may not be achieved. It is preferable not to allow people to enter a trial if they are likely to be exposed regardless of the intervention.

7:9B   In order to achieve the purpose of randomization, all subjects assigned to receive beta carotene supplements should be considered as exposed (intention-to-treat analysis). Thus, if subjects assigned to receive beta carotene would not take the supplements, some of those considered as exposed would actually be unexposed and the relative risk is biased towards $RR = 1$.

In an effort to avoid this source if bias, subjects might be considered as exposed only if they had actually taken their beta carotene supplements (on-teatment analysis). But then the result would not be based on the random assignments, and the purpose of avoiding confounding by randomization may not be achieved. It is preferable not to allow people to enter a trial if they are likely to be unable or unwilling to participate in the intervention. In addition, efforts should be made to monitor and maintain a high degree of compliance in all randomized subjects.

Greenberg ER, Baron JA, Stukel TA, et al. A clinical trial of beta carotene to prevent basal-cell and squamous-cell cancers of the skin. *N. Engl. J. Med.* 323(1990):789–795.

7:10A   Bias towards $RR = 1$.

7:10B Bias towards RR = 1. (But in addition, confounding may be present in an on-treatment analysis, and this may result in an overestimation or underestimation of the relative risk.)

Hong WK, Lippman SM, Itri LM, et al. Prevention of second primary tumors with isotretinoin in squamous-cell carcinoma of the head and neck. *N. Engl. J. Med.* 323(1990): 795–801.

Steering Committee of the Physicians' Health Study Research Group. Final report on the aspirin component of the ongoing Physicians' Health Study. *N. Engl. J. Med.* 321(1989):129–135.

Norell SE. Methods in assessing drug compliance. *Acta Med. Scand.* Suppl 683(1984):35–40.

7:11A The principles discussed in Chapter 3 apply to experimental as well as to nonexperimental studies, except that subjects selected for an experimental study should:

a) *not be exposed regardless of the intervention.* If study subjects would have the water-sanitation behaviors regardless of the intervention, the relative risk is biased towards RR = 1 (cf. Exercise 7:9A). In a nonexperimental study, on the other hand, the study population should be selected to include a sufficiently large proportion (up to 50% at RR = 1) of exposed subjects (cf. Chapter 3).

b) *be able and willing to participate in the intervention.* Noncompliance with the intervention will bias the relative risk towards RR = 1 (cf. Exercises 7:9B and 7:10). This may be taken into account when selecting a study population.

7:11B None. The principles discussed in Chapter 4 apply to experimental as well as to nonexperimental studies. (But when analyzing the data from an experimental study, exposure classification is based on assignments: intention-to-treat analysis.)

7:11C None. The principles discussed in Chapter 5 apply to experimental as well as to nonexperimental studies.

Clemens JD, and Stanton BF. An educational intervention for altering water-sanitation behaviours to reduce childhood diarrhea in urban Bangladesh: I. Application of the case-control method for development of an intervention. *Am. J. Epidemiol.* 125(1987):284–291.

Stanton BF, and Clemens JD. An educational intervention for altering water-sanitation behaviours to reduce childhood diarrhea in urban Bangladesh: II. A randomized trial to assess the impact of the intervention on hygienic behaviours and rates of diarrhea. *Am. J. Epidemiol.* 125(1987):292–301.

7:12A The possibility of avoiding confounding by unknown risk factors.

7:12B A lower cost-efficiency, since the cost per study subject is likely to be considerably higher in an experimental study.

> Shekelle RB, and Stamler J. Dietary cholesterol and ischemic heart disease. *Lancet* 1(1989):1177–1179.

7:13 Placebo and blinding are used to avoid that the intervention introduces: 1) confounding (e.g., if treatment with fish oil, or awareness of such treatment, would influence other treatments or influence diet and smoking habits); 2) differences in disease misclassification (e.g., if treatment with fish oil, or awareness of such treatment, would influence a subject's perception and description of symptoms, or the physicians' interpretation of exercise tests and angiograms); 3) differences in selective loss to follow-up (e.g., if treatment with fish oil, or awareness of such treatment, would influence withdrawals due to symptoms of the disease).

> Reis GJ, Boucher TM, Sipperly ME, et al. Randomised trial of fish oil for prevention of restenosis after coronary angioplasty. *Lancet* 2(1989): 177–181.

7:14A Confounding is introduced if staff members' awareness of a subject's exposure status would influence other aspects of preventive care or advice that affect the risk of common cold.

7:14B Confounding is introduced if the study subjects' awareness of their own exposure status would influence aspects of their living that affect the risk of common cold. For instance, subjects could be more (or less) careful to avoid close contact with infected people if they know that they receive "active" treatment.

7:14C Differential disease misclassification is introduced if staff members' awareness of a subject's exposure status would influence the intensity of follow-up or the evaluation of symptoms or diagnostic signs and tests.

7:14D Differential disease misclassification is introduced if the study subjects' awareness of their own exposure status would influence their evaluation and recording of symptoms in the diary, or their tendency to call the study nurse for further examination.

7:14E Differential selection is introduced if staff members' awareness of a subject's exposure status would influence their efforts to continue follow-up, and thus prevent withdrawals that are influenced by the disease.

7:14F Differential selection is introduced if the study subjects' awareness of their own exposure status would prevent withdrawals that are influenced by the disease. For instance, subjects who know that they are receiving "active" treatment could be less likely than others to withdraw because they have fallen ill.

7:14G By selecting an unexposed group that is "placebo exposed"—that is, exposed to a factor that appears to be similar to the exposure under study but does not influence the risk of developing the disease (e.g., Exercise 3:25C). This is not always feasible, but neither is the use of placebo and blinding in experimental research. In addition, there are several other strategies (discussed in previous chapters) to deal with confounding, selection bias, and differential disease misclassification in nonexperimental as well as in experimental studies.

Douglas RM, Moore BW, Miles HB, et al. Prophylactic efficacy of intra-nasal alpha$_2$-interferon against rhinovirus infections in the family setting. *N. Engl. J. Med.* 314(1986):65–70.

7:15 The blinding had been broken (unless the higher dropout rate in the placebo group was due to chance). This was confirmed by data from a routine end-of-study questionnaire, which showed that the study subjects had been able to guess if they had received placebo or ascorbic acid. It was noticed that the taste of the contents of the placebo capsules was different from that of the ascorbic acid capsules.

The trial was stopped because the blinding had been broken and did no longer serve its purpose of avoiding confounding, differential disease misclassification, and differences in selective loss to follow-up. Continuous monitoring of withdrawals during a trial, and information on the subjects lost during follow-up (in the final report), may be useful in evaluating several aspects of validity.

Karlowski TR, Chalmers TC, Frenkel LD, et al. Ascorbic acid for the common cold: a prophylactic and therapeutic trial. *JAMA* 231(1975): 1038–1042.

7:16A The side effects of the drug could (in principle at least) introduce confounding, differential disease misclassification, and differences in selective loss to follow-up. This is similar to the consequences of breaking the blinding. (However, in the present study the side effects were unlikely to introduce any bias since similar side effects were reported by a similar proportion of the subjects on placebo treatment). Continuous monitoring of side effects during a trial, and information on side effects in each treatment group (in the final report), may be useful in evaluating several aspects of validity.

7:16B As pointed out by the investigators, this could have influenced the blinding of the clinical staff.

Pedersen C, Sandström E, Petersen CS, et al. The efficacy of inosine pranobex in preventing the aquired immunodeficiency syndrome in patients with human immunodeficiency virus infection. *N. Engl. J. Med.* 322(1990):1757–1763.

7:17 A difference in compliance between the groups could indicate that the blinding was broken (or that there was a difference in side effects). This has potential consequences with regard to confounding, differential disease misclassification, and differences in selective loss to follow-up.

Frick MH, Elo O, Haapa K et al. Helsinki Heart Study: primary-prevention trial with gemfibrozil in middle-aged men with dyslipidemia. Safety of treatment, changes in risk factors, and incidence of coronary heart disease. *N. Engl. J. Med.* 317(1987):1237–1245.

7:18 Yes. Differences between the two groups with regard to potential confounders, such as blood pressure, could be introduced by the intervention. For instance, awareness of a strict diet could make the patient or his physician more conscious of the need for strict blood pressure control. Similarly, protein restriction may lead to changes with regard to other dietary factors. This would introduce confounding by blood pressure and other dietary factors. (In the present study, each subject was examined at certain intervals during follow-up with regard to potential confounders, including blood pressure, diet, and nutritional status.)

Ihle BU, Becker GJ, Whitworth JA, et al. The effect of protein restriction on the progression of renal insufficiency. *N. Engl. J. Med.* 321(1989): 1773–1777.

7:19   Differences between the exposed (ranitidine) and unexposed (placebo) with regard to:

- loss to follow-up (cf. Exercise 7:15);
- noncompliance (cf. Exercise 7:17);
- side effects (cf. Exercise 7:16A).

A difference in loss to follow-up or noncompliance may indicate that the blinding has been broken (or it could be due to chance). A difference in side effects may have consequences similar to broken blinding. In addition, study subjects may be asked to guess their exposure status in an end-of-study questionnaire (cf. Exercise 7:15). In principle, a similar inquiry could be made among staff members involved in treatment and follow-up. A check of different sources of information available to study subjects or staff members may be useful (cf. Exercise 7:16B). In principle, study subjects could also be examined with regard to potential confounders during follow-up (cf. Exercise 7:18).

Van Deventer GM, Elashoff JD, Reedy TJ, et al. A randomized study of maintenance therapy with rantidine to prevent the recurrence of duodenal ulcer. *N. Engl. J. Med.* 329(1989):1113–1119.

7:20A   The study subjects may be examined with regard to potential confounders during follow-up, and confounding may be controlled in the data analysis.

7:20B   Differential misclassification may be avoided by using strict diagnostic criteria and by blinding of the physicians involved in the identification of cases, although symptoms are still perceived and reported by study subjects who are not blinded. (In the present study, all CHD events were "diagnosed by two cardiologists who were not involved in the study and did not know to which group the men belonged. The diagnostic criteria used were strictly defined before the start of the study . . .").

7:20C   Selective withdrawal may be avoided by several strategies used to improve the completeness of follow-up; cf. Chapter 5. (In the present study, there were only five men for whom no information was available at the end of the 5-year follow-up period.)

Hjermann I, Velve Byre K, Holme I, and Leren P. Effect of diet and smoking intervention on the incidence of coronary heart disease. Report from the Oslo Study Group of a Randomised Trial in Healthy Men. *Lancet* 2(1981):1303–1310.

7:21A In principle, lack of blinding (awareness of the intervention) may introduce bias due to confounding, differential disease misclassification, and differences in selective loss to follow-up.

7:21B In the present study, however, the lack of blinding is not likely to have introduced much bias. The identification of stillbirths and deaths within 7 days after birth is unlikely to be influenced by the lack of blinding. Similarly, the four women lost to follow-up could not have introduced any substantial bias. Awareness of participation in the program could lead to changes in other aspects of care or personal habits affecting perinatal mortality. Depending upon how the "exposure" is defined, this may be considered as effects of the exposure (program)—or as confounding. Such potential confounders may be listed, and their occurrence in each group examined.

Saari-Kemppainen A, Karjalainen O, Ylöstalo P, and Heinonen OP. Ultrasound screening and perinatal mortality: controlled trial of systematic one-stage screening in pregnancy. The Helsinki Ultrasound Trial. *Lancet* 336(1990):387–391.

7:22A Yes, since the randomization involved a large number of women (with randomization at the individual level) the purpose of avoiding confounding is likely to be achieved—provided that the results are based on all women according to their assignment (intention-to-treat analysis), and that the randomization was carried out properly. (But information on potential confounders may still be presented for each group and, if necessary, taken into account in the data analysis.)

7:22B Placebo and blinding were used to avoid such confounding. But confounding could be introduced by any differences in side effects between the calcium group and the placebo group, or if the blinding was broken (cf. Exercise 7:19).

7:22C Noncompliance in taking the calcium supplements may bias the relative risk towards RR = 1 (intention-to-treat analysis). This source of exposure misclassification could be dealt with by using information only on those taking their supplements (on-treatment analysis), but this would interfere with the purpose of randomization (to avoid confounding). The problem may, at least to some extent, be avoided if only women considered able and willing to participate in the intervention are included in the trial. In addition, efforts should be made to maintain a high degree of compliance during the trial.

Dietary intake of calcium is another potential source of exposure misclassification. Women assigned to receive placebo are considered as unexposed, even if they have a high dietary intake of calcium. When considering calcium intake as the exposure of interest, this will bias the relative risk towards RR = 1. Such bias may be avoided if women who are exposed (have a high calcium intake) regardless of the intervention are not included in the trial.

7:22D The sources of disease misclassification include errors in the measurement of blood pressure, and in the analysis of urinary protein. In addition, misclassification may be introduced by a gap between a theoretical and empirical definition (diagnostic criteria). Unless the blinding was broken (cf. Exercise 7:19), any disease misclassification is likely to be nondifferential and the relative risk may be biased towards RR = 1. (Strategies used to avoid such misclassification are as discussed in Chapter 5.)

7:22E Placebo and blinding were used to avoid differences in selective loss to follow-up. This is likely to be achieved, unless there were differences in side effects between the calcium group and the placebo group, or the blinding was broken (cf. Exercise 7:19). Nondifferential selection (resulting in overestimation or underestimation of the absolute effect) is not prevented by randomization, placebo, or blinding.

Belizán JM, Villar J, Gonzalez L, et al. Calcium supplementation to prevent hypertensive disorders of pregnancy. *N. Engl. J. Med.* 325 (1991):1399–1405.

7:23A In principle, a bias towards RR = 0 could be introduced by confounding, differential misclassification, or selection bias. In the present study, confounding may have been avoided by randomization, although the number of units involved in the randomization was limited (261 wards). In addition, confounding (by the intervention), differential misclassification, and differences in selective loss to follow-up were prevented by the use of placebo and blinding—unless the blinding was broken (or there were differences in side effects between vitamin A and placebo).

7:23B Nondifferential exposure misclassification (bias towards RR = 1) may be introduced by sources of vitamin A intake other than the supplementation, or by noncompliance in taking the supplements. A similar bias could be introduced by failure to take the induction time into account. Exposure misclassification is also introduced if, by mistake, children assigned vitamin A would be given placebo (or vice versa). In principle, overestimation of the relative risk could also be introduced by the sources of bias mentioned above (A).

West KP Jr, Pokhrel RP, Katz J, et al. Efficacy of vitamin A in reducing preschool child mortality in Nepal. *Lancet* 338(1991):67–71.

7:24A The disadvantage of the first approach is that the willingness to participate could be associated with risk factors for polio. This would introduce confounding, when excluding those who were unwilling to participate from the exposed but not from the unexposed. The second approach avoids such confounding by not excluding any children who were unwilling to participate.

7:24B The disadvantage of the second approach is that the unvaccinated second graders are included as if they had been vaccinated. This will tend to bias the result towards RR = 1. The first approach avoids such "dilution" of the effect, but may introduce confounding, that is, bias towards RR = 0 or RR = ∞ (see A, above).

7:24C Both of the above disadvantages would be avoided by excluding children who were unwilling to participate from the unexposed (first and third graders) as well as from the exposed (second graders). This approach was discussed as "the ideal," but was not used because the information about willingness to participate (parental consent form) among the first and third graders was not considered to be accurate and complete.

7:24D Considering the large number of children involved, the randomization is likely to make the vaccine and placebo group equal with regard to potential confounders including socioeconomic status. Thus, there is unlikely to be any confounding by socioeconomic status in the randomized part of the trial.

7:24E   Even in the nonrandomized part of the trial, there is unlikely to be any differences in socioeconomic status between those selected to receive vaccine (second graders) and placebo (first and third graders). However, socioeconomic status could very well be related to the willingness to participate. This would introduce confounding when those who were unwilling to participate are excluded from the exposed but not from the unexposed (cf. A, above).

7:24F   Nondifferential disease misclassification, where children with diseases other than polio were included among the cases when the diagnosis was based only on clinical examination (bias towards RR = 1).

7:24G   Bias towards RR = 1.

> Francis T, Korns RF, Voight RB, et al. An evaluation of the 1954 poliomyelitis vaccine trials. *Am. J. Pub. Health* 45(May suppl.)(1955): 1–63. Copyright: American Public Health Association.

7:25   By using the case-referent strategy (Chapter 6) in the randomized trial. If a serum sample from each study subject was kept frozen until the end of follow-up, the analyses of several lipids could then be performed only for the cases and a random sample of the study base (referents). In the present study, 378 cases of myocardial infarction were identified. If, for instance, five times as many referents were selected (r = 5), the laboratory analyses would include only 2,268 (about 10%) of the 22,071 serum samples.

> Steering Committee of the Physicians' Health Study Research Group. Final report on the aspirin component of the ongoing Physicians' Health Study. *N. Engl. J. Med.* 321(1989):129–135.

7:26A   Yes. The precursor lesions identified at the end of the treatment period may already have been present at the time of randomization (although this was not verified, since only one endoscopy per subject was acceptable). If so, the result would suggest that the supplementation does not induce regression of (but could still prevent) precursor lesions of cancer of the esophagus.

7:26B   The result is biased towards RR = 1, and this could conceal an effect of retinol in the present study.

Muñoz N, Wahrendorf J, Bang LJ, et al. No effect of riboflavine, retinol, and zinc on prevalence of precancerous lesions of oesophagus. Randomised double-blind intervention study in high-risk population of China. *Lancet* 2(1985):111–114.

7:27A These men were included in the intervention group although they did not participate in the intervention. Any effect of the intervention (or exposure) of interest is likely to be "diluted" (biased towards RR = 1) by their inclusion. On the other hand, they should not be excluded from the intervention group since this could introduce a difference between the groups. (These men were found to have an unusually high morbidity and mortality, and their exclusion from the intervention group would thus have biased the result towards RR = 0.) This problem may be avoided, if only subjects who are willing and able to participate are selected for the study and included in the randomization.

7:27B Again, these men were included in the intervention group although they did not participate in the intervention program. Any effect of the intervention (or exposure) of interest is likely to be "diluted" (biased towards RR = 1) by their inclusion. This may be avoided, if only subjects who are eligible for the intervention program are selected for the study and included in the randomization.

Wilhelmsen L, Berglund G, Elmfeldt D, et al. The multifactor primary prevention trial in Göteborg, Sweden. *Eur. Heart J.* 7(1986): 279–288.

7:28A The randomization involved only four units (fire districts), which gives little assurance against confounding (cf. Exercise 7:1A).

7:28B Randomization would make no difference. Regardless of randomization, confounding is introduced by differences between the two districts with regard to risk factors for injuries. The magnitude of these differences (and thus confounding) are not influenced by random assignment of the two districts.

Hilyer JC, Brown KC, Sirles AT, and Peoples L. A flexibility intervention to reduce the incidence and severity of joint injuries among municipal firefighters. *J. Occup. Med.* 32(1990):631–637.

7:29 Randomization is used to avoid confounding. But in the present study, the randomization only involved the three intervention groups. Thus, confounding may have been avoided by randomization in comparisons between the three intervention groups—but not in any comparison with the nonintervention group. (Comparisons with the nonintervention group are confounded by any risk factors associated with bone density at baseline.)

Placebo and blinding are used to avoid certain sources of bias (cf. Exercise 7:14). In the present study, this may have been achieved in comparisons between the three intervention groups—but not in any comparison with the nonintervention group, since placebo and blinding could not be used for the nonintervention group.

Prince RL, Smith M, Dick IM, et al. Prevention of postmenopausal osteoporosis. A comparative study of exercise, calcium supplementation, and hormone-replacement therapy. *N. Engl. J. Med.* 325(1991): 1189–1195.

7:30A Prevent confounding due to differences in risk factors between men assigned to receive clofibrate and placebo, respectively. This is likely to be achieved with the large number of men involved in the randomization, provided that the randomization was carried out properly and that the results were based on all randomized men according to their assignments (intention-to-treat analysis).

7:30B As for A (above) when studying the effect of the change in serum cholesterol induced by clofibrate. (Provided that any effect of clofibrate on the risk of MI is mediated by serum cholesterol.)

7:30C The randomization in the present study does not improve the accuracy of these results. (No random assignment of intervention to alter blood pressure.)

7:30D Prevent confounding by the intervention (or by awareness of the intervention), differential disease misclassification, and bias due to differences in selective loss to follow-up (cf. Exercise 7:13–14). But this may not be achieved if the blinding is broken, or if there are differences in side effects (cf. Exercises 7:15–16).

7:30E As for D (above) when studying the effect of the change in serum cholesterol induced by clofibrate.

7:30F The use of placebo (and blinding with regard to assignment) in the present study does not improve the accuracy of these results.

7:30G Clofibrate could, in principle at least, affect the risk of MI by lowering serum cholesterol—or by some other pathway. The latter possibility would introduce confounding (by clofibrate) when evaluating the effect of serum cholesterol on the risk of MI. In addition, failure of clofibrate to lower serum cholesterol would tend to bias the result for serum cholesterol towards RR = 1 (intention-to-treat analysis).

> Green KG, Heady A, and Oliver MF. Blood pressure, cigarette smoking and heart attack in the WHO co-operative trial of clofibrate. *Int. J. Epidemiol.* 18(1989):355–360.

■■ CHAPTER 8

Exercise 8:1

8:1A:1 Type of estrogen, dose (quantity) and frequency of administration, patterns of use (e.g., constant vs. intermittent use), timing (e.g., in relation to menopause), and duration of use.

8:1A:2 The effect (if any) may be different in different subgroups of the population. If so, there is an interest in the separate effects rather than in an average effect (cf. Chapter 1).

8:1A:3 Effect measures, disease, and induction time (cf. Chapter 2).

8:1B:1 Restriction to avoid confounding by previous CVD.

8:1B:2 *Advantages:* reduce confounding by age, and improve the comparability, accuracy, and completeness of information that can be obtained.
Disadvantage: a further restriction could lead to a shortage in available study subjects (although this would not be a problem when considered before the initial enrollment of subjects).

8:1B:3 No. In order to improve validity, it may be preferable to use restrictions with regard to potential confounders and factors that are likely to influence the comparability, accuracy, and completeness of information (cf. Chapters 1 and 3).

8:1B:4 No. In order to improve precision (at any particular study size), it may be preferable to use restrictions to influence the occurrence of the exposure and the disease (cf. Chapters 1 and 3).

8:1B:5 No. The generalizability is improved by restrictions with regard to modifiers, and is not influenced by the occurrence of other characteristics (cf. Chapters 1 and 3).

8:1C:1 Towards RR = 1, if the risk of CVD was affected by a certain duration of estrogen use, dose of estrogen, or type of estrogen.

8:1C:2 Towards RR = 1, if the risk of CVD was affected by current use and some of the women classified as exposed did not use estrogens during follow-up (or vice versa).

8:1C:3 Towards RR = 1, if the risk of CVD was affected only during a certain time interval ("time window") following exposure—for example, 5–15 years after exposure.

8:1C:4 Towards RR = 1, unless the use of some other drug that affects the risk of CVD was reported as estrogen use.

8:1D:1 Yes. Some of the "postmenopausal cardiovascular symptoms" treated with estrogen could be early symptoms of (undiagnosed) CVD. If so, confounding by this indication would introduce a bias towards RR = ∞.

8:1D:2 Yes. Women at "high risk of thrombosis" are at high risk of certain cardiovascular diseases. Confounding by this contraindication would introduce a bias towards RR = 0.

8:1D:3 No, not in the present study where women were classified as exposed if they had ever used postmenopausal estrogen. But in a study where women are classified as exposed only if they use estrogens currently (or during a certain period of time), this would introduce a bias (confounding) towards RR = 0.

8:1D:4 Yes. The number of cigarettes per day, and the duration of smoking, were not taken into account. These aspects affect the risk of CVD, and could also be related to estrogen use. If so, the smoking-adjusted relative risks could still be confounded by smoking.

8:1D:5 Yes. Women who smoked regularly during 1 year were classified as smokers, regardless of how much they had smoked. But heavy smokers could be more (or less) likely to use estrogen than other regular smokers. If so, confounding by smoking would introduce a bias towards RR = ∞ (or RR = 0) when estimating the effect of estrogen use among smokers.

8:1E:1   a) No, nondifferential disease misclassification due to low sensitivity does not bias the relative risk (cf. Chapter 1).

b) Yes. If, for some reason, incident cases of CVD were less likely to be identified in women who had used estrogen than in women who had not used estrogen, the relative risk would be biased towards RR = 0 (in the previous studies).

c) No. If, for some reason, incident cases of CVD were less likely to be identified in women who had not used estrogen than in women who had used estrogen, the relative risk would be biased towards RR = ∞ (in the previous studies).

8:1E:2   Bias towards RR = ∞. This potential source of error may have been avoided by the biennial examinations of all women during follow-up.

8:1E:3   Bias towards RR = 0. This potential source of error may have been avoided by the biennial examinations of all women prior to follow-up.

Wilson PWF, Garrison RJ, and Castelli WP. Postmenopausal estrogen use, cigarette smoking, and cardiovascular morbidity in women over 50. The Framingham Study. *N. Engl. J. Med.* 313(1985):1038–1043.

Exercise 8:2

8:2A:1   The number of women (and cases) may not be sufficient to answer, with adequate precision, questions concerning:

• the effect of certain levels (or other aspects) of alcohol intake. For example, the number of women in NHANES I who had a high alcohol intake may not be sufficient to estimate the effect of a high alcohol intake.

• the effect in different subgroups of the study population. The number of women in NHANES I may not be sufficient to allow restrictions with regard to potential modifiers.

• the effect on the risk of different types of breast cancer. For example, premenopausal and postmenopausal breast cancer may differ from an etiologic point of view, but the number of women in NHANES I may not be sufficient to answer questions concerning the separate effects.

8:2A:2 Several questions may not be addressed if the available information only includes certain aspects of alcohol intake. Limitations may include the quantity, frequency, patterns, and duration of alcohol intake. (For example, only information on alcohol intake during 1 year prior to follow-up was available from NHANES I).

8:2B:1 *Advantage:* reduces the cost and time necessary to complete the study, since information had already been collected for NHANES I.
    Disadvantages: the study population of NHANES I was a sample selected to represent the U.S. population whereas, for the purpose of the present study, a much more restricted study population would be preferable with regard to validity and generalizability. In addition, information on some potential confounders may not be available from a general survey such as NHANES I.

8:2B:2 Restriction to avoid confounding by previous breast cancer.

8:2B:3 Confounding may be increased or reduced, depending upon how the variability of confounders is influenced. Misclassification and loss to follow-up is likely to be reduced (if the women who did not provide information were less motivated to participate).

8:2B:4 Selection bias is introduced, if nonparticipation in the follow-up examination was influenced by the occurrence of breast cancer.

8:2B:5 a) Observed RR $= (0.70*a)*(0.86*D)/(0.86*b)*(0.86*C)$
    But $a*D/b*C = 1$. Thus, RR $= 0.70*0.86/0.86*0.86 = 0.81$
    b) Observed RR $= (0.86*a)*(0.86*D)/(0.70*b)*(0.86*C)$
    But $a*D/b*C = 1$. Thus, RR $= 0.86*0.86/0.70*0.86 = 1.23$
    (In the present study, the crude relative risk was 1.23 at the highest level of alcohol consumption.)

8:2C:1 Yes, but this is not likely. Differential exposure misclassification may be introduced if the exposure information is influenced by a risk indicator for breast cancer, that is not controlled in the data analysis. Another possible source of differential exposure misclassification (that may be avoided by blinding) is handling of exposure information after the cases have been identified.

8:2C:2 Nondifferential exposure misclassification may be introduced by a gap between the empirical definition (average alcohol intake per day during 1 year prior to follow-up) and the theoretical definition (where different aspects of alcohol intake during a longer period of time may be relevant), and by errors in measuring alcohol intake during the past year. Failure to take the induction time into account may result in a bias similar to that introduced by non-differential exposure misclassification.

8:2C:3 Towards RR = 1, if some exposed women were classified as unexposed. But the effect of a low alcohol intake may be overestimated, if some women with a high intake were classified as having a low alcohol intake.

8:2D:1 It should be associated with alcohol consumption in the study base, and be a risk factor (or risk indicator) for breast cancer among the unexposed—that is, among women with no alcohol intake.

8:2D:2 Towards RR = 0.

8:2D:3 Towards RR = ∞.

8:2D:4 a) It should be positively associated with alcohol intake in the study base—that is, women exposed to ionizing radiation (or postmenopausal estrogens, or benign breast disease) should use alcohol more often than other women.
  b) It should be negatively associated with alcohol intake in the study base—that is, women exposed to ionizing radiation (or postmenopausal estrogens, or benign breast disease) should use alcohol less often than other women.

8:2D:5 Yes, there are several sources of confounder misclassification. Total fat intake may vary considerably from one day to another, and the intake during one day may not reflect the intake during a longer period of time. This is likely to introduce confounder misclassification, since the risk of breast cancer is influenced by fat intake over a longer period of time (rather than by a 24-hour intake). In addition, the confounding effect may depend upon the type of fat (and other aspects of fat intake) and on the time elapsed (induction time). Finally, there could be measurement errors and limitations introduced by the categories used for classification.

8:2E:1 A differential disease misclassification could be introduced if a woman's alcohol consumption would influence her tendency to seek medical advice for symptoms of breast cancer, or influence the diagnosis of breast cancer. But a delay in the diagnosis of breast cancers related to alcohol use may not be sufficient to introduce differential misclassification, unless some of the cases would remain unidentified due to their exposure status.

8:2E:2 A differential disease misclassification could be introduced if a woman's alcohol consumption would influence her tendency to attend a screening examination. Prevalent cases of early, asymptomatic breast cancer detected at screening may or may not have been identified as incident cases of symptomatic disease at a later stage.

8:2E:3 A differential disease misclassification could be introduced if the autopsy rate, or examination routines, would be related to a woman's alcohol intake. In addition, it may be useful to separate incident cases of symptomatic disease (E:1) and prevalent cases of asymptomatic disease (E:2), from women dying from breast cancer (incident cases of fatal disease) or with breast cancer (prevalent cases at the time of death).

8:2E:4 If, from an etiologic point of view, premenopausal and postmenopausal breast cancer are two different disease entities, the study may be restricted to one of these diseases. Alternatively, there should be a sufficient number of cases of each disease entity (within each exposure category) for separate analyses. This would require information on menopausal status at the time when the disease occurred, and during each woman-year of follow-up.

Schatzkin A, Jones DY, Hoover RN, et al. Alcohol consumption and breast cancer in the epidemiologic follow-up study of the first National Health and Nutrition Examination Survey. *N. Engl. J. Med.* 316 (1987):1169–1173.

Exercise 8:3

8:3A:1 There is a primary interest in serum selenium, provided that factors other than dietary intake may influence serum selenium. If so, serum selenium could be a mediator of the effect of such factors (rather than of dietary selenium intake) on the risk of thyroid cancer.

8:3A:2 Separate questions should be asked concerning the effects of dietary intake and serum levels of selenium. To the extent that serum selenium reflects dietary intake, the answers to these questions will be similar.

8:3B:1 The study population used to study the effect of dietary intake of selenium may be defined as all subjects who answered the diet questionnaire at entry, and had their sera stored in the JANUS serum bank between 1972 and the end of 1985.

8:3B:2 a) The study period was from 1972 (when the first subject entered JANUS), until the end of 1985.
b) Individual follow-up periods were from the time when a subject entered JANUS (subjects entering at different times during the period 1972–1985), until the end of 1985.

8:3B:3 a) The person-time at risk contributed by (the individual follow-up periods of) all subjects who had their sera stored in the JANUS serum bank between 1972 and the end of 1985.
b) The person-time at risk contributed by (the individual follow-up periods of) all subjects who answered the diet questionnaire at entry and had their sera stored in the JANUS serum bank between 1972 and the end of 1985.

8:3B:4 Ten unexposed cases.
There were 5 cases/100,000 person-years, both in the exposed and in the unexposed (since RR = 1). The unexposed contributed 200,000 (20% of one million) person-years at risk. Thus, there would be 200,000 * 5/100,000 = 10 cases in the unexposed.

8:3C:1 The purpose of selecting referents is to improve cost-efficiency— that is, the relation between precision and cost.

8:3C:2 a) By 4.99 million USD.
All subjects: 100,000 * 50 USD = 5 million USD
Cases and referents: (50+150) * 50 USD = 10,000 USD
Cost reduced by (5,000,000 − 10,000) = 4.99 million USD
b) By 499 000 USD.
All subjects: 100,000 * 5 USD = 500,000 USD
Cases and referents: (50+150) * 5 USD = 1,000 USD
Cost reduced by (500,000 − 1,000) = 499,000 USD

8:3C:3 By about 25%. There were three times as many referents as cases (r = 3). The precision is about $r/(r+1) = 3/(3+1) = 0.75$, or 75% of the highest possible with that number of cases.

8:3C:4 None, if the referents are selected as a random sample of the study base (or, as in the present study, as a matched sample with the matching taken into account in the data analysis). But, regardless of whether or not referents are selected, a differential exposure misclassification may be introduced when serum samples or questionnaires are analyzed only after the cases have been identified (cf. D:1, below).

8:3D:1 Differential misclassification introduced by differences between laboratories or examiners can be avoided by using only one laboratory and examiner, or by having a similar proportion of the cases and referents examined by each laboratory and examiner (and by ensuring comparability between laboratories and examiners). Differential misclassification introduced by time of examination can be avoided, for example, by having the serum samples (or questionnaires) of cases and the corresponding referents examined at the same time. Differential misclassification introduced by awareness of case-referent status can be avoided by blinding—that is, by keeping the examiner unaware of whether a questionnaire (or serum sample) belongs to a case or a referent.

8:3D:2 Nondifferential misclassification may be introduced by a gap between the empirical and theoretical definition of the exposure. For instance, the selenium level in a single serum sample may not reflect the serum level of selenium during an etiologically relevant period of time. Similarly, the questionnaire provided information on rather crude measures of three sources of current selenium intake. This may not reflect a subject's dietary intake of selenium during a relevant period of time (regardless of any measurement errors). In addition, nondifferential misclassification may be introduced by errors in the measurement of the selenium concentration in a serum sample, and by inaccurate answers to the questionnaire.

8:3D:3 Towards RR = ∞. Such bias could be avoided by disregarding the first part of the follow-up period (corresponding to the time it would take for such tumors to be diagnosed).

8:3D:4 Yes, if the loss of information (questionnaires, serum samples) was influenced by the disease. But this may be unlikely, depending upon the way in which the information was lost.

8:3E:1 To introduce confounding, exposure to radiation should be associated with selenium intake (or serum levels) in the study base.

8:3E:2 By restriction when selecting the study population (or the cases and referents).

8:3E:3 By obtaining information on iodine intake, and taking it into account as a confounder in the data analysis.

8:3F:1 The possibility of incompleteness and errors in the reporting and registration of diagnosed cancers. Possible errors in the record linkage due to incomplete or incorrect personal identification numbers (used for the linkage).

8:3F:2 No bias is introduced by a nondifferential disease misclassification with sensitivity < 1 and specificity $= 1$. (But since there would be fewer cases, the precision is reduced).

8:3F:3 The effect would be "diluted" (and perhaps missed in the study) due to the absence of effect on the other types of thyroid cancer. This can be avoided by subdivision of thyroid cancers, in a study of sufficient size to investigate (with adequate precision) the effect of selenium on the risk of different types of thyroid cancer.

8:3F:4 The examiner (and those who make the decisions concerning the classification and exclusion of tumors) should be kept unaware of the selenium intake and serum levels of those initially identified as cases. In the absence of such blinding, decisions concerning the classification and exclusions could be influenced by exposure status.

Glattre E, Thomassen Y, Thoresen SØ, et al. Prediagnostic serum selenium in a case-control study of thyroid cancer. *Int. J. Epidemiol.* 18(1989): 45–49.

Exercise 8:4

8:4A:1 General question: Does the use of NANSAIDs increase the risk of developing a bleeding peptic ulcer—and if so, by how much? However, the question to be addressed by the present study was limited to the effect of current use of NANSAID in subjects aged $\geq$ 60 years.

8:4A:2 The questions should be specified with regard to:

Effect measures: As for any drug or other treatment, the benefits of NANSAIDs must be weighed against their side effects and risks. Thus, there may be an interest in the absolute effect as well as in the relative effect.

Exposure: Non-aspirin non-steroidal anti-inflammatory drugs (NANSAID) include more than one drug. If there could be differences between their effects, there would be an interest in the effect of each drug. In addition, the effect (if any) is likely to depend upon other aspects of the exposure, such as the daily dose of NANSAID.

Induction time: The risk of bleeding peptic ulcer may be affected by current or past use of NANSAID, or both. The present study was desinged to evaluate the effect of current use of NANSAID.

Disease: There are different kinds of peptic ulcers—for example, gastric ulcer and duodenal ulcer. NANSAID use may affect the risk of certain kinds of peptic ulcer, but not others. If so, questions should be specified in this respect.

Modifiers: Age could be a modifer, and the present study was limited to subjects aged $\geq$ 60 years. If there is modification by other factors, questions should be specified in these respects.

8:4B:1 In principle, there are two different alternatives (I and II):

I. The study population may be defined as subjects aged $\geq$ 60 years recorded in the practice registers of the general practices within the catchment areas of the two hospitals. If so, the study base is the person-time at risk contributed by these subjects during the 2-year period. The community referents were selected from this study base (matched to the cases by age, sex, and practice register).

II. Alternatively, the study population may be defined as subjects aged $\geq$ 60 years who, if they had developed a bleeding peptic ulcer during the 2-year period, would have been identified at the two hospitals. If so, the study base is the person-time at risk contributed by these subjects during the 2-year period. The cases identified at the two hospitals are (by definition) all cases that occurred in this study base. However, it may be difficult to select referents that are representative (with regard to NANSAID use) of a study base defined in this way.

8:4B:2 Restriction may be used to prevent *confounding* by previous episodes of peptic ulcer, and perhaps by other risk factors that could be associated with NANSAID use. *Misclassification* may be reduced, for example, by an upper age limit if very old people are more likely to be misclassified (with regard to exposure, disease, or potential confounders). An upper age limit could also reduce *selection bias* (if selective nonparticipation in the interviews increases with age).

8:4B:3 Yes, if using some other study population could increase cost-efficiency, or reduce confounding, misclassification, or selection bias (cf. Chapter 3, Introduction). In addition, for a case-referent study, it may be useful if the study base is easily accessible for sampling (selection of referents) from a register or similar source.

8:4C:1 No referent selection bias is introduced by the community referents, if the study base is defined according to B:1, alternative I (and the matching was taken into account in the data analysis).

However, if the study base is defined secondary to the cases (i.e., according to B:1, alternative II), a referent selection bias is introduced by the community referents to the extent that there are differences in NANSAID use between study base (I) and study base (II).

8:4C:2 Yes, the hospital referents may introduce a referent selection bias regardless of how the study base was defined. The hospital referents were not selected as a sample of the study base, but rather as a sample of other patients admitted to the same hospitals as the cases. Such patients could differ from the study base with regard to drug use (including NANSAID). If so, a referent selection bias is introduced by the hospital referents.

8:4C:3 The purpose is to improve efficiency (rather than to control confounding, which may be achieved in the data analysis regardless of matching). Efficiency may be improved if there is a strong association between the matching factor (e.g., age) and the disease under study. Otherwise matching may reduce efficiency (so-called over-matching).

8:4C:4 Matched referents do not reflect the occurrence of the exposure in the source from which they were selected—for example, the study base. When this is taken into account in the data analysis (matched pairs are analyzed together), the loss due to nonresponse may increase considerably, since a pair is lost unless both members have responded. Any replacements for lost referents will introduce a bias, if they differ in exposure from those who were lost.

In studies including two or more diseases, individual matching means that new referents have to be matched to the cases of each disease (whereas the same unmatched referents may be used for cases of different diseases). In addition, the study cannot be utilized to investigate how the risk of disease is influenced by the matching factor, for example, age. Finally, the efficiency may be reduced if there is not a strong association between the matching factor and the disease under study (overmatching).

8:4D:1 When exposure information is collected only after the cases have been identified, a subject's disease status could influence the exposure information, resulting in differential exposure misclassification (e.g. recall bias, interviewer bias). On the other hand, exposure information collected prior to follow-up may not reflect current exposure during follow-up (which is likely to introduce considerable nondifferential misclassification when studying the effect of current NANSAID use).

8:4D:2 Although all interviews were conducted by the same interviewer using the same questionnaire, there were differences in other respects: 1) Cases and hospital referents (but not community referents) were interviewed after being admitted for an acute medical condition. 2) Cases and hospital referents were interviewed in the hospital, but community referents were interviewed in their homes (where they might have access to medicine bottles or other family members as sources of information). 3) Cases and hospital referents were asked about their drug use on the day of the event causing admission, but community referents were asked about their drug use on the day of the interview. If this day is selected at the convenience of the community referent, it may be a day when there is less pain and less use of analgesic drugs (including NANSAID).

8:4D:3 It may be useful to know why 21% of the cases (and 10% of the community referents) did not participate in the interviews. In addition, some information on the nonparticipants may be available from other sources—for example, the medical records of cases.

In the present study, cases were lost to interviews because they refused (1%), were unable to reply clearly (7%), died before interview was possible (5%), or because of "early discharge/interviewer unavailable" (7%). A review of the medical records of all cases showed that NANSAID use was documented in the records of a similar proportion of participants and nonparticipants.

8:4E:1 Drugs that are often used together with NANSAID and may affect the risk of bleeding peptic ulcer. (This applies, for instance, to aspirin.)

8:4E:2 By restricting the study to include only subjects with medical conditions for which some (but not all) take NANSAID. (There may still be some confounding by specific indications, which could be avoided only in a randomized trial.)

8:4E:3 a) That subjects are more likely to use NANSAID if they had a previous peptic ulcer. b) That subjects are less likely to use NANSAID if they had a previous peptic ulcer.

8:4E:4 As a confounder, age would introduce a bias (towards RR = 0 or RR = ∞). To introduce confounding, age should be associated with the exposure (NANSAID use) in the study base and affect the risk of bleeding peptic ulcer in the unexposed.

As a modifier, age would not introduce any bias. But the effect of NANSAID use on the risk of bleeding peptic ulcer (as measured by, e.g., the relative risk) would be different in different age groups.

8:4F:1 Yes. Cases identified at the two hospitals during the 2-year period, did not occur in the study base unless they could be identified in the practice register of a general practice in the catchment areas of the two hospitals. Any such cases could, however, easily be excluded from the study.

Furthermore, some cases occurring in the study base could have been lost to the study, for example, if they were identified and treated in a private clinic or if they died before entering the hospital. The relative risk is biased if NANSAID use among these cases was different from that among the cases identified. (But such bias, if any, is not likely to be compensated by including additional cases identified at the two hospitals.)

8:4F:2 No. This bias would appear as a referent selection bias, when using the community referents (cf. C:1, above. The hospital referents may introduce a referent selection bias, regardless of how the study base is defined. Cf. C:2, above).

8:4F:3 Yes. If subjects seeing a doctor regularly would be more likely to be referred to a hospital for minor bleedings from a peptic ulcer, this would introduce a detection bias.

> Somerville K, Faulkner G, and Langman M: Non-steroidal anti-inflammatory drugs and bleeding peptic ulcer. *Lancet* 1(1986): 462–464.

Exercise 8:5

8:5A:1 The occurrence of smoking, hypertension, and elevated serum cholesterol among the high risk men. The risk score (used to define "high risk") was based on all three factors. Thus, men could have a high risk score due to their smoking, blood pressure, serum cholesterol, or any combination of these. As an example, suppose that only the intervention against smoking would reduce the risk of death from CHD. If so, the overall intervention effect would be small if only a small proportion of the high risk men were smokers. But the overall intervention effect would increase with an increasing proportion of smokers (among high risk men, as defined by the same total risk score).

8:5A:2 The extent to which a) the intervention against smoking results in a change in smoking habits, b) the intervention against hypertension results in a change in blood pressure, and c) the intervention against high serum cholesterol results in a change in serum cholesterol. (In addition, an intervention could affect the risk of death from CHD by some other pathway. For example, intervention against smoking could result in both smoking cessation and weight gain.)

8:5A:3 Yes, if smoking, hypertension, and elevated serum cholesterol are risk factors for CHD death, the effect (absolute, or relative, or both) of one factor is modified by the others. Thus, there may be an interest in the separate effects, for instance in the effect of smoking in men with hypertension (but not elevated serum cholesterol), elevated serum cholesterol (but not hypertension), both, or neither.

8:5B:1 a) No. b) Yes. (Efficiency is, of course, not the only aspect worth considering when selecting a suitable age interval.)

8:5B:2 Restrictions to avoid confounding by these conditions.

8:5B:3 Because these subjects could introduce bias due to noncompliance with the intervention or loss to follow-up.

8:5B:4 Towards RR = 1. (Of all study subjects, 19.3% were already under treatment with antihypertensive medications and their mortality from CHD was almost identical in the intervention and nonintervention group.)

This may be avoided in a trial not including subjects who are undergoing (or intend to undergo) treatments or interventions aimed at reducing elevated blood pressure (or elevated serum cholesterol, or smoking).

8:5B:5 a) The effect would be apparent throughout the 6-year follow-up period (provided that the intervention resulted in an instant change in exposure status that persisted during the entire period).

b) There would be no effect during the first 2 years of follow-up. Thus, the effect would be most readily apparent when the first 2 years of follow-up are disregarded.

c) There would be no effect during the first 5 years of follow-up. When disregarding the first 5 years of follow-up, the remaining number of CHD deaths in each group may be small. Thus, it may be necessary to prolong the follow-up in order to improve precision.

d) No effect would be apparent during the 6 years of follow-up in the present study.

8:5C:1 The principal advantage is the possibility of avoiding confounding due to unidentified factors. The principal disadvantage is a low cost-efficiency. (In addition, there may be limitations due to ethical concerns or practical problems, such as noncompliance with the intervention.)

8:5C:2 Blocked randomization was used to assure that, within each stratum (clinic), a similar number of men would be allocated to each group.

a) If the block size would be considerably smaller (e.g., 2), those who recruit study subjects could be able to predict the next assignment (cf. C:3, below).

b) If the block size would be considerably larger (e.g., 20), the blocking may not serve its purpose of assuring that, at each clinic, the two groups are of similar size. (Cf. Chapter 7).

8:5C:3 If the clinic staff would be informed about the next assignment in advance, the assignments could be influenced by the staff—for example, by order of enrollment of study subjects. If so, the purpose of randomization would not be achieved.

8:5C:4 To achieve the purpose of randomization, results should be based on all study subjects with exposure status according to assignment (intention-to-treat analysis). But the intervention may fail to change the exposure status. If so, the result is biased towards RR = 1. This is avoided in an analysis based only on those who complied with the intervention, and changed their exposure status. The latter approach will, however, introduce confounding (bias towards RR = 0 or RR = ∞) if the tendency to change exposure status (e.g., quit smoking) is associated with a risk factor for death from CHD.

8:5C:5 Placebo (sham intervention) is used, together with blinding, to avoid three sources of bias: confounding introduced by the intervention (or by awareness of the intervention), differential disease misclassification, and differences in selective loss to follow-up.

8:5D:1 Towards RR = 1 (intention-to-treat analysis).

8:5D:2 a) No blinding was used (but informed consent was obtained). Thus, these men (and their physicians) knew that they had been allocated to the nonintervention group in a study of CHD in high risk men. (In addition, data collected at the annual follow-up examinations were made available to the physicians.) There may also have been a general trend to reduce smoking and so on during the study period.

b) Towards RR = 1 (intention-to-treat analysis).

8:5D:3 Yes. Subjects who complied with the intervention may be more likely to participate in the annual examinations. This would result in overestimation of the proportion who quit smoking and so on in the intervention group. (However, in the present study, a high proportion participated in the annual examinations: 88–95% in the intervention group, and 87–94% in the nonintervention group.)

8:5D:4 Yes. Prior to scheduled visits, subjects may increase their compliance with a prescribed antihypertensive medication or low cholesterol diet. This would exaggerate the effects of the intervention on blood pressure and serum cholesterol, since the blood pressure and serum cholesterol levels at scheduled annual examinations during follow-up would not reflect the levels during follow-up. Subjects participating in the MRFIT intervention against smoking could, in addition, tend to exaggerate their success with regard to smoking cessation. (Among current cigarette smokers at baseline, 43% in the intervention group and 14% in the nonintervention group said that they had quit smoking 1 year later. But when serum thiocyanate levels were used as an objective measure of smoking, the corresponding figures were 31% and 12%, respectively.)

8:5E:1 a) Yes, but this is very unlikely if the randomization is carried out properly—and involves a large number of subjects (or other units of randomization), as in the present study.
b) Yes, confounding is introduced when such factors are associated with the tendency to change exposure status.

8:5E:2 a) Yes. Confounding is introduced if such factors are influenced by the intervention, or by awareness of the intervention.
b) Yes, for two reasons (cf. E:1b and E:2a).

8:5E:3 Yes, any effect of the intervention against elevated serum cholesterol is mixed with (confounded by) the effect of the intervention against hypertension.

8:5F:1 A differential disease misclassification could be introduced if the cardiologists knew to what group the deceased had been allocated. To avoid this source of bias, cardiologists who were not associated with any MRFIT center were chosen for the panel, and the reviews were made blind—that is, without knowledge of the allocation of the deceased.

Another possible source of differential disease misclassification is differences between the groups with regard to the information that was available for review (e.g., death certificates, medical records). However, there was no indication of such differences. For instance, autopsies were performed in a similar proportion (31–33%) of the deaths in each group.

8:5F:2　When estimating the effect on total CHD mortality, the effect on MI mortality would be "diluted" by the absence of effect on other CHD mortality. Depending upon study size, low precision (few cases) may limit the possibility of studying the effects on death from different kinds of CHD separately.

8:5F:3　No. Relatively few subjects were lost to follow-up in each group. Although death could influence the loss differently in each group, this is unlikely to result in any substantial bias due to differences in the loss of CHD deaths. (In the intention-to-treat analysis, the subjects lost to follow-up were included as survivors.)

Multiple Risk Factor Intervention Trial Research Group. Multiple Risk Factor Intervention Trial: risk factor changes and mortality results. *JAMA* 248(1982):1465–1477.

REFERENCES

Ahlbom A, and Norell SE. Introduction to modern epidemiology. Chestnut Hill, Mass.: Epidemiology Resources Inc., 1984 (second ed. 1990).

Austin DF, and Werner SB. Epidemiology for the health sciences: a primer on epidemiologic concepts and their uses. Springfield, Ill.: Charles C. Thomas Pub., 1974.

Barker DJP, and Rose G. Epidemiology in medical practice. Edinburgh: Churchill Livingstone, 1976 (fourth ed. 1990).

Breslow NE, and Day NE. Statistical methods in cancer research: vol. 1—the analysis of case-control studies. Lyon: International Agency for Research on Cancer, 1980.

Breslow NE, and Day NE. Statistical methods in cancer research: vol. 2—the design and analysis of cohort studies. Lyon: International Agency for Research on Cancer, 1987.

Bulpitt CJ. Confidence intervals. *Lancet* 1(1987):494–497.

Christie D, Gordon I, and Heller R. Epidemiology: an introductory text for medical and other health science students. Kensington: New South Wales University Press, 1987.

Dosemeci M, Wacholder S, and Lubin JH. Does nondifferential misclassification always bias the true effect toward the null value? *Am. J. Epidemiol.* 132(1990):746–748.

Elandt-Johnson RC. Definition of rates: some remarks on their use and misuse. *Am. J. Epidemiol.* 102(1975):267–271.

Elwood JM. Causal relationships in medicine: a practical system for critical appraisal. Oxford: Oxford University Press, 1988.

Feinstein AR. Clinical epidemiology: the architecture of clinical research. Philadelphia: WB Saunders Co., 1985.

Flegal KM, Brownie C, and Haas JD. The effects of exposure misclassification on estimates of relative risk. *Am. J. Epidemiol.* 123(1986):736–751.

Flegal KM, Keyl M, and Nieto FJ. Differential misclassification arising from nondifferential errors in exposure measurement. *Am. J. Epidemiol.* 134(1991): 1233–1244.

Fletcher RH, Fletcher SW, and Wagner EH. Clinical epidemiology: the essentials. Baltimore: Williams & Wilkins, 1982 (second ed. 1988).

Fletcher W. Rice and beri-beri: preliminary report of an experiment conducted at the Kuala Lumpur Lunatic Asylum. *Lancet* 1(1907):1776–1779.

Freeman J, and Hutchinson GB. Prevalence, incidence and duration. *Am. J. Epidemiol.* 112(1980):707–723.

Friedman GD. Primer of epidemiology. New York: McGraw-Hill Book Co., 1974 (third ed. 1987).

Friedman LM, Furberg CD, and DeMets DL. Fundamentals of clinical trials. Littleton: PSG Publishing Co, 1981 (second ed. 1985).

Goldberger J, Wheeler GA, Lillie RD, and Rogers LM. A further study of butter, fresh beef, and yeast as pellagra preventives, with consideration of the relation of factor P-P of pellagra (and black tongue of dogs) to vitamin B. Public Health Reports 41(1926): 297–318.

Gordis L (ed.). Epidemiology and health risk assessment. New York: Oxford University Press, 1988.

Greenland S (ed.). Evolution of epidemiologic ideas. Chestnut Hill, Mass.: Epidemiology Resources Inc., 1987.

Greenland S. Randomization, statistics, and causal inference. *Epidemiology* 1(1990):421–429.

Greenland S, and Robins JM. Confounding and misclassification. *Am. J. Epidemiol.* 122(1985):495–506.

Greenland S, and Robins JM. Conceptual problems in the definition and interpretation of attributable fractions. *Am. J. Epidemiol.* 128(1988):1185–1197.

Hennekens CH, and Buring JE. Epidemiology in medicine. Boston: Little, Brown and Co., 1987.

Jenner E. An inquiry into the causes and effects of the variolae vaccinae. London: Sampson Low, 1798.

Jones WHS (ed.). Hippocrates: airs, waters, places. Cambridge: Harvard University Press, 1948.

Kahn HA. An introduction to epidemiologic methods. New York: Oxford University Press, 1983.

Kahn HA, and Sempos CT. Statistical methods in epidemiology. New York:Oxford University Press, 1989.

Kelsey JL, Thompson WD, and Evans AS. Methods in observational epidemiology. New York: Oxford University Press, 1986.

Kish L. Statistical design for research. New York: John Wiley & Sons, 1987.

Kleinbaum DG, Kupper LL, and Morgenstern H. Epidemiologic research: principles and quantitative methods. New York: Van Nostrand Reinhold, 1982.

Kramer MS. Clinical epidemiology and biostatistics: a primer for clinical investigators and decision-makers. Berlin: Springer-Verlag, 1988.

Last JM (ed.). A dictionary of epidemiology. New York: Oxford University Press, 1983 (second ed. 1988).

Lind J. A treatise of the scurvy. Edinburgh: Kincaid & Donaldson, 1753. Reprinted in Stewart CP, and Guthrie D (eds.), Lind's treatise on scurvy. Edinburgh: Edinburgh University Press, 1953.

MacMahon B, and Pugh TF. Epidemiology: principles and methods. Boston: Little, Brown and Co., 1970.

Mausner JS, and Bahn AK. Epidemiology: an introductory text. Philadelphia: WB Saunders Co., 1974.

McMichael AJ. Standardized mortality ratios and the "Healthy worker effect": scratching beneath the surface. *J. Occup. Med.* 18(1976):165–168.

Meinert CL. Clinical trials: design, conduct, and analysis. New York: Oxford University Press, 1986.

Miettinen OS. Proportion of disease caused or prevented by a given exposure, trait or intervention. *Am. J. Epidemiol.* 99(1974):325–332.

Miettinen OS. Estimability and estimation in case-referent studies. *Am. J. Epidemiol.* 103(1976):226–235.

Miettinen OS. Design options in epidemiologic research. An update. *Scand. J. Work Environ. Health* 8(suppl.)(1982):7–14.

Miettinen OS. Theoretical epidemiology: principles of occurrence research in medicine. New York: John Wiley & Sons, 1985.

Miettinen OS, and Cook EF. Confounding: essence and detection. *Am. J. Epidemiol.* 114(1981):593–603.

Morgenstern H, Kleinbaum DG, and Kupper LL. Measures of disease incidence used in epidemiologic research. *Int. J. Epidemiol.* 9(1980):97–104.

Morgenstern H, and Winn DM. A method for determining the sampling ratio in epidemiologic studies. *Stat. Med.* 2:(1983):387–396.

Morrison AS. Sequential pathogenic components of rates. *Am. J. Epidemiol.* 109(1979):709–718.

Norell SE. A short course in epidemiology. New York: Raven Press, 1992.

Pocock SJ. Clinical trials: a practical approach. Chichester: John Wiley & Sons, 1983.

Rothman KJ. Causes. *Am. J. Epidemiol.* 104(1976):587–592.

Rothman KJ. Induction and latent periods. *Am. J. Epidemiol.* 114(1981): 253–259.

Rothman KJ. Modern epidemiology. Boston: Little, Brown and Co., 1986.

Rothman KJ (ed.). Causal inference. Chestnut Hill, Mass.: Epidemiology Resources Inc., 1988.

Sackett DL, Haynes RB, and Tugwell P. Clinical epidemiology: a basic science for clinical medicine. Boston: Little, Brown and Co., 1985.

Schlesselman JJ. Case-control studies: design, conduct, analysis. New York: Oxford University Press, 1982.

Schuman SH. Practice-based epidemiology: an introduction. New York: Gordon and Breach Science Pub., 1986.

Semmelweis IP. The etiology, concept, and prophylaxis of childbed fever. 1861. Translated and republished by The University of Wisconsin Press, Madison, 1983.

Snow J. On the mode of communication of cholera. London: Churchill, 1855. Reproduced in Snow on cholera. New York: Commonwealth Fund, 1936. Reprinted by Hafner, New York, 1965.

Streiner DL, and Norman GR. Health measurement scales: a practical guide to their development and use. Oxford: Oxford University Press, 1989.

Streiner DL, Norman GR, and Blum HM. PDQ epidemiology. Toronto: BC Decker Inc., 1989.

Terris M (ed.). Goldberger on pellagra. Baton Rouge: Louisiana State University Press, 1964.

Weiss NS. Clinical epidemiology: the study of the outcome of illness. New York: Oxford University Press, 1986.

White E. The effect of misclassification of disease status in follow-up studies: Implications for selecting disease classification criteria. *Am. J. Epidemiol.* 124(1986):816–825.

World Health Organization. International statistical classification of diseases and related health problems. 10th revision. Geneva 1992–1993.

INDEX

Absolute effect, *11*, 12, 30, 37–38, 43, 54, 126, 153
Accuracy, 4, 15, *16–37*, 39–41, 53–57, 75–79, 99–103, 123–28, 149–53
Assignment of exposure, 4, 41, *149–153*
Association, 12, 13, 17–21, 37, 44, 126
Attributable fraction, *11–13*, 15, 43

Base, 123–28
Bias, *16*, 17–33, 39–41, 54–56, 76–79, 101–103, 124–28, 149–53
Blinding, 4, 21, 29–30, 33, 40–41, 78, 102–103, 127, 151–53
Blocked randomization, 150

Case-control study. *See* Case-referent study
Case-referent study, 40–41, *123–28*
Cases, *4*, 5ff
Causation, 3–4, 9, *12–14*, 41, 44ff
Causes, 3, *9–10*, *12–14*, 42ff
Comparability of information
  on exposure, 26–27. *See also* Exposure misclassification, differential
  on disease, 29. *See also* Disease misclassification, differential
Confidence interval, 34–35
Confounder, 17–20. *See also* Confounding bias
Confounder misclassification, 21, 54, 56. *See also* Exposure misclassification; Misclassification bias
Confounding. *See* Confounding bias

Confounding bias, 12, *16–21*, 34, 38–41, 54, 56–57, 100, 126, 149–53
Confounding factor. *See* Confounder
Contributing cause, 12, *13*, 42
Controls. *See* Referents; Nonintervention group; Unexposed
Cost-efficiency, 36. *See also* Efficiency
Cumulative incidence. *See* Incidence proportion

Definitions, *21–22*, 24, 27, 30, 33, 40, 43–46, 55, 75–76, 99–102
Descriptive epidemiology, *3–4*, 44
Detection bias, 102. *See also* Disease misclassification, differential
Differential misclassification. *See* Disease misclassification; Exposure misclassification
Differential selection, 30–32. *See also* Selection bias
Disease, *3*, 4ff
Disease misclassification, *21–24*, *27–30*, 40, 54, 56, 101–102, 151–53
  differential, *28–29*, 30, 101–102, 149, 151–53
  nondifferential, *27–28*, 30, 101, 153
Double-blind, 151

Effect modification, *37–39*, 45, 54, 57
Efficiency, *35–37*, 39–41, 53–54, 57, 123–28, 150
Empirical definition, 21–22. *See also* Definitions
Epidemiology, *3–4*, 10ff
Equal randomization, 150

RR. *See* Relative risk

Random error, 26, *33–37*. *See also* Precision

Randomization, 33, 41, 103, 149–53

Randomization list, 151

Randomized experiment. *See* Randomized trial

Randomized trial, 149–53

Rate difference. *See* IR difference

Rate ratio. *See* IR ratio

Recall bias, *26*, 30, 40, 77, 125

Referents, 37, 40–41, *123–28*

Referent selection bias, 41, *125*

Relative effect, *10–11*, 15, 43, 53, 126

Relative risk, *10–11*, 12ff

Restriction, 20, 38–40, 53–57, 151

Risk difference. *See* IP difference

Risk factor, *12–13*, 17ff

Risk indicator, *12*, 13ff

Risk ratio. *See* IP ratio

Sample size, 125–26

Sampling fraction, 126

Selection. *See* Selection bias

Selection bias, 16, *30–33*, 34, 39–40, 54–56, 77–79, 102–103, 149, 152–53

Selective lack of information, 32. *See also* Selection bias

Selective loss of information, 31–32. *See also* Selection bias

Selective loss to follow-up, 31. *See also* Selection bias

Sensitivity, *22–23*, 24–29, 40, 76, 101

Sham treatment. *See* Placebo

Simple randomization, 150

Single-blind, 151

Size-efficiency, 36. *See also* Efficiency

Specificity, *22–23*, 24–29, 40, 76, 101

Spill-over effect, 150

Stratified analysis, 21, 126

Stratified randomization, 150

Study base, *15–16*, 17ff

Study period, *14*, 22ff

Study population, 4, *14*, 15ff

Study size, 35–36, 39, 56, 123

Sufficient cause, 13

Systematic error. *See* Bias

Theoretical definition, 21–22. *See also* Definitions

Timing, 26, 33, 40, 43, 55, 77–79

Trial, 149–53. *See also* Experimental study

True negatives, 23

True positives, 23

Unexposed, 10, 43–44, 75–76, 149, 152

Unit of randomization, 150

Validity, 16. *See also* Bias